Clinical Tuberculosis

Clinical Tuberculosis

Editor: Megan Durham

AMERICAN
MEDICAL PUBLISHERS
www.americanmedicalpublishers.com

AMERICAN
MEDICAL PUBLISHERS
www.americanmedicalpublishers.com

Cataloging-in-Publication Data

Clinical tuberculosis / edited by Megan Durham.
p. cm.
Includes bibliographical references and index.
ISBN 978-1-63927-458-1
1. Tuberculosis. 2. Tuberculosis--Treatment. 3. Lungs--Diseases. 4. Chest--Diseases.
5. Mycobacterium tuberculosis. I. Durham, Megan.
RC311.1 .C55 2022
616.995--dc23

American Medical Publishers,
41 Flatbush Avenue,
1st Floor, New York,
NY 11217, USA

ISBN 978-1-63927-458-1 (Hardback)

Contents

Preface

Tuberculosis or TB is an infectious disease, which generally affects the lungs, but may affect other parts of the body as well. It is caused by the bacteria called Mycobacterium tuberculosis. Fever, night sweats, blood-containing sputum and weight loss are primary symptoms of TB. Most cases of TB do not exhibit symptoms and are called latent. However, nearly 10% of such latent infections lead to active disease, which can be fatal if not treated. A diagnosis of active TB requires culture and microscopic examination of bodily fluids, and chest X-rays. Latent TB can be diagnosed with the Mantoux tuberculin skin test. It is treated with isoniazid alone or in combination with rifampicin or rifapentine. Active TB treatment requires multiple antibiotics over a long period of time. This book provides a fair idea about tuberculosis and the recent advances in its diagnosis and treatment. It presents researches and studies performed by experts across the globe. For all those who are interested in this disease, this book can prove to be an essential guide.

This book is a result of research of several months to collate the most relevant data in the field.

When I was approached with the idea of this book and the proposal to edit it, I was overwhelmed. It gave me an opportunity to reach out to all those who share a common interest with me in this field. I had 3 main parameters for editing this text:

1. Accuracy – The data and information provided in this book should be up-to-date and valuable to the readers.
2. Structure – The data must be presented in a structured format for easy understanding and better grasping of the readers.
3. Universal Approach – This book not only targets students but also experts and innovators in the field, thus my aim was to present topics which are of use to all.

Thus, it took me a couple of months to finish the editing of this book.

I would like to make a special mention of my publisher who considered me worthy of this opportunity and also supported me throughout the editing process. I would also like to thank the editing team at the back-end who extended their help whenever required.

Editor

1

18-fluorodeoxyglucose positron emission tomography for tuberculosis diagnosis and management

Scott K Heysell[1*], Tania A Thomas[1], Costi D Sifri[1,2], Patrice K Rehm[3] and Eric R Houpt[1]

Abstract

Background: F-fluorodeoxyglucose positron emission tomography (FDG-PET) is increasingly used to investigate for malignancy in the evaluation of pulmonary nodules, yet both active tuberculosis (TB) and malignancy have high uptake of FDG. Definitive diagnosis of TB can be further hindered in patients without growth of the organism from sputum.

Case presentations: We describe a series of four representative cases of TB in varying disease state originally imaged by FDG-PET during evaluation for malignancy. Decisions regarding treatment for active TB in the presence of negative cultures and the evolving understanding of the spectrum of the TB disease state are discussed.

Conclusions: FDG-PET may possess a role in the diagnosis of active TB infection in settings where conventional microbiological methods are unavaiable and holds particular promise for monitoring response to therapy in cases of unsettled treatment duration such as multidrug-resistant TB or in extrapulmonary TB.

Keywords: Positron emission tomography, Tuberculosis, Multidrug-resistant tuberculosis, Pulmonary nodule

Background

Diagnosis of tuberculosis (TB) can be challenging in patients without growth of *Mycobacterium tuberculosis* in sputum or in patients with atypical extrapulmonary presentations. Tuberculin skin tests (TST) or serum interferon-gamma release assays can determine TB exposure but cannot distinguish between latent and active disease. Chest x-rays are performed as part of traditional evaluation for active disease, but in the modern era many individuals undergo chest computed tomography (CT) scans which reveal significantly more abnormalities. A common scenario is the patient with a pulmonary nodule diagnosed by CT, who is then referred for ^{18}F-fluorodeoxyglucose positron emission tomography (FDG-PET), most commonly combined FDG-PET/CT, in order to evaluate for malignancy [1]. Yet, when imaged by FDG-PET, both malignant lesions and those with active *M. tuberculosis* infection may have high uptake of FDG [2]. We describe four challenging but representative cases evaluated for active pulmonary TB based on FDG-PET/CT performed for the work-up of malignancy and explore the potential niche for FDG-PET in TB management. Age, gender, country of origin and other identifiers have been removed for confidentiality, and cases were obtained from across the state.

* Correspondence: skh8r@virginia.edu
[1]Division of Infectious Diseases and International Health, University of Virginia, PO Box 801337, Charlottesville, VA 29908-1337, USA
Full list of author information is available at the end of the article

Case presentations

Case 1

An elderly patient was born in a country non-endemic for TB, but had been exposed to active TB as a teenager and despite a positive TST, had never received latent TB infection treatment. The patient presented with 1–2 - months of fatigue and cough. Radiograph revealed right and left upper lobe nodules with hilar and mediastinal lymphadenopathy. FDG-PET/CT scan found the left lung nodule with maximum SUV of 2.5 and a more intensely FDG-avid adjacent lymph node with maximum SUV of 5.1 (Figure 1A). Smear microscopy for acid-fast bacilli and mycobacterial culture of the sputum were negative. Ultimately a videoscopic wedge resection of the left lung found multiple granulomas and a mediastinal

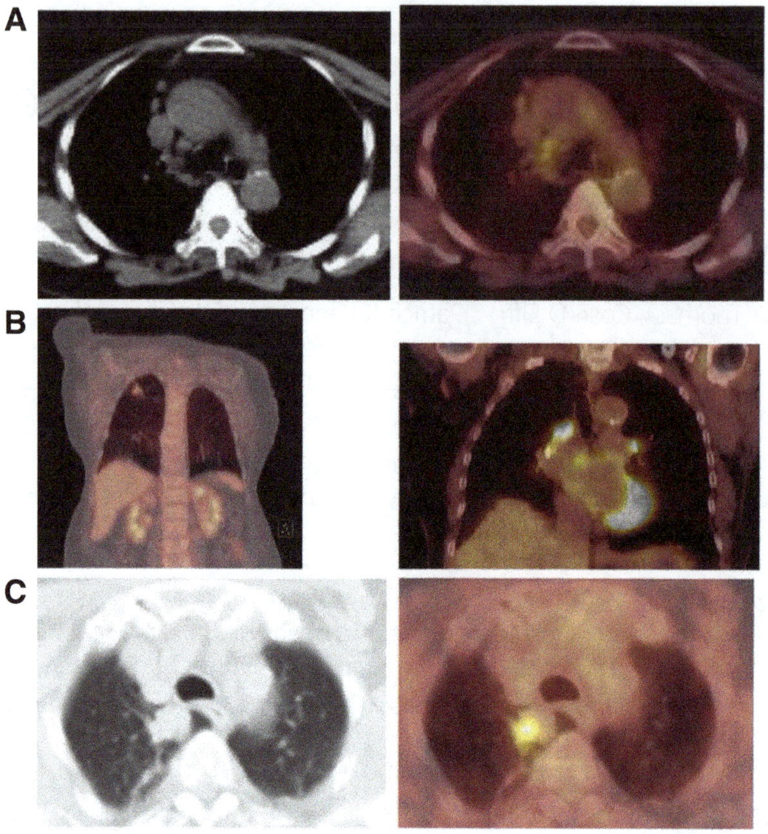

Figure 1 Representative FDG-PET/CT images. A. Case 1: axial CT (left) and fused FDG-PET/CT, with abnormal FDG uptake in the mediastinal lymph nodes. **B.** Case 2: fused FDG-PET/CT highlighting abnormal uptake in the right upper lobe nodule and more intense uptake in mediastinal lymph nodes. **C.** Case 3: axial CT (left) and fused FDG-PET/CT (right) with abnormal uptake in the right upper lobe nodule.

lymph node biopsy grew pan-susceptible *M. tuberculosis*. The patient was started on four-drug anti-tuberculosis therapy, but was intolerant of pyrazinamide, thus ultimately completed a total of 9 months of treatment with complete symptom and radiographic resolution. There was no evidence of disease recurrence at 1 year of follow-up after treatment completion.

Case 2

An elderly patient emigrated from a TB endemic country five years prior and had known TB contacts, was found to have a poorly differentiated squamous cell carcinoma of the cervix. The patient endorsed fatigue, a non-productive cough and 10 pound weight loss in the antecedent 4 months. Pre-chemotherapy work-up included a positive TST. FDG-PET/CT was performed for cancer staging and demonstrated the cervix mass as well as an FDG avid, peripheral nodular lesion in the right upper lobe of the lung, measuring approximately 1.6 × 1.4 cm and prominent hypermetabolic mediastinal lymph nodes adjacent to the right upper lobe bronchus, the largest with a maximum standardized uptake value (SUV) of 11 (Figure 1B). Three sputum samples were negative for acid fast bacilli by smear microscopy. Given that the pulmonary imaging was atypical for metastatic cervical cancer and favored to represent TB infection, and that active TB could not be ruled out which carried significant patient care and infection control implications while hospitalized for urgent cancer therapy, the patient was started on 4-drug treatment for active pulmonary TB. After two months of therapy, excessive nausea precluded continuation of her TB treatment, all cultures remained negative, and thus no further therapy was immediately pursued. To date, the patient has not had return of TB symptoms, now greater than 6 months after conclusion of therapy.

Case 3

An elderly patient from a non-endemic TB country was incidentally found to have a right upper lobe lung mass detected on a CT scan of the head/neck performed for evaluation of transient ischemic attacks. He was a lifetime non-smoker and had no symptoms of active TB. However, the patient was treated for TB as a young adult with 6 months of isoniazid and 4-aminobenzoic acid. To further evaluate the lung mass FDG-PET/CT scan of the chest was performed and revealed a hypermetabolic nodular lesion measuring 3.0 cm with a peak SUV of 5.75; no metabolically active perihilar or mediastinal lymph nodes were seen (Figure 1C). While a videoscopic wedge resection of the mass was negative for malignancy, gross pathology revealed a central cavity abutting the pleura. Histology found granulomatous inflammation and immunohistochemical staining for *M. tuberculosis* demonstrated rare intracellular rod forms. Bacterial, fungal and mycobacterial cultures as well as *M. tuberculosis* PCR of the tissue were negative. Given the histopathology and FDG-PET findings, anti-tuberculosis treatment was recommended but the patient refused and was lost to follow-up.

Case 4

An elderly patient from a TB endemic country who had been treated for active TB 50 years prior, presented with fever and cough of one week's duration following an international flight from the patient's country of origin. Chest x-ray revealed biapical pleural thickening, bronchiectasis and a patchy right hilar consolidation. Expectorated sputum samples and bronchioalveolar lavage were unremarkable and negative for acid fast bacilli. The patient was planning on returning to the home country by plane as soon as medically cleared. The patient also had a history of multiple urological malignancies. In this setting FDG-PET/CT was performed which confirmed the biapical thickening and linear densities of the apices, but was without any significant FDG uptake in the lungs or adjacent lymph nodes. He was discharged without TB treatment and all cultures finalized as negative.

Conclusions

FDG-PET/CT is an increasingly accessed technology for evaluation of malignancy in areas of both high and low TB prevalence [3] and therefore understanding the potential impact for its use in TB diagnosis and management is important for clinicians ordering and interpreting FDG-PET/CT. FDG uptake reflects cell glycolysis and is found in activated macrophages and lymphocytes [4], both of which are prominent in TB and other granulomatous inflammatory processes, as well as in neoplastic cells. The rate of uptake is reported as a standardized uptake value (SUV), the regional radioactivity concentration divided by the total injected dose and adjusted to the patient weight [5]. The maximum SUV is elevated in active TB. For instance, in a study of 150 subjects undergoing work-up for pulmonary nodules at a South Korean hospital, 10 cases of active pulmonary TB were identified and 9 (90%) had nodules with a maximum SUV above the threshold of 2.5 [6]. In a separate study of 25 subjects with culture-confirmed pulmonary TB, the mean maximum SUV was 4.96 ± 1.61 [7]. In addition, the maximum SUV declines on treatment, as demonstrated by a series of 21 HIV uninfected TB patients in whom the maximum SUV decreased by a median of 31% at one month of therapy [8]. Extrapulmonary sites of disease, particularly lymph nodes [9], may have an even higher maximum SUV, as was observed in Case 2. While quantitative assessment of SUV cannot distinguish active tuberculosis from malignancy [10], use of adjunctive tracers such as ^{11}C-choline and ^{18}F-fluorothymidine may provide improved discrimination. In a study of 97 patients with lung cancer, 14 with active pulmonary TB and 5 with non-tuberculous mycobacteria, the SUV of ^{11}C-choline was low in active TB compared to lung cancer, and values of FDG and ^{11}C-choline were both low in the patients with non-tuberculous mycobacteria [5].

Studies in humans examining FDG-PET for distinguishing latent and active TB are limited, but in one report of 25 patients, pulmonary TB disease activity was scored based on histopathology, culture and response to anti-tuberculosis treatment [11]. FDG-PET/CT revealed a

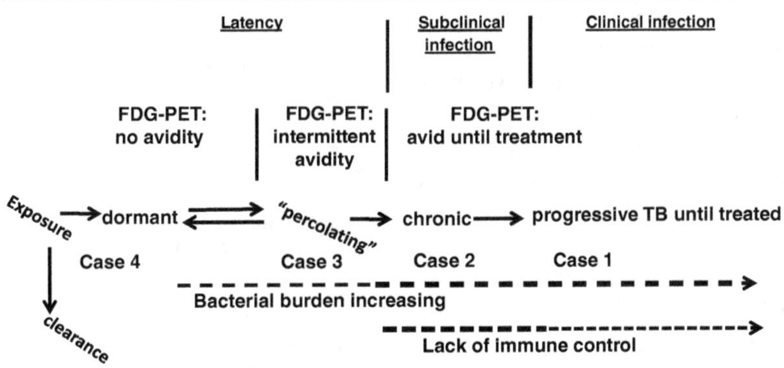

Figure 2 Spectrum of tuberculosis infection with proposed relationship to FDG-PET findings. Following exposure to *M. tuberculosis* an unknown percentage will clear infection entirely, while the vast majority develop latency (adapted from [10, 11]). Treatment of TB may eradicate all bacteria or leave a small population in a dormant non-replicating state. Populations with occasional replication termed "percolating" can be held under immunological control (noted by the dotted line) [10, 11]. Yet as bacterial burden increases, the risk of progression to active infection increases (noted by the hashed line). Cases 1–4 are presumptively placed along the proposed spectrum based on clinical, histopathological and microbiological studies and ^{18}F-fluorodeoxyglucose positron emission tomography (FDG-PET) avidity.

significantly higher early and late phase SUV (60 and 120 - minutes post-injection respectively) in patients with active compared to inactive TB [11]. Therefore a pulmonary nodule with high uptake on FDG-PET in a patient with evidence of TB exposure by positive TST or interferon-gamma release assay may tip the balance of treatment toward active TB, particularly if resection with histopathology and culture cannot be performed or if further immunosuppressing chemotherapy is immediately planned, as in Case 2.

Complicating the matter, however, is recent work in non-human primates that suggests the TB disease state may be more dynamic than previously believed [12,13]. Rather than simply latent or active, TB infection occupies a more diverse spectrum (Figure 2). In certain individuals a robust acquired immune response with T-cell priming may have eliminated infection completely while in others a quiescent infection remains with some mycobacteria persisting in non-replicating form [13,14]. In a small proportion of patients, the immune response has kept active infection of replicating mycobacteria at the sub-clinical level, while in other patients, active inflammation, TB replication, and symptoms propagate [13, 14]. Therefore, high uptake of FDG by PET may represent ongoing active disease, as demonstrated by Case 1, or simply the host immune system activity that will ultimately prevail, such as could be argued for Case 3 (Figure 2). Given such emerging evidence from non-human primates, we would not advocate for the immediate adoption of FDG-PET/CT in treatment decisions regarding TB latency. However the implications of FDG-PET/CT findings must be considered in patients for whom this modality was employed for another clinical indication, as exemplified by Case 2, in whom low-grade TB symptoms may have been masked by the concurrent malignancy.

Perhaps the most promising role of FDG-PET/CT is in the monitoring of therapeutic response in select cases of extrapulmonary TB where sputum culture is unavailable, or in multidrug-resistant (MDR)-TB where second-line drugs are less efficacious and definitive treatment duration is not known [15]. Extrapulmonary tuberculoma may persist with little change for years if imaged with conventional radiology [16]. Uncontrolled case series have described the benefit of decreased FDG uptake following treatment in extrapulmonary sites of disease. In a series of 30 patients with TB of the spine for instance, the percent change in maximum SUV discriminated residual infection from successful treatment [17]. Another conceivable issue is that if imaged too early in the course of treatment, a paradoxical increase in FDG uptake may be observed due to immune reconstitution, however, this has not been observed in animal models [14]. The use of FDG-PET/CT has only begun to be reported for MDR-TB [18], but in a murine model of TB treatment FDG uptake correlated with mycobacterial burden in the lung and decreased proportional to the degree of bactericidal activity of the drug regimen [19]. Furthermore, in a promising series of HIV co-infected TB patients from South Africa, the number of lymph node bastions was found predictive of response to drug-susceptible TB treatment and a surrogate marker for clinical MDR-TB [18]. Given that the cost of treating MDR-TB may be 100 times more expensive than drug-susceptible TB, the decision to extend or shorten treatment, in some cases upward of 24 months, may defray the cost of FDG-PET/CT in certain well-resourced settings. Despite conceptual appeal for the use of FDG-PET/CT in assessment of transmissibility or even relapse following therapy, as was done in part for Case 4, further data are required to support these applications.

In summary, FDG-PET/CT is an increasingly employed modality and TB clinicians should become familiar with its use. FDG-PET/CT may need to be interpreted in the context of distinguishing latent versus active disease, and it has the potential to become a tool in monitoring treatment response in select cases of extrapulmonary TB or multidrug-resistance.

Consent

The Institutional Review Board at the University of Virginia approved this report.

Abbreviations

TB: Tuberculosis; TST: Tuberculin skin test; CT: Computed tomography; FDG-PET: ^{18}F-fluorodeoxyglucose positron emission tomography; SUV: Standardized uptake value..

Competing interests

The authors declare that they have no competing interest.

Authors' contributions

SKH conceived of the study, performed literature review and analysis, and drafted the manuscript. TAT participated in chart review and provided critical revision of the manuscript. CDS cared for cases, provided oversight of infection control, interpretation of the literature and critical revision of the manuscript. PKR analyzed the imaging and provided critical revision of the manuscript. ERH cared for cases, conceived of the study, and provided critical revision of the manuscript. All authors read and approved the final manuscript.

Acknowledgements

SKH was supported by National Institutes of Health grant K23AI099019 and the Burroughs Wellcome Fund/ American Society of Tropical Medicine and Hygiene, TAT by National Institutes of Health grant K23AI097197 and ERH in part by National Institutes of Health grant R01AI093358. Funders had no role in study design, data collection or analysis, decision to publish, or preparation of the manuscript.

Author details

[1]Division of Infectious Diseases and International Health, University of Virginia, PO Box 801337, Charlottesville, VA 29908-1337, USA. [2]Office of Hospital Epidemiology/Infection Prevention and Control, University of Virginia Health System, Charlottesville, USA. [3]Department of Radiology and Medical Imaging, University of Virginia, Charlottesville, USA.

References

1. Lillington GA, Caskey CI: **Evaluation and management of solitary and multiple pulmonary nodules.** *Clin Chest Med* 1993, **14:**111–119.
2. El-Haddad G, Zhuang H, Gupta N, Alavi A: **Evolving role of positron emission tomography in the management of patients with inflammatory and other benign disorders.** *Semin Nucl Med* 2004, **34**(4):313–329.
3. Sathekge MM, Maes A, Pottel H, Stoltz A, van de Wiele C: **Dual time-point FDG PET/CT for differentiating benign from malignant solitary pulmonary nodules in a TB endemic area.** *S Afr Med J* 2010, **100:**598–601.
4. Malik K, Dedhia HV, Bishop H, *et al*: **Clinical utility of PET-FDG imaging in detecting malignancy in pulmonary lesions.** *Chest* 1996, **110**(suppl):95S.
5. Hara T, Kosaka N, Suzuki T, Kudo K, Niino H: **Uptake rates of 18-Fluorodeoxyglucose and 11C-choline in lung cancer and pulmonary tuberculosis: a positron emission tomography study.** *Chest* 2003, **124:**893–901.
6. Goo JM, Im JG, Do KH, Yeo JS, Seo JB, Kim HY, Chung JK: **Pulmonary tuberculoma evaluated by means of FDG PET: findings in 10 cases.** *Radiology* 2000, **216:**117–121.
7. Demura Y, Tsuchida T, Uesaka D, Umeda Y, Morikawa M, Ameshima S, Ishizaki T, Fujibayashi Y, Okazawa H: **Usefulness of 18 F-fluorodeoxyglucose positron emission tomography for diagnosing disease activity and monitoring therapeutic response in patients with pulmonary mycobacteriosis.** *Eur J Nucl Med Mol Imaging* 2009, **36:**632–639.
8. Martinez V, Castilla-Lievre MA, Guillet-Caruba C, Grenier G, Fior R, Desarnaud S, Doucet-Populaire F, Boué F: **(18)F-FDG PET/CT in tuberculosis: an early non-invasive marker of therapeutic response.** *Int J Tuberc Lung Dis* 2012, **16**(9):1180–1185.
9. Soussan M, Brillet PY, Mekinian A, Khafagy A, Nicolas P, Vessieres A, Brauner M: **Patterns of pulmonary tuberculosis on FDG-PET/CT.** *Eur J Radiol* 2012, **81**(10):2872–2876.
10. Treglia G, MD, Taralli S, Calcagni ML, Maggi F, Giordan A, Bonomo L: **Is there a role for fluorine 18-fluorodeoxyglucose positron emission tomography and positron emission tomography/computed tomography in evaluating patients with mycobacteriosis? A systematic review.** *J Comput Assist Tomogr* 2011, **35:**387–393.
11. Kim IJ, Lee JS, Kim SJ, Kim YK, Jeong YJ, Jun S, Nam HY, Kim JS: **Double phase 18 F-FDG PET-CT for determination of pulmonary tuberculoma activity.** *Eur J Nucl Med Mol Imaging* 2008, **35:**808–814.
12. Barry CE, Boshoff HI, Dartois V, Dick T, Ehrt S, Flynn J, Schnappinger D, Wilkinson RJ, Young D: **The spectrum of latent tuberculosis: rethinking the biology and intervention strategies.** *Nature Reviews* 2009, **7:**845–855.
13. Lin PL, Flynn JL: **Understanding latent tuberculosis: a moving target.** *J Immunol* 2010, **185:**15–22.
14. Via LE, Schimel D, Weiner DM, *et al*: **Infection dynamics and response to chemotherapy in a rabbit model of tuberculosis using [18 F]2-Fluoro-Deoxy-D-Glucose Positron Emission Tomography and Computed Tomography.** *Antimicrob Agents Chemother* 2012, **56**(8):4391.
15. Gandhi NR, Nunn P, Dheda K, Schaaf HS, Zignol M, van Soolingen D, Jensen P, Bayona J: **Multidrug-resistant and extensively drug-resistant tuberculosis: a threat to global control of tuberculosis.** *Lancet* 2010, **375:**1830–1843.
16. Tian G, Xiao Y, Chen B, Xia J, Guan H, Deng Q: **FDG PET/CT for therapeutic response monitoring in multi-site non-respiratory tuberculosis.** *Acta Radiologica* 2010, **9:**1002–1006.
17. Kim SJ, Kim IJ, Suh KT, Kim YK, Lee JS: **Prediction of residual disease of spine infection using F-18 FDG PET/CT.** *Spine* 2009, **34:**2424–2430.
18. Sathekge M, Maes A, Kgomo M, Stoltz A, Van de Wiele C: **Use of 18 F-FDG PET to predict response to first-line tuberculostatics in HIV-associated tuberculosis.** *J Nucl Med* 2011, **52:**880–885.
19. Davis SL, Nuermberger EL, Um PK, Vidal C, Jedynak B, Pomper MG, Bishai WR, Jain SK: **Noninvasive pulmonary [18 F]-2-fluoro-deoxy-D-glucose positron emission tomography correlates with bactericidal activity of tuberculosis drug treatment.** *Antimicrob Agents Chemother* 2009, **53:**4879–4884.

2

Retrospective observational study of diagnostic accuracy of the Xpert® MTB/RIF assay on fiberoptic bronchoscopy sampling for early diagnosis of smear-negative or sputum-scarce patients with suspected tuberculosis

Pierre Le Palud[1], Vincent Cattoir[2,3], Brigitte Malbruny[2^], Romain Magnier[1], Karine Campbell[1,3], Youssef Oulkhouir[1], Gérard Zalcman[1,3] and Emmanuel Bergot[1,3,4*]

Abstract

Background: Fiberoptic bronchoscopy (FOB) is a useful diagnosis tool in low-burden countries for patients with suspected pulmonary tuberculosis (TB) who are smear-negative or sputum-scarce. This study sought to determine the accuracy of the Xpert® MTB/RIF (XP) assay using FOB samples.

Methods: We retrospectively reviewed clinical, radiological, and microbiological characteristics of 175 TB-suspected patients requiring diagnostic FOB (bronchial aspirate or bronchoalveolar lavage) with XP assay. Polymerase chain reaction (PCR) and smear microscopy (SM) performances were first compared to culture, then to the final diagnosis, established based on clinical or radiological evolution when cultures were negative.

Results: Of the total 162 included patients, 30 (18.5%) had a final diagnosis of pulmonary TB, with positive cultures reported in 23. As compared to culture, sensitivity and specificity values were 80.0% and 98.6% for the XP assay, and 25.0% and 95.8% for SM, respectively. As compared to final diagnosis, the corresponding performance values were 60.0% and 100.0% for the XP assay, and 16.7% and 95.5% for SM, respectively. The sensitivity of the XP assay was significantly higher than that of SM in both cases ($p = 0.003$ and $p = 0.001$). Concerning the final diagnosis, both XP assay and culture sensitivities were similar (60% *vs.* 66.7%). PCR assay enabled pulmonary TB to be diagnosed earlier in 13 more cases, compared to SM.

Conclusion: Our study has confirmed the clinical benefits provided by XP assay compared to SM for the early diagnosis of suspected pulmonary TB cases requiring FOB, on *per* procedure samples, especially in a low TB-burden country.

Keywords: Tuberculosis diagnosis, Fiberoptic bronchoscopy, Xpert® MTB/RIF assay, Smear microscopy

* Correspondence: bergot-e@chu-caen.fr
^Deceased
[1]CHU de Caen, Service de Pneumologie et Oncologie thoracique, F-14000 Caen, France
[3]Université de Caen-Basse Normandie, F-14000 Caen, France
Full list of author information is available at the end of the article

Background

Tuberculosis (TB) still constitutes a major health problem worldwide, with an 8.8% incidence and 1.3% mortality rate reported in 2010 [1]. In the same year, TB incidence was reported at 8.1 cases per 100,000 in France [2], defining it as a low TB-burden country. It is worth noting that 73% of TB cases were pulmonary infections, with almost 50% producing a negative smear microscopy (SM) [2].

By detecting active pulmonary TB early, an appropriate treatment can be initiated, and disease transmission can then be preemptively blocked. Some patients presenting with active pulmonary TB may, however, exhibit negative sputum acid-fast bacilli (AFB) smears. In developed countries, fiberoptic bronchoscopy (FOB) is considered a good option for these cases that pose a diagnostic challenge [3], although SM is still exhibiting low sensitivity on FOB samples, with 5-35% on bronchial aspirates (BA) and 10-30% on bronchoalveolar lavages (BAL) [4-9]. Furthermore, while mycobacterial culture remains the gold standard for laboratory diagnosis of TB, it requires 2–6 weeks to confirm a diagnosis. This results in delays in initiating appropriate treatment while waiting for this confirmation, except for cases where there is strong enough clinical suspicion to initiate a presumptive anti-TB therapy.

Several polymerase chain reaction- (PCR-) based molecular methods have recently been developed for early TB diagnosis and rapid detection of drug resistance from clinical specimens [10-14]. The Xpert® MTB/RIF assay (Cepheid, Sunnyvale, CA, USA) is one of these methods, and consists of a hemi-nested real-time PCR test that simultaneously identifies *Mycobacterium tuberculosis* and detects rifampicin resistance, as a surrogate of multidrug resistance (MDR), directly from clinical specimens. This assay requires less than 2 hours, and its key advantage over other PCR methods is that it is a fully-automated process, designed to run on the GeneXpert Dx system (Cepheid). This system incorporates DNA extraction, often considered the critical step [15], along with real-time PCR amplification and detection in a single hands-free process, thus acting as a real "lab-on-chip" device.

Since December 2010, WHO has recommended the Xpert® MTB/RIF assay as a *bona fide* follow-on test due to its high-quality performance [16], compared to microscopy, whenever MDR-TB or HIV are of lesser concern, and especially in cases of smear-negative specimens [17]. This conditional recommendation does, in fact, exclusively concern sputum samples [17], whereas no specific recommendations for FOB samples have yet been formulated. Finally, there have only been two recent studies that have assessed the Xpert® MTB/RIF assay performance using FOB samples for TB diagnosis in high TB-burden countries [18,19].

This study sought to evaluate the clinical value of the Xpert® MTB/RIF assay using FOB samples for an early diagnosis of pulmonary TB in either patients with negative sputum AFB smears or those who could not produce an expectorated sputum sample. Patients were treated in a French university hospital in a low TB-burden region (5.9 cases per 100,000 in 2010).

Methods

Study population

We retrospectively reviewed the medical records of patients with suspected TB requiring a diagnostic FOB at the Caen University Hospital (Basse-Normandie region, North-Western France) from October 2009 to April 2013. TB was suspected based on clinical features (*e.g.*, cough, hemoptysis, fever, asthenia, loss of weight, and night sweats) or radiological features (*e.g.*, nodule, pneumonia, excavation, and pleurisy). All included patients either produced a negative sputum AFB SM prior to FOB procedure or were unable to produce sputum.

Our institution, a regional center of reference for TB diagnosis and treatment, has adopted the Xpert® MTB/RIF assay since 2009. Patients were included in the ongoing retrospective survey if one or more Xpert® MTB/RIF assays had been performed on their FOB samples, in addition to SM and mycobacterial culture procedures. Samples were excluded if culture results were unavailable or if the Xpert® MTB/RIF assay produced invalid results (see below). Patients who had previously received anti-TB drugs were also excluded from analysis.

Bronchoscopic procedures

Bronchoscopy was performed using a flexible fiberscope of either 4.9 mm (model BF-P180, Olympus Optical) or 5.1 mm in diameter (model F1-16RB, Pentax) by trained lung specialists who first inspected the bronchial tree and then collected BA or BAL specimens. The type of sample was chosen at the specialist's discretion and depending on the patient's tolerance of the procedure. The lung section sample was generally chosen based on chest X-ray or CT-scan abnormalities. BA samples were obtained by the aspiration of pure bronchial secretions or following the instillation of 20-50 mL isotonic saline solution. For the BAL samples, 100-150 mL isotonic saline solution was instilled by 50 mL aliquots in a lung segment, and then aspirated.

Microbiological diagnosis

All samples were digested, decontaminated by means of N-acetyl-cysteine-2% NaOH, concentrated by centrifugation (at 3,500 rpm for 20 min), and tested with SM, culture (used as the reference technique), and PCR.

For the smear test, fixed preparations were stained with auramine and visualized under a fluorescence microscope (at × 400 magnification). Each slide was observed for 5 min, corresponding to 200 fields examined. Sample aliquots of 500 μL and 200 μL were inoculated in an MGIT liquid medium (BD Diagnostics, Le Pont-de-Claix, France) or on Coletsos slants (Bio-Rad, Marnes-la-Coquette, France), respectively. Liquid cultures were automatically monitored by the BACTEC MGIT 960 system (BD Diagnostics) for up to 6 weeks, while solid media were studied for up to 12 weeks. Positive cultures were those with the presence of *M. tuberculosis* confirmed by means of the TB Ag MPT64 Rapid® assay (Standard Diagnostics, Yongin, South Korea), and rifampicin susceptibility was tested using the MGIT 960 SIRE kit (BD Diagnostics) [20]. The different species of nontuberculous mycobacteria (NTM) were identified using the GenoType® *Mycobacterium* CM/AS (HainLifescience, Nehren, Germany).

For the Xpert® MTB/RIF assay, a 500 μL aliquot was poured into a single-use disposable cartridge that was placed into the GeneXpert™ Dx module, with the results produced in less than 2 hours. Each PCR run comprised an internal control for sample processing (DNA extraction) and PCR validity (presence of inhibitors), with positive and negative controls tested every day. The system automatically interpreted all results from measured fluorescent signals, with embedded calculation algorithms, into the following categories: invalid, if PCR inhibitors were detected with amplification failure; negative or positive. If positive, the strain was categorized as susceptible or resistant to rifampicin [21,22].

Pulmonary TB diagnosis

The final diagnosis of active pulmonary TB was primarily based on the *M. tuberculosis* culture taken from a respiratory specimen. Additional cases were classified as definitive TB, taking into account both the clinical symptoms and histological/radiological findings compatible with active pulmonary TB, as well as improvement observed with anti-TB specific therapy.

Ethical considerations

According to the WHO recommendations on the Xpert® MTB/RIF assay [16], the use of this diagnosis TB test has been routinely implemented in our University hospital. According to French laws, a formal agreement from an ethics committee is not required for retrospective collection of data dealing with usual standard medical care *(ref: law n°2004-806 from August, 9th 2004, modified by government ordinance n°2066-477 from April 26th 2006, article R1121-3, Journal officiel de la République Française)*. All collected data from the charts of the Microbiology Department were anonymous and therefore complied with the restrictive requirements of the *Commision Nationale de l'Informatique et des Libertés (CNIL)*, the organization that ensures the application of

Table 1 Demographic, clinical, and radiological characteristics of the 162 included patients

Characteristic	**N (%)**
Median age, years (range)	**54 (34–74)**
Gender	
Male	102 (63.0)
Female	60 (37.0)
HIV	
Positive	7 (4.3)
Negative	98 (60.5)
NA	57 (35.2)
Symptoms	
Cough	84 (51.9)
Hemoptysis	17 (10.5)
General symptoms[a]	73 (45.1)
Fever	43 (26.5)
Night sweats	26 (16.0)
NA	11 (6.8)
Chest radiography	
Nodules	87 (53.7)
Pneumonia	44 (27.1)
Excavation	14 (8.6)
Pleurisy	21 (13.0)
NA	13 (8.0)
Chest CT scan	
Nodules	98 (60.5)
Pneumonia	49 (30.2)
Excavation	27 (16.7)
Pleurisy	21 (13.0)
NA	29 (17.9)
Final diagnosis	
Pulmonary Tuberculosis	30 (18.5)
Pleural Tuberculosis	2 (1.2)
Tuberculosis sequelae	11 (6.8)
NTM[b] infection	9 (5.6)
Non-mycobacterial lung infection[c]	28 (17.3)
Bronchial disease exacerbation	7 (4.3)
Non-mycobacterial granulomatosis disease	7 (4.3)
Lung cancer	21 (13.0)
Other[d]	23 (14.2)
No diagnosis	18 (11.1)
NA	6 (3.7)

[a]General symptoms: asthenia and/or loss of appetite and/or loss of weight.
[b]*NTM*: Nontuberculous mycobacteria (including four *M. avium*, two *M. xenopi*, one *M. szulgai*, one *M. malmoense*, and one other).
[c]Including 24 infectious pneumonia, two lung abscesses, and two invasive aspergillosis.
[d]Including eight non-infectious pneumonia, five acute pulmonary edema, five idiopathic hemoptysis, two interstitial lung disease exacerbations, one pulmonary infarction, one intra-alveolar hemorrhage, and one inflammatory pseudo-tumor lung.

data privacy laws in France. Moreover, the study protocol was evaluated and approved by the institutional review board of the French Society for Respiratory Medecine ("Société de Pneumologie de Langue Française") for observational studies (CEPRO). Finally, all patients were informed of our TB diagnostic strategy, received written information about the FOB procedure and gave there oral consent (as recommended by the French Society of Respiratory Diseases).

Statistical analysis

Sensitivity, specificity, positive predictive value (PPV), and negative predictive value (NPV) were calculated, along with the corresponding 95% confidence intervals. Sensitivity and specificity values were compared by means of the McNemar's test. A *p*-value inferior to 0.05 was considered statistically significant. Statistical analysis was performed using the SPSS Statistics 20.0 software (Armonk, NY, USA).

Results

Patient characteristics

From October 2009 to April 2013, 175 consecutive patients presenting with suspected active pulmonary TB underwent FOB with an Xpert® MTB/RIF assay using respiratory samples. A total of 13 samples from 13 different patients were excluded from our study for the following reasons: 1) two due to PCR failure; 2) 10 due to unavailable culture; 3) one due to recent anti-TB treatment. A total of 229 FOB samples taken from 162 patients (median age: 54 years; male/female ratio: 1.7) were included.

The principal clinical symptoms were cough (51.9%) and general symptoms, such as asthenia, loss of appetite, and loss of weight for half of the patients (Table 1). The most common lesions detected by chest imaging were nodules (CT-scan: 60.5%) and pneumonia (CT-scan: 30.2%) (Table 1). It should be noted that 18, 9, and 80 patients had 1, 2, and 3 sputum samples, respectively, that were collected before FOB, with the number of Xpert® MTB/RIF assays performed on the sample ranging from 0 to 3 for each patient (0: 110 patients; 1: 21; 2: 22; 3: 9). No sputum could be collected before the FOB procedure for 55 patients (34%) due to their inability to expectorate sputum.

Xpert® MTB/RIF assay was performed on BA (n = 48), BAL (n = 47), or a BA/BAL mix (n = 67) (Figure 1). Out of the 162 patients, 30 TB cases were finally diagnosed, corresponding to a prevalence of 18.5% (Figure 1). Of these cases, positive cultures were reported on FOB and sputum samples for 20 and 3, respectively, including one TB case caused by *"Mycobacterium canetti"*. For the remaining seven patients, diagnosis was based on clinical and histological/radiological features, with favorable evolution under anti-TB therapy serving as confirmation. The final diagnoses for the other patients are detailed in Table 1.

Performances of microbiological methods

In comparison with culture used as reference, the overall sensitivity, specificity, PPV, and NPVs for the Xpert® MTB/RIF assay were 80.0% (95% CI: 57.8-92.5), 98.6% (95% CI: 94.7-99.9), 88.9% (95% CI: 66.0-98.1), and 97.2%

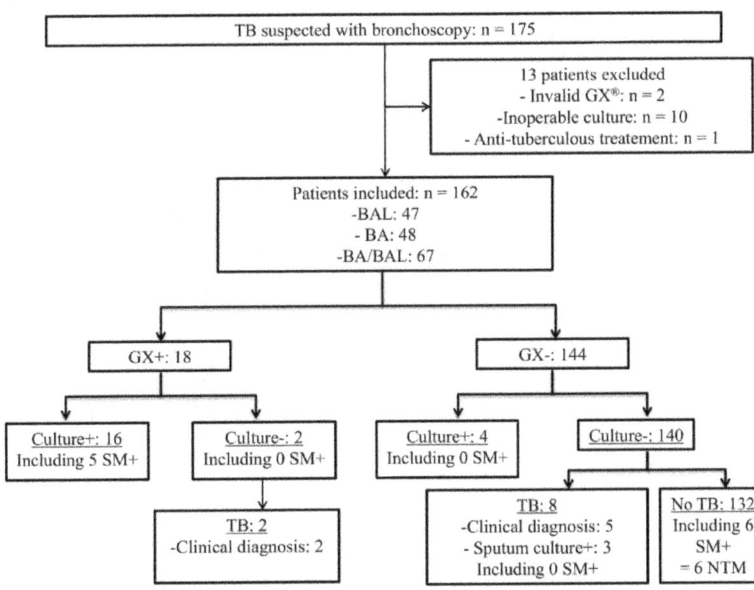

Figure 1 Flow diagram of patients included in the study. BA: bronchial aspirate; BAL: bronchoalveolar lavage; SM: smear microscopy; GX: Xpert®MTB/RIF assay; NTM: nontuberculous mycobacteria; TB: tuberculosis.

(95% CI: 92.8-99.2), respectively. The corresponding values for SM were recorded as 25.0% (95% CI: 10.8-47.3), 95.8% (95% CI: 90.9-98.3), 45.5% (95% CI: 21.3-72.0), and 90.1% (95% CI: 84.2-94.0), respectively (Table 2). It is interesting to note that the sensitivity of the Xpert® MTB/RIF assay was found to be significantly higher than that of SM ($p = 0.003$; Table 2).

When considered relative to the final diagnosis, the performances of both sensitivity (60%; 95% CI: 42.3-75.4) and specificity (100%; 95% CI: 96.6-100.0) of the Xpert® MTB/RIF assay were also shown to be significantly higher than those of SM (16.7%; 95% CI: 6.9 to 34.0; 95.5%; 95% CI: 90.2 to 98.1) ($p = 0.001$ and $p = 0.041$) (Table 2). PPV and NPV were 100.0% (95% CI: 79.3-100.0) and 91.7% (95% CI: 85.9-95.3) for the Xpert® MTB/RIF assay, respectively, while these values were measured at 45.5% (95% CI: 21.3-72.0) and 83.4% (95% CI: 76.6-88.6) for SM, respectively. It is worth noting that all six samples with a positive SM and a negative PCR assay were seen to grow an NTM species. Regarding the final diagnosis, no significant difference was observed between Xpert® MTB/RIF assay and culture sensitivities (60%; 95% CI: 42.3-75.4 *vs.* 66.7%; 95% CI: 48.7-80.9; $p = 0.683$).

The Xpert® MTB/RIF assay also enabled earlier TB diagnosis and treatment for 13 more patients than was possible with SM (Table 3). In addition, the Xpert® MTB/RIF assay led to the early detection of one MDR-TB case in our series, which was subsequently confirmed using phenotypic tests.

Table 3 Gain in early pulmonary tuberculosis diagnosis with the Xpert® MTB/RIF assay

N = 162 patients	TB + (N = 30 patients)	TB- (N = 132 patients)
Xpert®MTB/RIF (XP)+	18	0
Smear microscopy (SM) +	5	6 (=6 NTM[a])
Gain in early TB[b] diagnosis (XP-SM)	13	0

[a]*NTM*: Nontuberculous mycobacteria.
[b]*TB*: Tuberculosis.

Discussion

FOB constitutes an interesting alternative for TB diagnosis in smear-negative or sputum-scarce patients, especially in developed countries where this procedure is widely available. Given that WHO recommendations on the Xpert® MTB/RIF assay only pertain to sputum samples [17], further investigation must be conducted regarding the use of this PCR on FOB samples. To the best of our knowledge, there has been no publication specifically describing the clinical interest and accuracy of the Xpert® MTB/RIF assay using FOB samples for TB diagnosis in a low-prevalence country.

Our study produced results in line with previous reports on respiratory samples [16,23-31], demonstrating that the Xpert® MTB/RIF assay significantly outperformed SM on FOB samples (sensitivities: 80.0% *vs.* 25.0%; $p = 0.003$) in a low TB-prevalence area. The sensitivity of the PCR assay was found to be lower when it was calculated relative to the final diagnosis, yet still remained

Table 2 Performances of the Xpert®MTB/RIF assay, smear microscopy, and culture using FOB samples for the diagnosis of pulmonary tuberculosis

	Performances relative to culture		Performances relative to final diagnosis	
	Sensitivity% (95% CI) n	Specificity% (95% CI) n	Sensitivity% (95% CI) n	Specificity% (95% CI) n
Xpert® MTB/RIF assay	80.0	98.6	60.0	100.0
	(57.8-92.5)	(94.7-99.9)	(42.3-75.4)	(96.6-100.0)
	16/20	140/142	18/30	132/132
Smear microscopy	25.0	95.8	16.7	95.5
	(10.8-47.3)	(90.9-98.3)	(6.9-34.0)	(90.2-98.1)
	5/20	136/142	5/30	126/132
Culture	-	-	66.7	100.0
			(48.7-80.9)	(96.6-100.0)
			20/30	132/132
p-value[a]	*0.003*	*0.288*	*0.001*[b]	*0.041*[b]
			0.683[c]	-
			0.0003[d]	*0.041*[d]

[a]*p*-values were calculated using the McNemar's test.
[b]*p*-value between Xpert®MTB/RIFassay *vs.* smear microscopy.
[c]*p*-value between Xpert®MTB/RIFassay *vs.* culture.
[d]*p*-value between culture *vs.* smear microscopy.

significantly higher than that achieved with SM (60.0% *vs.* 16.7%; $p = 0.001$). Our findings revealed similar performances to those reported by two recently published studies, which had previously explored the clinical usefulness of the Xpert® MTB/RIF assay on FOB samples, although this was conducted in high TB-prevalence areas [18,19]. In the Lee *et al.* retrospective study, 132 patients were recruited in a single South-Korean center. The study reported sensitivity and specificity values (relative to the culture) of 81.6% and 100.0% for the Xpert® MTB/RIF assay, compared to 13.2% and 98.8% for SM, respectively [18]. Theron *et al.* prospectively included 154 patients in a South-African single-center study and specifically analyzed BAL samples. The resulting sensitivity and specificity values compared to the culture were 92.6% and 96.0% for the Xpert® MTB/RIF assay, and 57.7% and 99.3% for SM, respectively [19].

We can therefore confirm that for suspected TB requiring bronchoscopic procedure, the Xpert® MTB/RIF assay is a potential alternative to SM using FOB samples. In our study, PCR allowed for early pulmonary TB diagnosis to be established, enabling appropriate treatment to be started early for 13 more patients as compared to SM (72%) ($p < 0.001$; Table 3). In these patients, the definitive TB diagnosis was secondarily confirmed either by culture or clinical evolution under specific antimicrobial therapy. These findings were similar to those of the Theron *et al.* study (>80%) [19], and are of particular significance in a low TB-incidence area, where there is a higher proportion of alternative diagnosis, such as lung cancer or pyogenic bacterial pneumonia.

Our study objectives did not include assessing the value of the GeneXpert® assay in detecting rifampicin resistance on FOB samples, since the incidence of such resistance was expected to be low, as seen in previous studies [18,19]. The unique case of MDR-TB was, however, unambiguously detected, and all PCR results were corroborated by those that were phenotypically determined.

Our study presented some limitations. Firstly, this was a retrospective study, despite all Xpert® MTB/RIF assays being performed on fresh FOB samples. Secondly, it was a single-center study. Finally the PCR assays were not systematically performed on the same FOB sample for all patients (BA or BAL). A prospective study should be designed with systematized and parallel FOB sampling (BA, BAL). This would provide a more proficient way of testing the Xpert® MTB/RIF assay in different types of per-endoscopic respiratory samples, an endpoint that we were unable to analyze due to our retrospective design. Cost-effectiveness studies should also be conducted in order to specify the rational use of the Xpert® MTB/RIF assay on FOB samples in novel diagnostic algorithms, including this PCR assay in well-resourced countries.

Conclusion

In summary, our study confirms the clinical usefulness of the Xpert® MTB/RIF assay, compared to SM, for the early diagnosis of suspected pulmonary TB requiring FOB, performed on *per* procedure samples. This is a reproducible commercial assay, and should especially be considered as a relevant option in low TB-burden countries.

Competing interests
The authors declare that they have no competing interests.

Authors' contributions
Study conception and design: PLP, VC, GZ, and EB. Acquisition of data: PLP, RM, KC and YO. Drafting of manuscript: PLP, VC, GZ, and EB. Analysis and interpretation of data: BM. Critical revision: VC, GZ, and EB. All authors read and approved the final manuscript.

Acknowledgements
The technical assistance of Gilles Le Marrec and Karine Courageux is gratefully acknowledged. This paper is dedicated to the memory of Dr. Brigitte Malbruny.

Author details
[1]CHU de Caen, Service de Pneumologie et Oncologie thoracique, F-14000 Caen, France. [2]CHU de Caen, Service de Microbiologie, F-14000 Caen, France. [3]Université de Caen-Basse Normandie, F-14000 Caen, France. [4]Groupe pour la Recherche et l'Enseignement en Pneumo-Infectiologie (GREPI) de la Société de Pneumologie de Langue Française (SPLF), F-75000 Paris, France.

References

1. World Health Organization: *WHO report 2011: global tuberculosis control. WHO/HTM/TB/2011.16.* Geneva, Switzerland: WHO; 2011.
2. Antoine D, Che D: **Les cas de tuberculose déclarés en France en 2010.** *Bull Epidémiol Hebd* 2012, **24–25:**285–287.
3. Mohan A, Sharma SK: **Fibreoptic bronchoscopy in the diagnosis of sputum smear-negative pulmonary tuberculosis: current status.** *Indian J Chest Dis Allied Sci* 2008, **50:**67–78.
4. de Gracia J, Curull V, Vidal R, Riba A, Orriols R, Martin N, Morell F: **Diagnostic value of bronchoalveolar lavage in suspected pulmonary tuberculosis.** *Chest* 1988, **93:**329–332.
5. Chawla R, Pant K, Jaggi OP, Chandrashekhar S, Thukral SS: **Fibreoptic bronchoscopy in smear-negative pulmonary tuberculosis.** *Eur Respir J* 1988, **1:**804–806.
6. Chan HS, Sun AJ, Hoheisel GB: **Bronchoscopic aspiration and bronchoalveolar lavage in the diagnosis of sputum smear-negative pulmonary tuberculosis.** *Lung* 1990, **168:**215–220.
7. Salzman SH, Schindel ML, Aranda CP, Smith RL, Lewis ML: **The role of bronchoscopy in the diagnosis of pulmonary tuberculosis in patients at risk for HIV infection.** *Chest* 1992, **102:**143–146.
8. Altaf Bachh A, Gupta R, Haq I, Varudkar HG: **Diagnosing sputum/smear-negative pulmonary tuberculosis: does fibre-optic bronchoscopy play a significant role?** *Lung India* 2010, **27:**58–62.
9. Shin JA, Chang YS, Kim TH, Kim HJ, Ahn CM, Byun MK: **Fiberoptic bronchoscopy for the rapid diagnosis of smear-negative pulmonary tuberculosis.** *BMC Infect Dis* 2012, **12:**141.
10. Brugière O, Vokurka M, Lecossier D, Mangiapan G, Amrane A, Milleron B, Mayaud C, Cadranel J, Hance AJ: **Diagnosis of smear-negative pulmonary tuberculosis using sequence capture polymerase chain reaction.** *Am J Respir Crit Care Med* 1997, **155:**1478–1481.
11. Liam CK, Chen YC, Yap SF, Srinivas P, Poi PJ: **Detection of Mycobacterium tuberculosis in bronchoalveolar lavage from patients with sputum smear-negative pulmonary tuberculosis using a polymerase chain reaction assay.** *Respirology* 1998, **3:**125–129.
12. Wong CF, Yew WW, Chan CY, Au LY, Cheung SW, Cheng AF: **Rapid diagnosis of smear-negative pulmonary tuberculosis via fibreoptic bronchoscopy:**

utility of polymerase chain reaction in bronchial aspirates as an adjunct to transbronchial biopsies. *Respir Med* 1998, **92**:815–819.
13. Chen NH, Liu YC, Tsao TC, Wu TL, Hsieh MJ, Chuang ML, Huang CC, Kuo AJ, Chen MC, Yang CT: **Combined bronchoalveolar lavage and polymerase chain reaction in the diagnosis of pulmonary tuberculosis in smear-negative patients.** *Int J Tuberc Lung Dis* 2002, **6**:350–355.
14. Tueller C, Chhajed PN, Buitrago-Tellez C, Frei R, Frey M, Tamm M: **Value of smear and PCR in bronchoalveolar lavage fluid in culture positive pulmonary tuberculosis.** *Eur Respir J* 2005, **26**:767–772.
15. Käser M, Ruf MT, Hauser J, Pluschke G: **Optimized DNA preparation from mycobacteria.** *Cold Spring Harb Protoc* 2010, **2010**(4):pdb.prot5408. doi:10.1101/pdb.prot5408.
16. Boehme CC, Nabeta P, Hillemann D, Nicol MP, Shenai S, Krapp F, Allen J, Tahirli R, Blakemore R, Rustomjee R, Milovic A, Jones M, O'Brien SM, Persing DH, Ruesch-Gerdes S, Gotuzzo E, Rodrigues C, Alland D, Perkins MD: **Rapid molecular detection of tuberculosis and rifampin resistance.** *New Engl J Med* 2010, **363**:1005–1015.
17. World Health Organization: *WHO report 2010: global tuberculosis control.* Geneva, Switzerland: WHO; 2010.
18. Lee HY, Seong MW, Park SS, Hwang SS, Lee J, Park YS, Lee CH, Lee SM, Yoo CG, Kim YW, Han SK, Yim JJ: **Diagnostic accuracy of Xpert MTB/RIF on bronchoscopy specimens in patients with suspected pulmonary tuberculosis.** *Int J Tuberc Lung Dis* 2013, **17**:917–921.
19. Theron G, Peter J, Meldau R, Khalfey H, Gina P, Matinyena B, Lenders L, Calligaro G, Allwood B, Symons G, Govender U, Setshedi M, Dheda K: **Accuracy and impact of Xpert MTB/RIF for the diagnosis of smear-negative or sputum-scarce tuberculosis using bronchoalveolar lavage fluid.** *Thorax* 2013, **68**:1043–1051.
20. Ismail NA, Baba K, Pombo D, Hoosen AA: **Use of an immunochromatographic kit for the rapid detection of *Mycobacterium tuberculosis* from broth cultures.** *Int J Tuberc Lung Dis* 2009, **13**:1045–1047.
21. Helb D, Jones M, Story E, Boehme C, Wallace E, Ho K, Kop J, Owens MR, Rodgers R, Banada P, Safi H, Blakemore R, Lan NT, Jones-López EC, Levi M, Burday M, Ayakaka I, Mugerwa RD, McMillan B, Winn-Deen E, Christel L, Dailey P, Perkins MD, Persing DH, Alland D: **Rapid detection of *Mycobacterium tuberculosis* and rifampin resistance by use of on-demand, near-patient technology.** *J Clin Microbiol* 2010, **48**:229–237.
22. Blakemore R, Story E, Helb D, Kop J, Banada P, Owens MR, Chakravorty S, Jones M, Alland D: **Evaluation of the analytical performance of the Xpert MTB/RIF assay.** *J Clin Microbiol* 2010, **48**:2495–2501.
23. Bowles EC, Freyée B, van Ingen J, Mulder B, Boeree MJ, van Soolingen D: **Xpert MTB/RIF®, a novel automated polymerase chain reaction–based tool for the diagnosis of tuberculosis.** *Int J Tuberc Lung Dis* 2011, **15**:988–989.
24. Malbruny B, Le Marrec G, Courageux K, Leclercq R, Cattoir V: **Rapid and efficient detection of Mycobacterium tuberculosis in respiratory and non-respiratory samples.** *Int J Tuberc Lung Dis* 2011, **15**:553–555.
25. Marlowe EM, Novak-Weekley SM, Cumpio J, Sharp SE, Momeny MA, Babst A, Carlson JS, Kawamura M, Pandori M: **Evaluation of the Cepheid Xpert MTB/RIF assay for direct detection of *Mycobacterium tuberculosis* complex in respiratory specimens.** *J Clin Microbiol* 2011, **49**:1621–1623.
26. Miller MB, Popowitch EB, Backlund MG, Ager EP: **Performance of Xpert MTB/RIF RUO assay and IS*6110* real-time PCR for *Mycobacterium tuberculosis* detection in clinical samples.** *J Clin Microbiol* 2011, **49**:3458–3462.
27. Moure R, Muñoz L, Torres M, Santin M, Martín R, Alcaide F: **Rapid detection of Mycobacterium tuberculosis complex and rifampin resistance in smear-negative clinical samples by use of an integrated real-time PCR method.** *J Clin Microbiol* 2011, **49**:1137–1139.
28. Rachow A, Zumla A, Heinrich N, Rojas-Ponce G, Mtafya B, Reither K, Ntinginya EN, O'Grady J, Huggett J, Dheda K, Boehme C, Perkins M, Saathoff E, Hoelscher M: **Rapid and accurate detection of Mycobacterium tuberculosis in sputum samples by Cepheid Xpert MTB/RIF assay–a clinical validation study.** *PLoS One* 2011, **6**:e20458.
29. Scott LE, McCarthy K, Gous N, Nduna M, Van Rie A, Sanne I, Venter WF, Duse A, Stevens W: **Comparison of Xpert MTB/RIF with other nucleic acid technologies for diagnosing pulmonary tuberculosis in a high HIV prevalence setting: a prospective study.** *PLoS Med* 2011, **8**:e1001061.
30. Theron G, Peter J, van Zyl-Smit R, Mishra H, Streicher E, Murray S, Dawson R, Whitelaw A, Hoelscher M, Sharma S, Pai M, Warren R, Dheda K: **Evaluation of the Xpert MTB/RIF assay for the diagnosis of pulmonary tuberculosis in a high HIV prevalence setting.** *Am J Resp Crit Care Med* 2011, **184**:132–140.
31. Chang K, Lu W, Wang J, Zhang K, Jia S, Li F, Deng S, Chen M: **Rapid and effective diagnosis of tuberculosis and rifampicin resistance with Xpert MTB/RIF assay: a meta-analysis.** *J Infect* 2012, **64**:580–588.

3

Association between toll-like receptors 9 (TLR9) gene polymorphism and risk of pulmonary tuberculosis

Zhi Chen, Wei Wang, Jianqin Liang, Jinhe Wang, Shisheng Feng and Guangyu Zhang*

Abstract

Background: Previous studies indicated that the single nucleotide polymorphisms (SNPs) in TLR9 gene might be associated with Tuberculosis (TB) risk. However, the results are inconsistent and inconclusive.

Methods: 1745 articles from four databases were involved in our study. A meta-analysis on the associations between the seven polymorphisms and TB risk was carried out by comparison using different genetic models.

Results: In this systematic review 8 studies from seven English articles were analyzed. Our results showed that rs352139 is significantly associated with TB risk (AA vs. AG, OR 0.77, 95% CI 0.65-0.92, P = 0.004). In the ethnic subgroup analysis, Indonesians with AA genotype had a decreased susceptibility while Mexicans with GG allele had an increased risk.

Conclusions: The meta-analysis indicated that rs352139 polymorphism might be associated with decreased TB risk in Indonesians whereas increased risk in Mexicans. Whether the observed association was due to causal effect needs to be further studied.

Keywords: Toll-like receptor 9, Polymorphism, Tuberculosis, Meta-analysis

Background

Pulmonary tuberculosis (TB) caused by *Mycobacterium tuberculosis* (MTB), is one of the most contagious diseases in humans. A recent report (2014) from WHO estimated that one third of the global population has been latently infected without clinical symptoms. In 2012, approximately 8.6 million people worldwide were diagnosed with TB and 1.3 million died from TB [1]. MTB could infect human by invading antigen presenting cell (Macrophages and Dendritic cells) in the lung. But only 5-10% of infected people developed clinical symptoms probably due to undermined immunity response [1].

Toll-like receptors (TLRs) are pattern recognizing receptors (PRRs) and play an important role in regulating human's immune system. The TLRs can recognize pathogen-associated molecular patterns (PAMPs) in both extracellular and intracellular environment. The TLRs have the ability to initiate signaling pathways that are responsible for activating both innate and acquired immune responses as well as the production of inflammatory cytokines. The members of TLRs family have been detected on human plasma membrane (TLR1, TLR2, TLR4-6) and in leukocyte endosome (TLR3, TLR7-9) [2]. For the risk of MTB infection, the most important TLRs are TLR1, TLR2, TLR4, TLR6 and TLR9 [3]. TLR1 combines with TLR2 as a heterodimer and recognizes triacylated lipopeptides of MTB. TLR2-TLR6 complex recognizes diacylated lipopeptides and bacterial LTA of Mycoplasmal compounds. TLR4 recognizes lipopolysaccharide (LPS) and TLR9 homodimer recognizes the exogenous MTB DNA as PAMPs [4]. Studies focusing on TLR1, 2, 4 and 6 have found that single nucleotide polymorphisms (SNPs) of these TLRs genes might be associated with differential TB risk. However, neither systematic review nor meta-analysis has been reported for TLR9 [3].

The gene of toll-like receptor 9 is located on chromosome 3p21.3. The total length of TLR9 gene is approximate 5 kb. Its coding gene has two exons, and the major

* Correspondence: chenzhidoctor@sina.com
Department of Tuberculosis, The 309th hospital of PLA, No. 17, Heishanhu Road, Haidian District, Beijing 100091, China

coding region is in the second exon [5]. Based on NCBI SNP database, twelve SNPs have been identified for TLR9 gene, in which NM_017442.3:c.-1486 T > C (rs187084) located at the upstream of promoter may be an important one [6]. Previous study it has shown that C genotype was associated with reduced TLR9 transcription activity when compared with T genotype [7], indicating population with C genotype may be susceptible to diseases related to TLR9 gene.

Researches have indicated certain race population with special genotype of TLR9 polymorphism might have higher risk for TB; however the findings are inconsistent and inconclusive. From public health perspective, given the widespread and severe nature of the disease, it is important to understand the association between TLR9 polymorphism and TB risk, so that individuals with higher risk genotype could be identified and receive targeted preventive care. In this study, we conducted a systematic review of current literature on this issue and analysis of the associations between TLR9 polymorphisms and TB risk.

Methods

Literature review

We searched the EMBASE, Web of science, PubMed and Chinese National Knowledge Infrastructure (CNKI) databases to identify the publications that reported the association between the TLR9 polymorphism and risk for pulmonary tuberculosis from April, 2004 to July, 2014. The key words used were 'toll like receptor 9, SNP, lung tuberculosis', 'toll like receptor 9, snp, pulmonary tuberculosis', 'toll like receptor 9, polymorphism, pulmonary tuberculosis', or 'toll like receptor 9, polymorphism, lung tuberculosis'. Only the articles in English or Chinese with an English abstract were selected. After excluding duplicates, titles and abstracts were reviewed. Studies would be selected if they: 1) were case-control studies; 2) reported genotype distribution in both cases and controls. The studies were excluded if they were: 1) review articles; 2) not related to TLR9; 3) not a human study; or 4) not related to the association between tuberculosis and host genetics. The study selection process was summarized in Figure 1. The study was approved by the Institutional Review Board of The 309th hospital of PLA.

Data extraction

For each study, the following information was extracted from original publication: the name of first author, the year of publication, country of origin, race of study population, genotypes distribution for each polymorphism in both cases and controls, statistical characteristics of each study (sample size, gender and age distribution of cases and controls, *P* values for HWE evaluation), source of controls, and genotyping methods (Table 1).

Statistical analyses

Hardy-Weinberg Equilibrium (HWE) was examined in controls by asymptotic Pearson's Chi-square test for

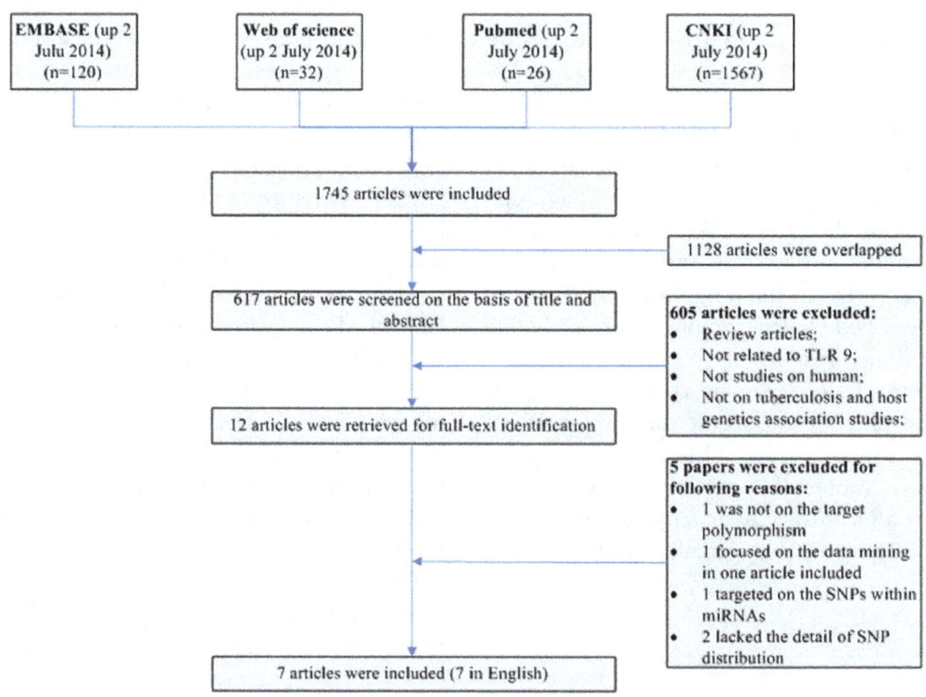

Figure 1 Flow chart showing the study selection procedure. CNKI: China National Knowledge Infrastructure.

Table 1 Characteristics of the 16 studies included in the meta-analysis

Authors	Year of publication	Country	Host ethnicity	Age, years Mean ± SD or Mean (Range)		Samples n		Genotyping method
				Cases	Controls	Cases	Controls	
Jahantigh, et al.	2013	Iran	Iranian population, Zahedan	51.1 ± 20	48.4 ± 14.7	124	149	PCR-RFLP
Kobayashi, et al.	2012	Indonesian	Javanese or Sundanese–Javanese	41.6 (16-92)	-	538	560	PCR-DNA chip
		Vietnam	Kinh	37.4 (15-60)	-	277	458	PCR-DNA chip
Olesen, et al.	2007	West African	West African	37.25	38.12	321	347	PCR-TaqMan SNP assays
Sa'nchez, et al.	2012	Colombia	Colombia population, Medellin	39 (26–51)	42 (25–54)	466	300	MALDI-TOF mass spectrometer
Yang, et al.	2013	China	Chinese	-	-	200	200	PCR-CHIP
Selvaraj, et al.	2010	India	south Indian population,	34.92 ± 11.42	32.33 ± 9.75	206	212	PCR-RFLP
Diana, et al.	2013	Mexico	Mexican Mazatecan	46.9 ± 17.8	42.9 ± 15.9	90	90	PCR-TaqMan assays

PCR = polymerase chain reaction; RFLP = restriction fragment length polymorphism; MALDI-TOF: chip-based matrix-assisted laser desorption/ionization time-of-flight.

each polymorphism in each study. The association between polymorphism and TB risk was estimated with odds ratios (OR) and corresponding 95% confidence intervals (CI). Between studies heterogeneity was tested using Q test and I^2 test, and the heterogeneity was considered significant if P-value was less than 0.05. Fixed-effects model was adopted when P-value was more than 0.05; otherwise random-effects models were used [8]. The publication bias was evaluated using Begg's test and Egger's test [9,10]. $P < 0.05$ was considered statistically significant. Statistical analyses were conducted with Stata 13.0 (College Station, TX).

We used 'Meta-analysis of Observational Studies in Epidemiology' [11] as guideline for conduction and reporting of this meta-analysis.

Results

Characteristics of included studies

A total of 1745 articles were obtained from the literature search. As shown in Figure 1, after excluding the duplicates, 617 abstracts were reviewed. A total of 12 research articles that reported the association of human TLR9 gene polymorphisms and TB risk were identified. Five of them were excluded after reviewing the full-text article due to studying irrelevant polymorphism, focusing on data mining, studying the SNPs within microRNAs, or lacking the detail of SNP distribution. Finally, 8 studies from 7 articles were included in this analysis. All articles were published in English [12-18]. Overall, 7 different TLR9 SNPs were studied. Among them, there were 3 studies for rs187084 [12,14,17], 1 study for rs352165 [15], 3 studies for rs5743836 [14,17,18], 1 study for rs5743842 [18], 4 studies for rs352139 [13,16,18] (Kobayashi et al did studies on Indonesian and Vietnamese), 1 study for rs352140 [16] and 1 study for rs352167 [15]. As shown in Table 1, the race of study population ranged from African, Asian to Latin American. No studies from Caucasian were included due to lack of detailed SNP distribution. The pooled study population consisted of 4538 subjects (2222 cases and 2316 controls). The genotype and allele distributions of all the polymorphisms are shown in Table 2. In 3 studies, the genotype distributions in controls were deviated from HWE. The location of each SNP was shown in Figure 2 based on information from CNBI SNPs database.

Data synthesis by polymorphism

TLR9 rs187084 polymorphism

The Human Genome Variation Society (HGVS) name of rs187084 is NM_017442.3:c.-1486 T > C [19,20]. Three case-control studies (987cases and 405 controls) addressed the relationship between rs187084 polymorphism and the risk of TB. As shown in Table 3, the heterogeneity was not significant (P = s 0.78, $I^2 = 0.0\%$). The overall OR (T vs. C alleles) using fixed-effect model was 0.93 (95% CI 0.79–1.10), P =0.43. Analyses of other genetic models were also performed, and no association was identified (Table 3). The publication bias was also negligible in these genetic models (Table 3). Subgroup analysis in allele comparison (T vs. C) was performed by ethnicity in Figure 3.

TLR9 rs5743836 polymorphism

The HGVS name of rs5743836 is NM_017442.3:c.-1237 T > C [19,21]. Three case-control studies (608 cases and 633 controls) were included for the analysis of the relationship between rs5743836 polymorphism and TB risk. As shown in Table 3, the heterogeneity between these studies was not significant (P = 0.72, $I^2 = 0.0\%$). The overall OR (T vs. C alleles) using fixed-effect model was 1.09 (95% CI 0.90–1.33), P =0.37. Analyses for other genetic models also did not identify significant association (Table 3). The publication bias was also insignificant (Table 3). Subgroup analysis in allele comparison (T vs. C) was performed by ethnicity in Figure 4.

Table 2 Genotype and allele distribution of TLR-9 polymorphisms in TB and controls

SNP	Study	Case					Control					HWE	
		TT	TC	CC	T	C	TT	TC	CC	T	C	χ^2	P
rs187084	P. Selvaraj. et. al.	75	91	27	241	145	84	92	32	260	156	0.66	0.42
	Jahantigh, et al.	63	51	10	177	71	82	59	8	223	75	0.39	0.53
	Olesen, et al.	171	122	25	464	172	186	132	21	504	174	0.14	0.71
rs352165	Sa'nchez, et al.	90	238	138	418	514	53	162	83	268	328	2.88	0.90
rs5743836	Olesen, et al.-a	104	154	62	362	278	101	175	66	377	307	0.40	0.53
	P. Selvaraj. et. al.	168	29	1	365	31	167	32	2	366	36	0.11	0.74
	Diana Torres-García, et. al.	82	8	0	172	8	78	12	0	168	12	0.46	0.50
rs5743842	Diana Torres-García, et. al.	0	2	88	2	178	0	0	90	0	180		
		AA	AG	GG	A	G	AA	AG	GG	A	G	χ^2	P
rs352139	Kobayashi, et. al.(Indonesian)	199	279	59	677	397	259	233	68	751	369	1.90	0.17
	Kobayashi, et. al.(Vietnamese)	123	125	28	371	181	232	183	40	647	263	0.20	0.65
	Yang, et al.	70	89	41	229	171	68	95	33	231	161	<0.00	0.98
	Diana Torres-García, et al.	23	48	19	94	86	14	41	35	69	111	0.12	0.73
rs352140	Yang, et al.	40	88	72	168	232	32	93	71	157	235	0.03	0.87
rs352167	Sa'nchez, et al.	101	238	127	440	492	60	162	76	282	314	2.44	0.12

HWE: Hardy-Weinberg Equilibrium.

TLR9 rs352139 polymorphism

The HGVS name of rs352139 is NM_017442.3:c.4-44A > G [19,22]. Four case-control studies (1103 cases and 1301 controls) were included in the analysis of the relationship between rs352139 polymorphism and TB risk. As shown in Table 3, the heterogeneity between these studies was significant (P = 0.012, I^2 = 72.5%). The overall OR (A vs. G alleles) using the random-effect model was 0.98 (95% CI 0.77–1.25), P =0.87. Analyses for other genetic models did not identify significant association (Table 3). Begg's test (P = 0.09) and Egger's test (P = 0.00) showed potential publication bias in the model of AA vs. AG + GG (Table 3). As shown in Figures 5 and 6, the Mexicans with homozygote gene AA might have higher risk TB whereas Indonesians with the same SNP genotype might have lower risk for TB. It is of note that there is only one study from each race.

TLR9 rs5743842, rs352165, rs352140 and rs352167polymorphism

There was only one study for each SNP, which limited further analysis. As shown in Table 4, the overall ORs for T vs. C or A vs. G were all around 1, indicating lack of association between these polymorphisms and risk of pulmonary tuberculosis. Analyses for other genetic models were also performed, and no association was found (Table 4).

Two individual researchers independently reviewed the studies. The inter-rater agreement, as measured by kappa statistics, was calculated with MedCalc® software [23]. The weighted kappa is 0.500; 95% CI is 0139 to 0.861, indicating a moderate agreement between 2 researchers.

Discussion

In this study, we performed a meta-analysis to assess the association between seven extensively studied TLR9 polymorphisms (rs187084, rs352165, rs5743836, rs5743842, rs352139, rs352140 and rs352167) and TB risk. The analysis revealed an association between certain TLR9 polymorphism and TB risk. In addition, 5 different genetic models (Allele, Heterozygote, Homozygote, Dominant and Recessive model) were analyzed in all polymorphisms. A subgroup analysis by race was also performed for rs187084, rs352139 and rs5743836 polymorphisms, the studies of which included Indians, Iranian and West African, Indonesians, Vietnamese, Chinese and Mexicans. The results showed that rs187084 and rs5743836 polymorphisms were not associated with TB risk, while the association between rs352139 polymorphism and TB risk may vary by race.

We chose TLR9 gene in our analysis because it's critical role in the incidence of TB from previous studies. Chen et al. demonstrated that cell apoptosis induced by *Mycobacterium Tuberculosis* required TLR9 in animal model [24]. Another study reported that the deficiency in a major adapter of TLR9 signaling pathway significantly increased the lethality of TB. The myeloid differentiation factor 88 knock-out mice (MyD88 −/−) died within 4 weeks after MTB infection [25]. All these evidences indicated the critical role of TLR9 in TB incidence and progression.

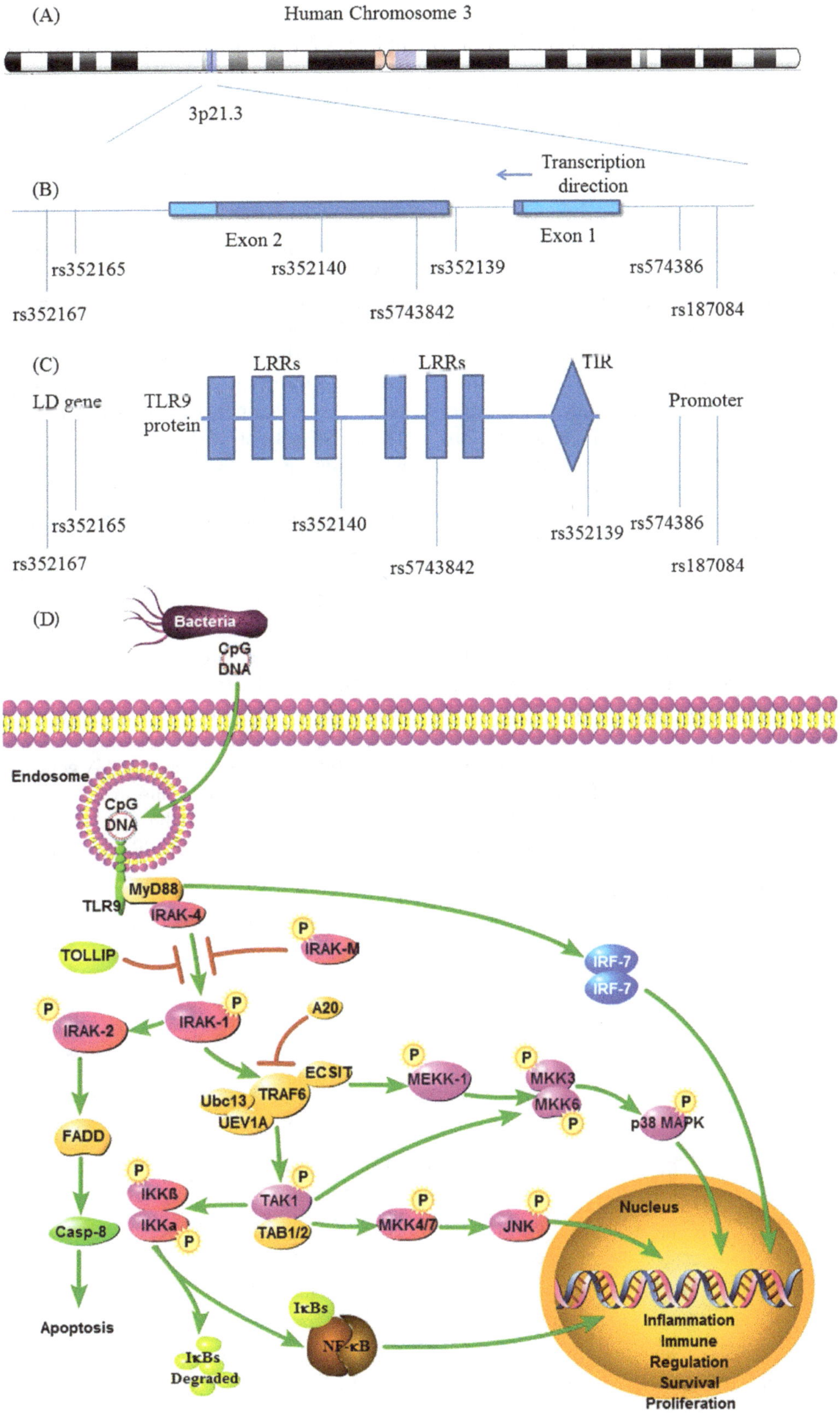

Figure 2 (See legend on next page.)

(See figure on previous page.)

Figure 2 The location of TLR9 SNPs and TLR9 signaling pathway. **(A)** Schematic representation of human chromosome 3 showing location of TLR9 gene. **(B)** Schematic representation of the selected single nucleotide polymorphisms (SNPs) in TLR9. Drak regions in exon 1&2: protein coding region. **(C)** Schematic representation of selected SNPs in TLR9 protein. TLR9: Toll-Like Receptor; LRR: Leucine-rich repeat; TIR: Toll-Interleukin-1 Receptor Domain; LD: linkage disequilibrium. **(D)** The signaling pathway of TLR9. TLR9 homodimer could recruit adaptor proteins MyD88. MyD88 recruits IRAK-4 and activates NF-κB through IRAKs, TRAF6, TAK1, and IκKs, resulting in cell apoptosis or inflammatory cytokine synthesis. TLR9: Toll-Like Receptor 9; MyD88: Myeloid Differentiation Primary Response Gene 88; NF-κB: nuclear factor kappa B; IRAK: Interleukin-1 Receptor associated kinase 1; TRAF 6: TNF Receptor Associated Factor 6; TAK1: TGF-b-Actiated Kinase 1; IκK: IκB kinase; IκB: Inhibitor of NF-κB.

TLR9 is a recognition receptor in leukocytes endosome, especially in B cells, plasmacytoid dendritic cells (pDCs) and macrophages. It is localized in the endosomal and lysosomal compartments. It is one of the most important receptors for the initiation of innate immune response against intracellular pathogens. The function of TLR9 is to recognize the unmethylated Cytosine-phosphate-Guanine (CpG) sequence which usually appears in bacterial DNA [5]. In recent study, hybrid RNA-DNA chains generated by viruses during reverse transcription were recognized by TLR9 [26]. The Toll-IL-1 receptor (TIR) domain of TLR9 in intracellular space associates with myeloid differentiation factor 88 (MyD88), and becomes the initiator component of TLR9 signaling pathway. Once bacterial CpG-DNA in lysosome combines with the nucleic acid ligand of TLR9, the signaling pathway is activated. MyD88, once stimulated, recruits IL-1 receptor associated kinase 4 (IRAK-4) to TLR9 through interaction of the functional domains. Then, IRAK-1 is phosphorylated and recruits Tumor necrosis factor receptor associated factor 6 (TRAF6). Consequently the inhibitor of nuclear factor kappa-B kinase (IKK) complex is activated, leading to the activation of Mitogen-activated protein (MAP) kinases (JNK, p38 MAPK). The nuclear factor inhibiter (IκB) is then phosphorylated and the level of nuclear factor kappa-B (NF-κB) is elevated [27]. NF-κBs translocate to the nucleus, and then bind to DNA sites to regulate relevant gene transcription. Finally, inflammatory cytokines are synthesized through host defense immune response by TLRs- NF-κB pathway. The signaling pathway of TLR9 was shown in Figure 2.

SNPs rs352165 and rs352167 were located in intron 5 of aminolevulinate delta-, synthase 1 (ALAS1) gene in the downstream of TLR9. Sanchez D et al. have reported that these two SNPs were in linkage disequilibrium (LD) with rs352139 and rs352140 SNPs of TLR9 [15]. Thus they chose rs352165 and rs352167 as proxies for TLR9 gene. Lack of significant association with TB risk from our analysis indicated there was no relationship between rs352165/ rs352167 and this disease.

In our study, the association of rs352139 with TB risk varied by race. In Indonesians AA genotype is associated with lower risk of TB, while in Mexicans it is associated with higher risk of TB. The Mexicans with AA allele had 2.73 times higher risk of TB than Indonesians with the

Table 3 Summary of different comparative meta-analysis results

Polymorphism	Genetic model	Participants	OR (95% CI)	Z	P value	I^2 %	P_{het}	Effect model	Begg's test p > |z|	Egger's test p > |t|
rs187084	TT vs. TC + CC	1331	0.93 (0.75, 1.15)	0.68	0.49	0.0	0.91	F	0.29	0.30
	CC vs. TC + TT	1331	1.12 (0.77, 1.63)	0.60	0.55	0.0	0.53	F	0.30	0.47
	TT vs. CC	784	0.85 (0.58, 1.27)	0.79	0.43	0.0	0.6	F	0.30	0.47
	TT vs. TC	1208	0.95 (0.75, 1.19)	0.50	0.63	0.0	0.91	F	0.30	0.17
	T vs. C	2660	0.93 (0.79, 1.10)	0.80	0.43	0.0	0.78	F	1.00	0.57
rs5743836	TT vs. TC + CC	1241	1.18 (0.90, 1.54)	1.18	0.24	0.0	0.82	F	0.30	0.36
	CC vs. TC + TT	1241	0.99 (0.68, 1.45)	0.06	0.95	0.0	0.58	F	1.00	_
	TT vs. CC	831	1.12 (0.72, 1.73)	0.5	0.62	0.0	0.63	F	1.00	_
	TT vs. TC	1110	1.19 (0.90, 1.57)	1.18	0.24	0.0	0.82	F	1.00	0.48
	T vs. C	2482	1.09 (0.90, 1.33)	0.89	0.37	0.0	0.72	F	0.30	0.15
rs352139	AA vs. AG + GG	2404	0.88 (0.65, 1.19)	0.83	0.40	62.1	0.049	R	0.09	0.00
	GG vs. AG + AA	2404	0.90 (0.60, 1.35)	0.51	0.61	61.9	0.049	R	0.73	0.59
	AA vs. AG	2081	0.84 (0.63, 1.12)	2.9	0.004	55.4	0.081	R	0.31	0.07
	AA vs. GG	1311	1.02 (0.65, 1.61)	0.1	0.92	62.0	0.048	R	0.73	0.24
	A vs. G	4808	0.98 (0.77, 1.25)	0.17	0.87	72.5	0.012	R	0.09	0.10

P_{het} = P value for heterogeneity; OR = odds ratio; CI = confidence interval; F = fixed-effect model; R = random-effect model.

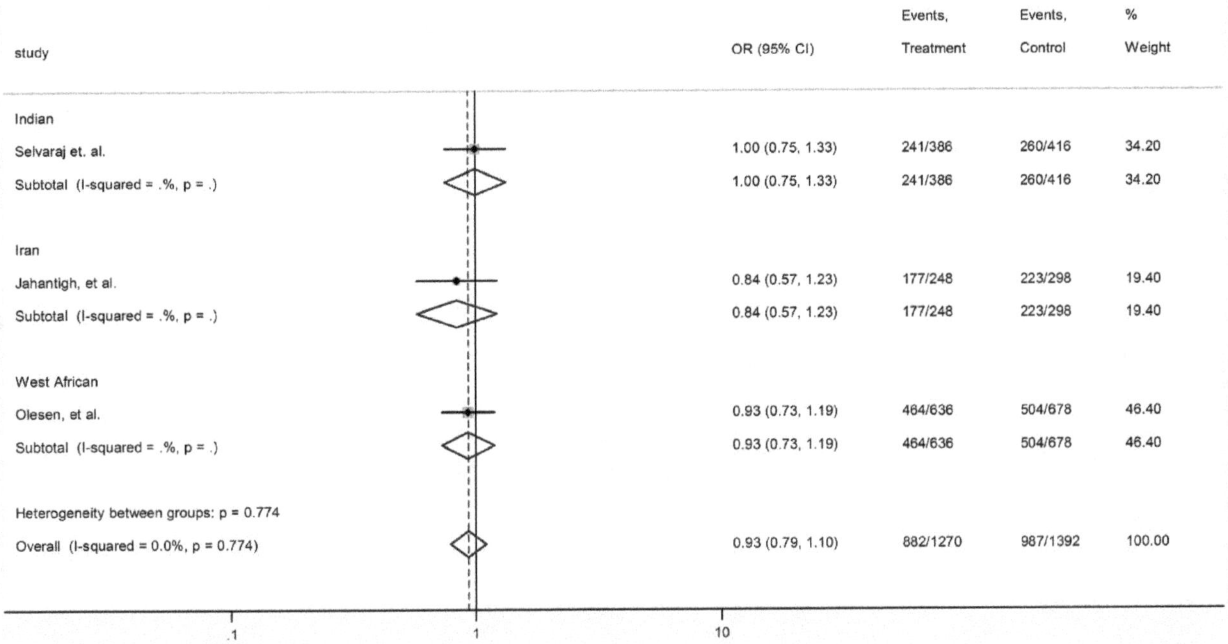

Figure 3 Forrest plot of the association between rs187084 and TB risk (T vs. C). Subgroup analysis was performed by ethnicity. OR: odds ratio; CI: confidence interval; df: degrees of freedom.

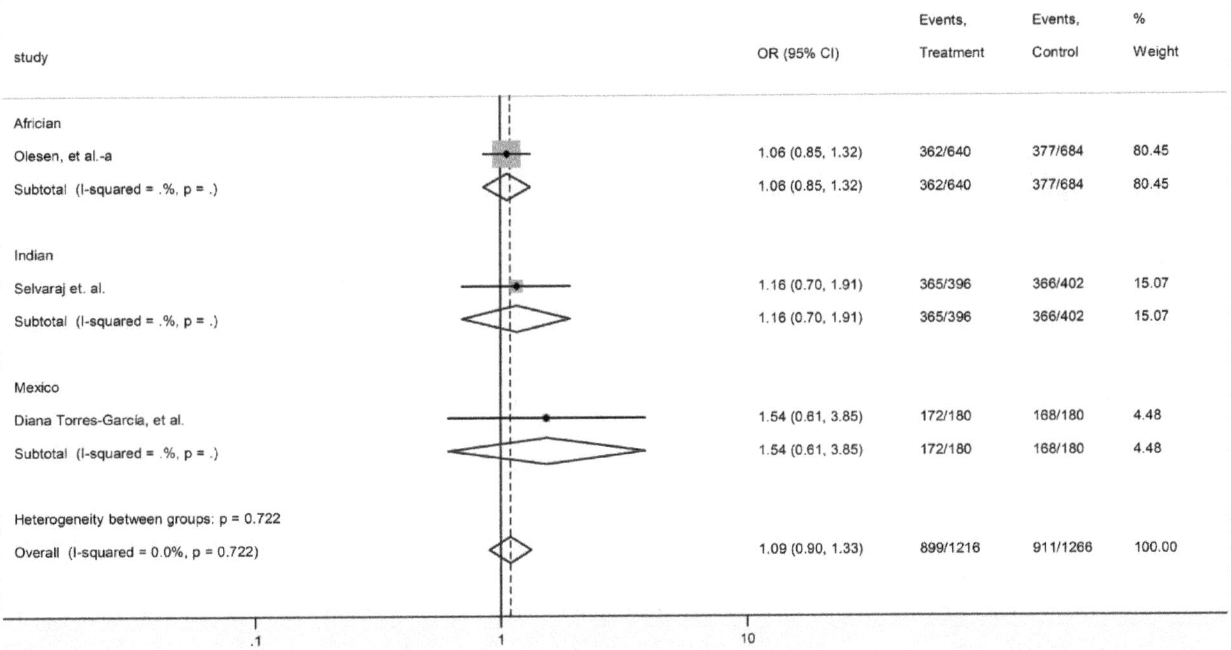

Figure 4 Forrest plot of the association between rs5743836 and TB risk (T vs. C). Subgroup analysis was performed by ethnicity. OR: odds ratio; CI: confidence interval; df: degrees of freedom.

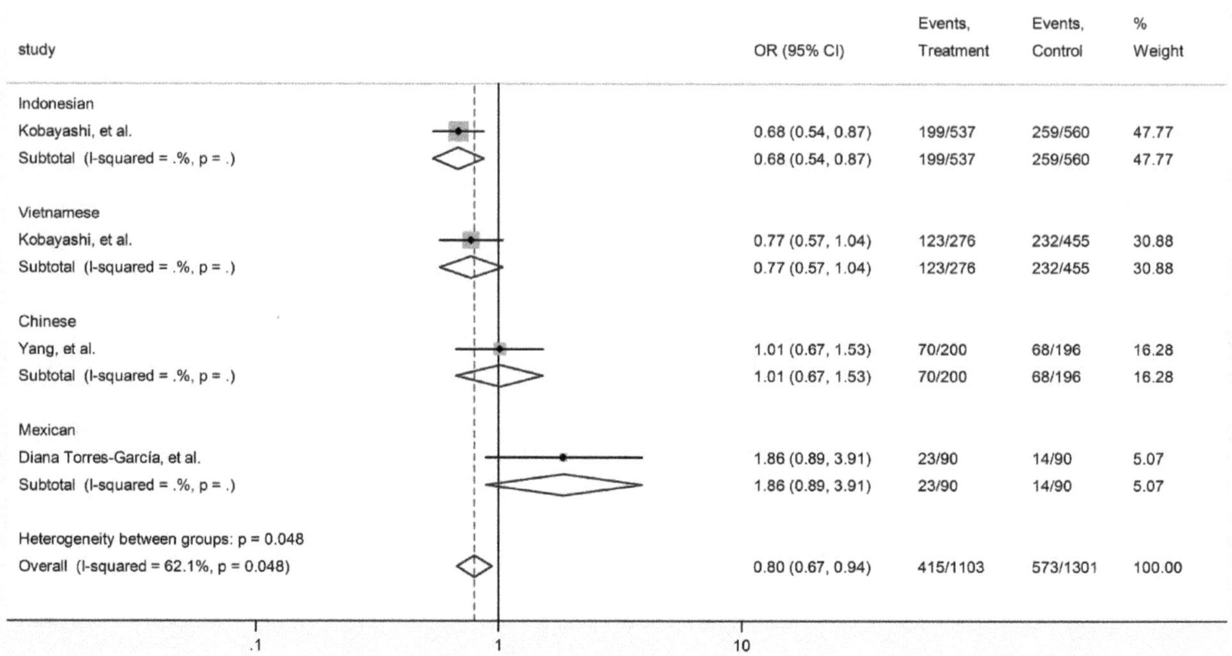

Figure 5 Forrest plot of the association between rs352139 and TB risk (AA vs. AG + GG). Subgroup analysis was performed by ethnicity. OR: odds ratio; CI: confidence interval; df: degrees of freedom.

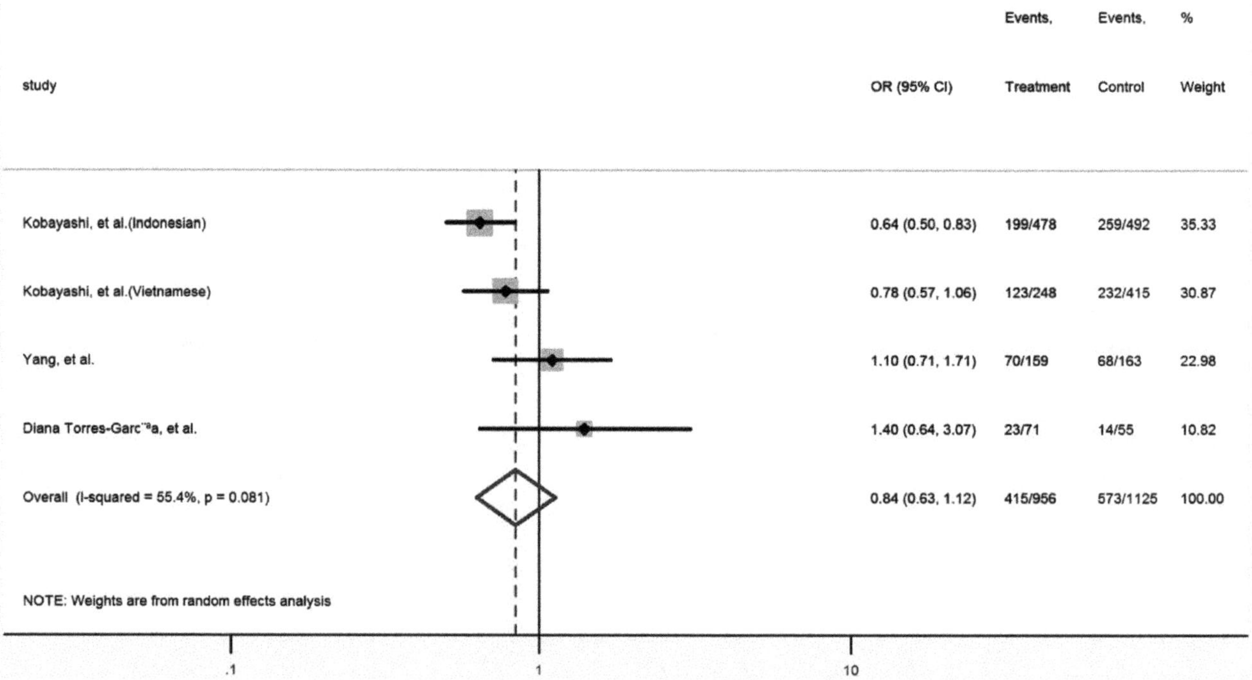

Figure 6 Forrest plot of the association between rs352139 and TB risk (AA vs. AG). Subgroup analysis was performed by ethnicity. OR: odds ratio; CI: confidence interval; df: degrees of freedom.

Table 4 Summary of different comparative SNPs results

Polymorphism	Genetic model	Participants	OR (95% CI)	Chi^2	P value
rs5743842	TT vs. TC + CC	180	–	–	–
	CC vs. TC + TT	180	0 (0, 1.91)	–	0.50
	TT vs. CC	178	–	–	–
	TT vs. TC	2	–	–	–
	T vs C	360	–	–	–
rs352165	TT vs. TC + CC	764	1.11 (0.75, 1.64)	0.28	0.60
	CC vs. TC + TT	764	1.09 (0.78, 1.53)	0.27	0.60
	TT vs. CC	364	1.02 (0.65, 1.62)	0.01	0.92
	TT vs. TC	543	1.16 (0.77, 1.75)	0.52	0.47
	T vs C	1528	1.00 (0.81, 1.23)	0.00	0.96
rs352140	AA vs. AG + GG	396	1.28 (0.74, 2.22)	0.90	0.34
	GG vs. AG + AA	396	0.99 (0.64, 1.52)	0.00	0.96
	AA vs. AG	253	1.32 (0.74, 2.38)	0.99	0.32
	AA vs. GG	215	1.23 (0.67, 2.27)	0.52	0.47
	A vs G	792	1.08 (0.81, 1.45)	0.31	0.58
rs352167	AA vs. AG + GG	764	1.10 (0.76, 1.60)	0.26	0.61
	GG vs. AG + AA	764	1.09 (0.78, 1.55)	0.29	0.59
	AA vs. AG	561	1.15 (0.77, 1.70)	0.50	0.48
	AA vs. GG	364	1.01 (0.64, 1.58)	0.00	0.97
	A vs G	1528	1.00 (0.81, 1.23)	0.00	0.97

OR = odds ratio; CI = confidence interval.

same genotype. There is no known explanation for the racial difference. Also, we observed a significant association between rs352139 polymorphism and TB risk in Indonesians for Allele, Heterozygote and Homozygote models. There was also a significant association between rs352139 polymorphism and TB risk in Mexicans for Allele, Dominant and Recessive models. Although 4 case-control studies of rs352139 were included in this analysis, there was only one study for each racial group. Therefore, our results should be interpreted with caution, and more studies with larger sample size should be considered to confirm this differential risk by race.

The SNP rs352139 is located in the intron of TLR9 gene (Figure 2). TIR domain consists of the end of exon 1, intron and a part of exon 2 which contains SNP rs352139. It is the only polymorphism located in the intron between two exons. The other polymorphisms are located in either the upstream of coding region or the exons. It is possible that the intron of TLR9 gene plays an important role in regulating the TLR-mediated immunologic response. However, it is currently unclear how this intronic SNP induces such a phenotype change. It is possible that it influences signaling by creating an alternative splicing site and thus, affecting the mRNA transcription and the final protein product. Similarly, the rs352139 SNP could be a likely marker in linkage disequilibrium with a polymorphic regulatory region that controls TLR9 expression or serve as a functional coding region SNP.

The SNP rs187084 is located in the promoter of TLR9 gene, which could create a Sp1 binding site [28]. Variant alleles of this SNP can alter the function of TLR9, impact the response to bacterial pathogens, and thereby change individual's disease risk [29,30]. In our analysis, several studies investigated the role of rs187084 in the development of tuberculosis, but none of them showed significant association.

The SNP rs5743836 is located in the promoter region of TLR9. This SNP was thought to be associated with increased transcriptional activity and function of TLR9 [31]. In our study, rs5743836 polymorphism showed no significant association with TB risk. Nevertheless in a study of Caucasian patients, Digna Rosa Velez et al reported that the rs5743836 polymorphism had significant association with dominant and recessive models (TT vs. CT&CC, OR = 0.50, 95% CI 0.28–0.87, p = 0.015). However, we did not include these data in our analysis because only the detail of additive model was presented in the original article.

Conclusions

This systematic review summarized the current literature on the association between TLR9 polymorphisms and TB risk. Our results indicated that rs187084, rs352165, rs5743836, rs5743842, rs352140 and rs352167 polymorphisms did not show significant association with TB risk. The rs352139 polymorphism might be associated with decreased TB risk in Indonesians whereas increased risk in Mexicans. However, the data were based on single study for each race. Whether the observed association was due to causal effect needs to be further studied.

Abbreviations

TB: Tuberculosis; MTB: *Mycobacterium Tuberculosis*; TLRs: Toll-like receptors; PRRs: Pattern recognizing receptors; PAMPs: Pathogen-associated molecular patterns; LPS: Lipopolysaccharide; SNPs: Single nucleotide polymorphisms; CNKI: Chinese national knowledge infrastructure; HWE: Hardy-Weinberg Equilibrium; OR: Odds ratios; CI: Confidence intervals; HGVS: Human genome variation society; pDCs: Plasmacytoid dendritic cells; CpG: Cytosine-phosphate-guanine; TIR: Toll-IL-1 receptor; MyD88: Myeloid differentiation factor 88; IRAK-4: IL-1 receptor associated kinase 4; TRAF6: Tumor necrosis factor receptor associated factor 6; IKK: Inhibitor of nuclear factor kappa-B kinase; MAP: Mitogen-activated protein; IκB: Nuclear factor inhibiter; NF-κB: Nuclear factor kappa-B; ALAS1: Aminolevulinate delta-, synthase 1; LD: Linkage disequilibrium.

Competing interests

The authors declare that they have no competing interests.

Authors' contributions

ZC carried out the study design, data analysis. WW carried out the manuscript review. JL participated in the literature research. JW participated in the literature research. SF participated in the literature research. GZ conceived of the study. All authors read and approved the final manuscript.

Acknowledgements

This work was supported by the National 12th Five-year special grand project for infectious diseases (No. 2012ZX10003009).

References

1. Global tuberculosis report 2013 [http://apps.who.int/iris/bitstream/10665/91355/1/9789241564656_eng.pdf]
2. Frazao JB, Errante PR, Condino-Neto A. Toll-like receptors' pathway disturbances are associated with increased susceptibility to infections in humans. Arch Immunol Ther Exp. 2013;61(6):427–43.
3. Zhang Y, Jiang T, Yang X, Xue Y, Wang C, Liu J, et al. Toll-like receptor -1, -2, and -6 polymorphisms and pulmonary tuberculosis susceptibility: a systematic review and meta-analysis. PLoS One. 2013;8(5), e63357.
4. Zhao S, Zhang Y, Zhang Q, Wang F, Zhang D. Toll-like receptors and prostate cancer. Front Immunol. 2014;5:352.
5. Hemmi H, Takeuchi O, Kawai T, Kaisho T, Sato S, Sanjo H, et al. A Toll-like receptor recognizes bacterial DNA. Nature. 2000;408(6813):740–5.
6. Coban C, Ishii KJ, Kawai T, Hemmi H, Sato S, Uematsu S, et al. Toll-like receptor 9 mediates innate immune activation by the malaria pigment hemozoin. J Exp Med. 2005;201(1):19–25.
7. Tao K, Fujii M, Tsukumo S, Maekawa Y, Kishihara K, Kimoto Y, et al. Genetic variations of Toll-like receptor 9 predispose to systemic lupus erythematosus in Japanese population. Ann Rheum Dis. 2007;66(7):905–9.
8. Kavvoura FK, Ioannidis JP. Methods for meta-analysis in genetic association studies: a review of their potential and pitfalls. Hum Genet. 2008;123(1):1–14.
9. Egger M, Davey Smith G, Schneider M, Minder C. Bias in meta-analysis detected by a simple, graphical test. BMJ. 1997;315(7109):629–34.
10. Begg CB, Berlin JA. Publication bias and dissemination of clinical research. J Natl Cancer Inst. 1989;81(2):107–15.
11. Stroup DF, Berlin JA, Morton SC, Olkin I, Williamson GD, Rennie D, et al. Meta-analysis of observational studies in epidemiology: a proposal for reporting. Meta-analysis Of Observational Studies in Epidemiology (MOOSE) group. Jama. 2000;283(15):2008–12.
12. Jahantigh D, Salimi S, Alavi-Naini R, Emamdadi A, Owaysee Osquee H, Farajian Mashhadi F. Association between TLR4 and TLR9 gene polymorphisms with development of pulmonary tuberculosis in Zahedan, southeastern Iran. Sci World J. 2013;2013:534053.
13. Kobayashi K, Yuliwulandari R, Yanai H, Naka I, Lien LT, Hang NT, et al. Association of TLR polymorphisms with development of tuberculosis in Indonesian females. Tissue Antigens. 2012;79(3):190–7.
14. Olesen R, Wejse C, Velez DR, Bisseye C, Sodemann M, Aaby P, et al. DC-SIGN (CD209), pentraxin 3 and vitamin D receptor gene variants associate with pulmonary tuberculosis risk in West Africans. Genes Immun. 2007;8(6):456–67.
15. Sanchez D, Lefebvre C, Rioux J, Garcia LF, Barrera LF. Evaluation of Toll-like receptor and adaptor molecule polymorphisms for susceptibility to tuberculosis in a Colombian population. Int J Immunogenet. 2012;39(3):216–23.
16. Yang Y, Li X, Cui W, Guan L, Shen F, Xu J, et al. Potential association of pulmonary tuberculosis with genetic polymorphisms of toll-like receptor 9 and interferon-gamma in a Chinese population. BMC Infect Dis. 2013;13:511.
17. Selvaraj P, Harishankar M, Singh B, Jawahar MS, Banurekha VV. Toll-like receptor and TIRAP gene polymorphisms in pulmonary tuberculosis patients of South India. Tuberculosis (Edinb). 2010;90(5):306–10.
18. Torres-Garcia D, Cruz-Lagunas A, Garcia-Sancho Figueroa MC, Fernandez-Plata R, Baez-Saldana R, Mendoza-Milla C, et al. Variants in toll-like receptor 9 gene influence susceptibility to tuberculosis in a Mexican population. J Transl Med. 2013;11:220.
19. den Dunnen JT, Antonarakis SE. Mutation nomenclature extensions and suggestions to describe complex mutations: a discussion. Hum Mutat. 2000;15(1):7–12.
20. Jia X, Cong B, Zhang J, Li H, Liu W, Chang H, et al. CCK8 negatively regulates the TLR9-induced activation of human peripheral blood pDCs by targeting TRAF6 signaling. Eur J Immunol. 2014;44(2):489–99.
21. Triantafilou K, Eryilmazlar D, Triantafilou M. Herpes simplex virus 2-induced activation in vaginal cells involves Toll-like receptors 2 and 9 and DNA sensors DAI and IFI16. Am J Obstet Gynecol. 2014;210(2):122 e121–10.
22. Yamaguchi M, Kitagawa Y, Zhou M, Itoh M, Gotoh B. An anti-interferon activity shared by paramyxovirus C proteins: inhibition of Toll-like receptor 7/9-dependent alpha interferon induction. FEBS Lett. 2014;588(1):28–34.
23. Fleiss JLLB, Paik MC. Statistical methods for rates and proportions. 3rd ed. 2003.
24. Chen L, Shi W, Li H, Sun X, Fan X, Lesage G, et al. Critical role of toll-like receptor 9 in morphine and Mycobacterium tuberculosis-Induced apoptosis in mice. PLoS One. 2010;5(2):e9205.
25. Fremond CM, Yeremeev V, Nicolle DM, Jacobs M, Quesniaux VF, Ryffel B. Fatal Mycobacterium tuberculosis infection despite adaptive immune response in the absence of MyD88. J Clin Invest. 2004;114(12):1790–9.
26. Rigby RE, Webb LM, Mackenzie KJ, Li Y, Leitch A, Reijns MA, et al. RNA: DNA hybrids are a novel molecular pattern sensed by TLR9. EMBO J. 2014;33(6):542–58.
27. Blasius AL, Beutler B. Intracellular toll-like receptors. Immunity. 2010;32(3):305–15.
28. Hamann L, Glaeser C, Hamprecht A, Gross M, Gomma A, Schumann RR. Toll-like receptor (TLR)-9 promotor polymorphisms and atherosclerosis. Clin Chim Acta. 2006;364(1-2):303–7.
29. Roszak A, Lianeri M, Sowinska A, Jagodzinski PP. Involvement of Toll-like Receptor 9 polymorphism in cervical cancer development. Mol Biol Rep. 2012;39(8):8425–30.
30. Ng MT, Van't Hof R, Crockett JC, Hope ME, Berry S, Thomson J, et al. Increase in NF-kappaB binding affinity of the variant C allele of the toll-like receptor 9–1237 T/C polymorphism is associated with Helicobacter pylori-induced gastric disease. Infect Immun. 2010;78(3):1345–52.
31. Mollaki V, Georgiadis T, Tassidou A, Ioannou M, Daniil Z, Koutsokera A, et al. Polymorphisms and haplotypes in TLR9 and MYD88 are associated with the development of Hodgkin's lymphoma: a candidate-gene association study. J Hum Genet. 2009;54(11):655–9.

4

The utility of Xpert MTB/RIF performed on bronchial washings obtained in patients with suspected pulmonary tuberculosis in a high prevalence setting

Dewald A. Barnard[1,2*], Elvis M. Irusen[1,2], Johannes W. Bruwer[1,2], Danté Plekker[3], Andrew C. Whitelaw[2,4,5], Jacobus D. Deetlefs[6] and Coenraad F. N. Koegelenberg[1,2]

Abstract

Background: Xpert MTB/RIF has been shown to have a superior sensitivity to microscopy for acid fast bacilli (AFB) in sputum and has been recommended as a standard first line investigation for pulmonary tuberculosis (PTB). Bronchoscopy is a valuable tool in diagnosing PTB in sputum negative patients. There is limited data on the utility of Xpert MTB/RIF performed on bronchial lavage specimens. Our aim was to evaluate the diagnostic efficiency of Xpert MTB/RIF performed on bronchial washings in sputum scarce/negative patients with suspected PTB.

Methods: All patients with a clinical and radiological suspicion of PTB who underwent bronchoscopy between January 2013 and April 2014 were included. The diagnostic efficiencies of Xpert MTB/RIF and microscopy for AFB were compared to culture for *Mycobacterium tuberculosis*.

Results: Thirty nine of 112 patients were diagnosed with culture-positive PTB. Xpert MTB/RIF was positive in 36/39 with a sensitivity of 92.3 % (95 % CI 78–98 %) for PTB, which was superior to that of smear microscopy (41 %; 95 % CI 26.0–57.8 %, $p = 0.005$). The specificities of Xpert MTB/RIF and smear microscopy were 87.7 % (95 % CI 77.4–93.9 %) and 98.6 % (95 % CI 91.6 %–99.9 %) respectively. Xpert MTB/RIF had a positive predictive value of 80 % (95 % CI; 65–89.9 %) and negative predictive value of 95.5 % (95 % CI 86.6–98.8 %). 3/9 patients with Xpert MTB/RIF positive culture negative results were treated for PTB based on clinical and radiological findings.

Conclusion: Xpert MTB/RIF has a higher sensitivity than smear microscopy and similar specificity for the immediate confirmation of PTB in specimens obtained by bronchial washing, and should be utilised in patients with a high suspicion of pulmonary tuberculosis.

Background

Early diagnosis and treatment of pulmonary tuberculosis is essential in reducing the spread, morbidity, mortality and the escalating costs associated with advanced disease [1]. Microbiological confirmation of *Mycobacterium tuberculosis* disease can be challenging in patients with a low bacterial load or in those who do not expectorate. Bronchoscopy with washings, with or without biopsy, can aid diagnosis by providing adequate samples for testing [2, 3].

Most of the evidence confirming the utility of the newly WHO endorsed Xpert MTB/RIF has been based on studies performed on sputum samples [4, 5]. The reported sensitivity of 90.4 % is significantly higher than that of smear microscopy, which is around 28 % [4, 6]. Recent studies have also suggested that Xpert MTB/RIF's sensitivity is not affected by HIV status [4, 7]. There is limited data validating the routine use of Xpert MTB/RIF on bronchial lavages, as the majority of cohorts

* Correspondence: dabarnard@live.com
[1]Divisions of Pulmonology, Department of Medicine, Stellenbosch University, PO Box 19063, 7505 Cape Town, South Africa
[2]Tygerberg Academic Hospital, Cape Town, South Africa
Full list of author information is available at the end of the article

contained low numbers of patients from whom bronchial lavages were obtained [4, 7–9].

The aim of this study was to evaluate the diagnostic efficiency of Xpert MTB/RIF performed on bronchial washing fluid obtained bronchoscopically from patients with a clinical and radiological suspicion of pulmonary tuberculosis.

Methods

Study population

We screened all smear negative/sputum scarce patients who underwent bronchoscopy as part of their work up for suspected pulmonary tuberculosis at Tygerberg Academic Hospital and Kuils River Hospital during the period from January 2013 to April 2014, and retrospectively included all patients with complete sets of medical, radiological and laboratory data. Tygerberg Academic Hospital is a tertiary hospital in Cape Town, South Africa. It is one of two referral centres and it renders a tertiary service to a population of approximately 3.6 million people. Kuilsrivier Hospital is a secondary hospital in Cape Town, offering private health care to patients. For the purposes of our study we considered a clinical suspicion of pulmonary tuberculosis if any two of the following were present: known HIV infection, persistent cough lasting > 3 weeks, haemoptysis, weight loss > 4 kg, intermittent fever > 3 weeks or drenching night sweats > 2 weeks. In addition, at least one of the following radiological criteria had to be present for inclusion: cavitation, diffuse infiltrates, hilar or mediastinal adenopathy. The study was approved by the Health Research Ethics Committee of Stellenbosch University (S13/04/063). A waiver of consent was approved due to the retrospective nature of the study.

Bronchoscopy procedure

Flexible bronchoscopies were performed in dedicated suites under conscious sedation. Washings were obtained by instilling 10 ml of 0.9 % saline into a segment of an affected lobe and aspirating available fluid (repeated three times). Transbronchial biopsies and transbronchial needle aspiration of lymph nodes were performed at the discretion of the endoscopist.

Microbiology

Samples were processed according to standard laboratory protocols by decontamination with N-acetyl-L-cysteine/NaOH, centrifugation and fluorescent microscopy for acid fast bacilli [10]. Decontaminated samples were inoculated in the BACTEC MGIT culture system, (Becton Dickinson, Sparks, Maryland, USA) and incubated for 6 weeks [11]. Positive cultures were identified as *M. tuberculosis* and tested for susceptibility to rifampicin and isoniazid using the MTBDRplus line probe assay (Hain LifeSciences, Nehren, Germany).

All Xpert MTB/RIF samples were processed according to the manufacturer's specifications [12]. Bronchial washing fluid was incubated, without prior decontamination, with sample reagent in a cartridge and loaded within 30 min of preparation. A test was positive if *Mycobacterium tuberculosis* was identified within 38 cycles [13]. Xpert MTB/RIF generated results (cycle threshold values) were categorised as either high positive (< 16), medium (16–21), low (22–28) or very low positive (> 28) [12].

Diagnosis of pulmonary tuberculosis

We use a positive culture of *Mycobacterium tuberculosis* as the gold standard for the diagnosis of pulmonary tuberculosis in our primary analysis. In a secondary analysis, we also included cases with histological or cytological features of caseating granuloma containing acid fast bacilli, or cases where at least three clinical and one radiological criterion were present in a patient who subsequently showed documented clinical and radiological improvement after six months of anti-tuberculosis treatment (despite negative microbiology).

Statistical analysis

Descriptive statistics were performed and a composite reference standard used. Analyses were conducted of data collected per patient. The sensitivity, specificity, positive predictive value (PPV) and negative predictive value (NPV) of Xpert MTB/RIF were calculated using standard methods and Xpert MTB/RIF generated results (cycle threshold values) listed. Unless stated otherwise, data is displayed as means and standard deviation (SD).

Results

Patients

We screened 184 patients with suspected pulmonary tuberculosis during the study period, and included 112 patients (age 44.4 +/− 15.9 years, 54 males) with complete records (Fig. 1). A total of 132 lobes were sampled in these patients.

A total of 44 patients were ultimately treated for pulmonary tuberculosis, based on positive culture ($n = 39$), histological or cytological features ($n = 2$) and on clinical and radiological grounds with clinical response to treatment ($n = 3$). Alternative diagnoses for the remaining 68 patients are summarised in Fig. 1.

Radiographic features observed in the study population included cavitatory disease ($n = 12$), consolidation ($n = 24$), diffuse nodular infiltrates ($n = 13$), alveolar infiltrates ($n = 35$), pulmonary mass lesions ($n = 13$), pleural effusions ($n = 9$) and isolated lymphadenopathy ($n = 6$).

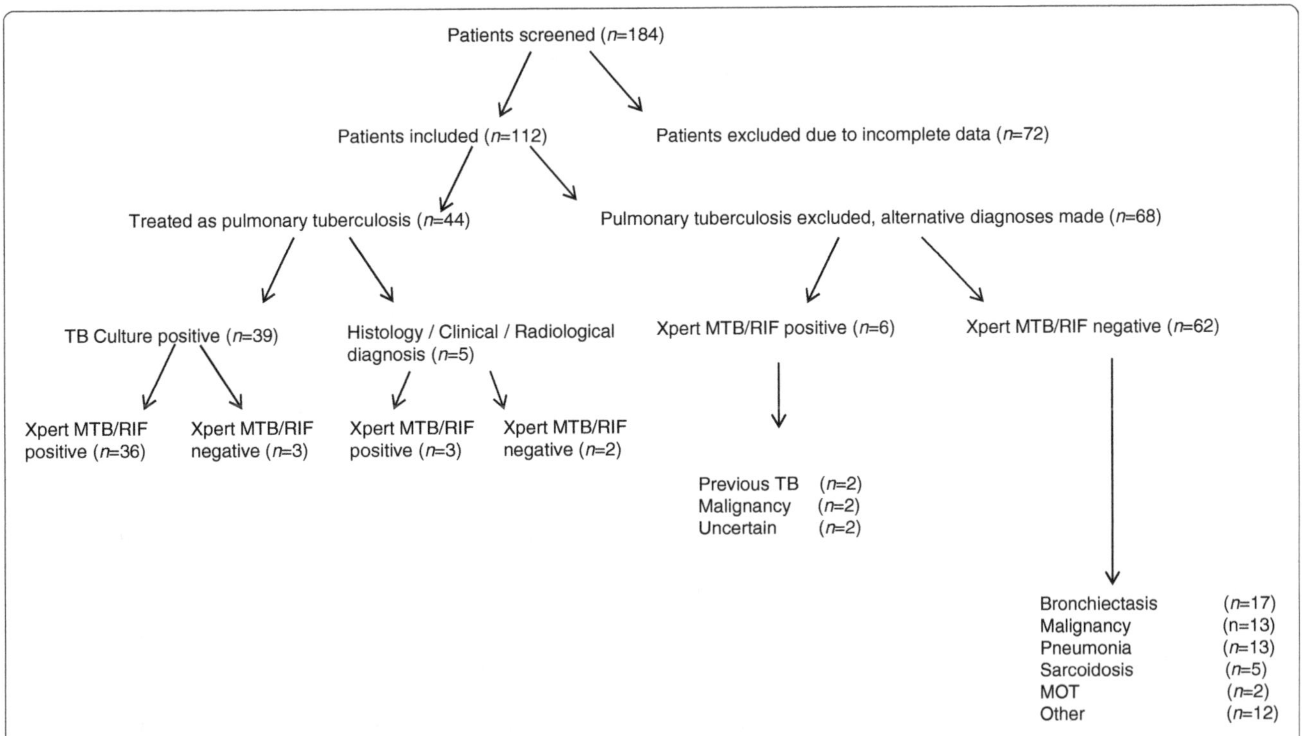

Fig. 1 Patients flow through the study. *MOT* Mycobacterium other than tuberculosis

Microbiology

Xpert MTB/RIF was positive in 36 of the 39 confirmed cases, compared to smear microscopy that was positive in 16. Only one case of isoniazid mono-resistance was identified in the 39 cases who were culture positive, with no cases of Rifampicin resistance. The sensitivities, specificities, PPVs and NPVs for culture, microscopy and Xpert MTB/RIF are summarised in Table 1. Xpert MTB/RIF had a sensitivity of 92.3 % (95 % CI 78–98 %) for PTB, which was superior to that of smear microscopy (41 %; 95 % CI 26–57.8 %, $p = 0.005$). The specificities of Xpert MTB/RIF and smear microscopy were 87.7 % (95 % CI 77.4–93.9 %) and 98.6 % (95 % CI 91.6 %–99.9 %) respectively. The diagnostic efficiency of Xpert MTB/RIF was 89.3 %. Cycle threshold values for the patients diagnosed with PTB varied between high positive ($n = 8$), medium ($n = 12$), low ($n = 11$), and very low positive ($n = 5$).

Nine Xpert MTB/RIF positive, culture negative cases were identified (Table 2). Of these, the majority had very low positive Xpert MTB/RIF results ($n = 7$) and only three were ultimately treated for suspected pulmonary tuberculosis.

Discussion

In this study, performed in a population with a high pretest probability for pulmonary tuberculosis, we found Xpert MTB/RIF to have a sensitivity, specificity and negative predictive value of around 90 %, and a positive predictive value of approximately 80 %. Xpert MTB/RIF had a very high diagnostic efficiency of 89.3 %. The majority of Xpert MTB/RIF positive, culture negative results were observed in cases with very low positive Xpert MTB/RIF results and a past history of pulmonary tuberculosis.

Table 1 Sensitivity, specificity, positive predictive value and negative predictive value of culture, microscopy and Xpert MTB/RIF performed on lavage specimens

	Smear Microscopy		Xpert MTB/RIF		Adjusted Xpert MTB/RIF[a]	
	%	95 % CI	%	95 % CI	%	95 % CI
Sensitivity	41.0	26 – 57.8	92.3	78 – 98	88.6	74.6 – 95.7
Specificity	98.6	91.6 – 99.9	87.7	77.4 – 93.9	91.2	81.1 – 96.4
PPV	94.1	69.2 – 99.7	80.0	64.9 – 89.9	86.7	72.5 – 94.4
NPV	75.8	65.7 – 83.7	95.5	86.6 – 98.8	92.5	82.7 – 97.2

95 % CI 95 % confidence interval, *PPV* positive predictive value, *NPV* negative predictive value
[a]Secondary analysis (including cases diagnosed on clinical, histological and radiological means)

Table 2 Xpert MTB/RIF positive, culture negative cases

Case	Previous PTB	Ct value	Treated for PTB	Alternative diagnoses/comments
1	Unknown	Low	Yes	Confirmed pleural tuberculosis
2	No	Very low	Yes	Takayashu's arteritis
3	Unknown	Very low	Yes	Clinical response to PTB treatment
4	Yes	Medium	No	Surveillance bronchoscopy to exclude bronchial stenosis 1 year after PTB
5	Yes	Very low	No	Repeat bronchoscopy culture and Xpert MTB/RIF negative
6	Unknown	Very low	No	Squamous cell carcinoma of the lung
7	No	Very low	No	Squamous cell carcinoma of the lung
8	No	Very low	No	Symptoms resolved with treatment
9	Yes	Very low	No	Culture positive for *Mycobacterium avium intracellulare*

PTB pulmonary tuberculosis, *Ct value* cycle threshold value

The sensitivity observed in the present study is on par with sensitivities recently reported in two studies (ranging from 82–93 %), but the specificity is marginally lower than the reported 96–100 % [7, 8]. The studies reported by Lee *et al.* and Theron *et al.* included similar numbers of patients diagnosed with pulmonary tuberculosis, and utilised comparable diagnostic criteria for the diagnosis of pulmonary tuberculosis [7, 8].

We identified 9 cases of Xpert MTB/RIF positive culture, negative cases, of which three were treated for pulmonary tuberculosis. Current evidence suggests that pulmonary tuberculosis treatment within the preceding 5 years can potentially RIF/RIF [14, 15]. Up to 27 % of patients have been reported to remain sputum Xpert MTB/RIF positive 26 weeks after successful anti-tuberculous treatment was initiated [16, 17]. Due to the nature of the polymerase chain reaction test, Xpert MTB/RIF amplifies any DNA whether it originates from alive or dead bacilli. Therefore it cannot be assumed, solely on the basis of the test, that a positive result equates to active disease [12, 18]. It is also unclear whether the bacterial load in bronchoscopy samples in patients with latent infection or recent exposure would reach this limit and potentially result in a very low positive Xpert MTB/RIF test result. More evidence is needed on the interpretation of Xpert MTB/RIF in the setting of recently treated tuberculosis, which may be the most important cause of false positive results.

No cross-reactivity has been reported between Xpert MTB/RIF and multiple bacteria, viruses, fungi or mycobacteria species other than tuberculosis and should therefore not be the reason for false positive results [19, 20]. We observed a single case of false positive Xpert MTB/RIF in a patient with confirmed *Mycobacterium avium intracellulare* infection. It is likely that dual pathology (including undiagnosed previous tuberculosis) and laboratory contamination may have been present in this case, as well as the other cases not treated as pulmonary tuberculosis, a finding that has been reported in similar settings with a high HIV prevalence [21-23].

It should be noted that 7 of the 9 Xpert MTB/RIF positive culture negative cases had very low positive test results. Some correlation between Xpert MTB/RIF generated quantitative information and bacterial load and disease severity has been described [21, 22]. Xpert MTB/RIF's calculated analytical limit of detection has been reported as 131 cfu/ml (95% CI 106.2–176.4). The relationship between Xpert MTB/RIF generated cycle threshold values, bacterial load and smear microscopy grades has shown that very low positive test results (cycle threshold values >28 cycles) correlate with negative microscopy and low positive values (22–28) with scanty positive smear microscopy [7, 21, 22]. This also correlated to the lower end of time-to-positivity of cultures. More research is required to aid in the interpretation of Xpert MTB/RIF with very low positive results, which in clinical practice, may be interpreted in the same light as a negative or, at best, scanty positive smear microscopy result. Our observations suggest that very low positive results require confirmation by culture or other means in cases with a low pre-test probability. Cut-off values for positivity should potentially vary between high and low endemic tuberculosis areas with lower cycle threshold values accepted as positive in high endemic areas. Moreover, clinicians practicing in high burden settings should be aware that past tuberculosis and dual pathology should be considered in cases with unexpected positive Xpert MTB/RIF.

The present study has several limitations. The retrospective nature limited the data collection to cases with complete clinical, radiological and microbiological data, and precluded any analyses on the excluded patient population. Some cases with false negative cultures may have gone undetected, and the true sensitivity may be different. We were also not able to document the true impact of Xpert MTB/RIF performed on bronchial lavages on the time to diagnosis or treatment, which is arguably of even greater clinical relevance.

Conclusion

Xpert MTB/RIF has a higher sensitivity than smear microscopy and similar specificity for the immediate confirmation of pulmonary tuberculosis on specimens obtained from bronchial washing, and should routinely be utilised in patients with a high clinical suspicion of pulmonary tuberculosis. Positive Xpert MTB/RIF, culture negative results should be interpreted in the clinical context, and ideally be confirmed with additional tests and/or follow-up.

Abbreviations

CI: Confidence Interval; DNA: Deoxyribonucleic acid; HIV: Human Immunodeficiency Virus; NaOH: Sodium Hydroxide; NPV: Negative Predictive Value; MTB/RIF: Mycobacterium tuberculosis/Rifampicin; PPV: Positive Predictive Value; PTB: Pulmonary tuberculosis; WHO: World Health Organisation.

Competing interests

The authors declare that they have no competing interests.

Authors contributions

DAB contributed to the study design, collection of data, analysis and interpretation of data, and writing the manuscript. EMI, JWB, ACW, JDD and DP contributed to the collection of data and editing the draft. CFNK contributed to the study design, study supervision, analysis and interpretation of data, and writing the manuscript. All authors read and approved the final manuscript.

Acknowledgements

We would like to thank Ms Kerry-Leigh Dennis from Ampath Laboratories (South Africa) and Dr Cornelia Rautenbach from the National Health Laboratory Services (South Africa) for assisting in data collection and interpretation of the technical aspects of Xpert MTB/RIF. No funding was received for the study.

Author details

[1]Divisions of Pulmonology, Department of Medicine, Stellenbosch University, PO Box 19063, 7505 Cape Town, South Africa. [2]Tygerberg Academic Hospital, Cape Town, South Africa. [3]Kuils River Hospital, Cape Town, South Africa. [4]Division of Medical Microbiology and Immunology, Department of Pathology, Stellenbosch University, Cape Town, South Africa. [5]National Health Laboratory Services, Cape Town, South Africa. [6]Ampath Laboratories, Cape Town, South Africa.

References

1. Keeler E, Perkins MD, Small P, Hanson C, Reed S, Cunningham J, et al. Reducing the global burden of tuberculosis: the contribution of improved diagnostics. Nature. 2006;444 Suppl 1:49–57. doi:10.1038/nature05446.
2. Shin JA, Chang YS, Kim TH, Kim HJ, Ahn CM, Byun MK. Fiberoptic bronchoscopy for the rapid diagnosis of smear-negative pulmonary tuberculosis. BMC Infect Dis. 2012;12(1):141. doi:10.1186/1471-2334-12-141.
3. Altaf Bachh A, Gupta R, Haq I, Varudkar HG. Diagnosing sputum/smear-negative pulmonary tuberculosis: Does fibre-optic bronchoscopy play a significant role? Lung India. 2010;27(2):58–62. doi:10.4103/0970-2113.63607.
4. Boehme CC, Nicol MP, Nabeta P, Michael JS, Gotuzzo E, Tahirli R, et al. Feasibility, diagnostic accuracy, and effectiveness of decentralised use of the Xpert MTB/RIF test for diagnosis of tuberculosis and multidrug resistance: a multicentre implementation study. Lancet. 2011;377(9776):1495–505. doi:10.1016/S0140-6736(11)60438-8.
5. Chang K, Lu W, Wang J, Zhang K, Jia S, Li F, et al. Rapid and effective diagnosis of tuberculosis and rifampicin resistance with Xpert MTB/RIF assay: a meta-analysis. J Infect. 2012;64(6):580–8. doi:10.1016/j.jinf.2012.02.012.
6. World Health Organisation. WHO Global Tuberculosis Report 2014. http://www.who.int/tb/publications/global_report/en (accessed 28 May 2015).
7. Theron G, Peter J, Meldau R, Khalfey H, Gina P, Matinyena B, et al. Accuracy and impact of Xpert MTB/RIF for the diagnosis of smear-negative or sputum-scarce tuberculosis using bronchoalveolar lavage fluid. Thorax. 2013;68(11):1043–51. doi:10.1136/thoraxjnl-2013-203485.
8. Lee HY, Seong MW, Park SS, Hwang SS, Lee J, Park YS, et al. Diagnostic accuracy of Xpert® MTB/RIF on bronchoscopy specimens in patients with suspected pulmonary tuberculosis. Int J Tuberc Lung Dis. 2013;17(7):917–21.
9. Le Palud P, Cattoir V, Malbruny B, Magnier R, Campbell K, Oulkhouir Y, et al. Retrospective observational study of diagnostic accuracy of the Xpert® MTB/RIF assay on fiberoptic bronchoscopy sampling for early diagnosis of smear-negative or sputum-scarce patients with suspected tuberculosis. BMC Pulm Med. 2014;14(1):137. doi:10.1186/1471-2466-14-137.
10. Steingart KR, Henry M, Ng V, Hopewell PC, Ramsay A, Cunningham J, et al. Fluorescence versus conventional sputum smear microscopy for tuberculosis: a systematic review. Lancet Infect Dis. 2006;6(9):570–81. doi:10.1016/S1473-3099(06)70578-3.
11. Bactec. MGIT For BACTEC ™ MGIT 960 ™ TB System. 2007. Available at: http://www.bd.com/ds/productCenter/MT-BactecMgit960.asp (accessed 28 May 2015).
12. Cepheid. Xpert MTB/RIF Brochure. 2010:1–4. Available at: http://www.cepheid.com/us/search?searchword=MTB+rif (accessed 28 May 2015).
13. Lawn S, Nicol M. Xpert® MTB/RIF assay: development, evaluation and implementation of a new rapid molecular diagnostic for tuberculosis and rifampicin resistance. Future Microbiol. 2011;1067–1082.
14. Boyles TH, Hughes J, Cox V, Burton R, Meintjes G, Mendelson M. False-positive Xpert® MTB/RIF assays in previously treated patients: need for caution in interpreting results. Int J Tuberc Lung Dis. 2014;18(7):876–8. doi:10.5588/ijtld.13.0853.
15. Metcalfe JZ, Makumbirofa S, Makamure B, Mutetwa R, Peñaloza RA, Sandy C, et al. Suboptimal specificity of Xpert MTB/RIF among treatment-experienced patients. Eur Respir J. 2015;111:1504–6. doi:10.1183/09031936.00214114.
16. Nicol MP. Xpert MTB/RIF: monitoring response to tuberculosis treatment. *lancet*. Respir Med. 2013;1(6):427–8. doi:10.1016/S2213-2600(13)70133-4.
17. Friedrich SO, Rachow A, Saathoff E, Singh K, Mangu CD, Dawson R, et al. Assessment of the sensitivity and specificity of Xpert MTB/RIF assay as an early sputum biomarker of response to tuberculosis treatment. Lancet Respir Med. 2013;1(6):462–70. doi:10.1016/S2213-2600(13)70119-X.
18. Van Rie A, Page-Shipp L, Scott L, Sanne I, Stevens W. Xpert(®) MTB/RIF for point-of-care diagnosis of TB in high-HIV burden, resource-limited countries: hype or hope? Expert Rev Mol Diagn. 2010;10(7):937–46. doi:10.1586/erm.10.67.
19. Blakemore R, Story E, Helb D, Kop J, Banada P, Owens MR, et al. Evaluation of the analytical performance of the Xpert MTB/RIF assay. J Clin Microbiol. 2010;48(7):2495–501. doi:10.1128/JCM.00128-10.
20. Helb D, Jones M, Story E, Boehme C, Wallace E, Ho K, et al. Rapid detection of Mycobacterium tuberculosis and rifampin resistance by use of on-demand, near-patient technology. J Clin Microbiol. 2010;48(1):229–37. doi:10.1128/JCM.01463-09.
21. Theron G, Peter J, van Zyl-Smit R, Mishra H, Streicher E, Murray S, et al. Evaluation of the Xpert MTB/RIF assay for the diagnosis of pulmonary tuberculosis in a high HIV prevalence setting. Am J Respir Crit Care Med. 2011;184(1):132–40. doi:10.1164/rccm.201101-0056OC.
22. Rachow A, Zumla A, Heinrich N, Rojas-Ponce G, Mtafya B, Reither K, et al. Rapid and accurate detection of Mycobacterium tuberculosis in sputum samples by Cepheid Xpert MTB/RIF Assay-A clinical validation study. PLoS One. 2011;6(6):1–8. doi:10.1371/journal.pone.0020458.
23. Hanrahan CF, Theron G, Bassett J, Dheda K, Scott L, Stevens W, et al. Xpert MTB/RIF as a measure of sputum bacillary burden. Variation by HIV status and immunosuppression. Am J Respir Crit Care Med. 2014;189(11):1426–34. doi:10.1164/rccm.201312-2140OC.

5

Radial endobronchial ultrasound in diagnosing peripheral lung lesions in a high tuberculosis setting

Adrian Chan[1*], Anantham Devanand[1,2], Su Ying Low[1,2] and Mariko Siyue Koh[1,2]

Abstract

Background: Current data for the utility of radial endobronchial ultrasound (EBUS) in investigating peripheral lung lesions (PLLs) has been restricted to populations with low pulmonary tuberculosis (TB) incidence. The aim of this study was to assess the diagnostic utility of radial EBUS with guide sheath in the diagnosis of peripheral lung lesions in Singapore, a high TB incidence setting.

Methods: A post-hoc database analysis was performed. 123 consecutive patients with computed tomographic evidence of PLLs who underwent radial EBUS guided bronchoscopy were included.

Results: The final diagnosis was malignancy in 76 cases and benign in 44 cases. Radial EBUS guided bronchoscopy had a sensitivity of 65.8 % for malignancy, positive predictive value of 100 %, negative predictive value of 62.9 %, and a diagnostic accuracy of 82.5 %. 22 patients had a final diagnosis of pulmonary TB. The diagnostic sensitivity for pulmonary TB was 77.3 %, with a positive predictive value of 100 %, negative predictive value of 95.2 % and a diagnostic accuracy of 95.8 %. Overall, 58.8 % of pulmonary TB cases relied on histology to make an early diagnosis.

Conclusion: Radial EBUS guided bronchosopy is useful in investigating PLLs in a high TB incidence setting. Our data also suggests that radial EBUS is a more rapid diagnosis technique for tuberculous lesions.

Background

Peripheral lung lesions (PLL) are defined as lesions that are not visualized within the bronchial tree during flexible bronchoscopy [1, 2]. Differential diagnoses can include both malignant causes and benign causes such as infection and inflammation. The diagnostic yield of flexible bronchoscopy in the biopsy of such lung lesions has been reported to be 54 % for malignant lesions and 41 % for benign lesions [3, 4]. To circumvent limitations of flexible bronchoscopy for such lesions, adjunct diagnostic tools have been proposed to guide bronchoscopic biopsies. Various studies have confirmed that radial EBUS is a modality that can improve diagnostic sensitivity [5–10]. The American College Of Chest Physicians Lung Cancer Guidelines has recommended using radial endobronchial ultrasound (EBUS) as an adjunct imaging modality for patients with peripheral lung nodules, where expertise and equipment are available. It can be used especially in cases where tissue diagnosis is required due to the uncertainty of diagnosis or poor surgical candidacy (Grade 1C evidence) [11]. Such guidelines are targeted at populations of an intermediate probability of lung cancer depending on clinical history, radiological stability and CT signs of malignancy such as size, spiculated borders, and absence of calcification.

However, pulmonary tuberculosis (TB) can also present as a peripheral lung lesion with varying disease activity: active infection, tuberculous granulomas, or inflammatory scars. In populations where tuberculosis is endemic, benign-looking lesions (based on clinical history and radiological characteristics) cannot always be managed with radiological surveillance because of both therapeutic implications and public health reasons. Delayed diagnosis and empiric tuberculosis treatment in an era of drug resistance will undermine the global control of TB [12, 13]. Percutaneous lung biopsy and surgical resection are options that offer a high diagnostic yield, but these will

* Correspondence: adrian.chan.k.w@sgh.com.sg
[1]Department of Respiratory and Critical Care Medicine, Singapore General Hospital, Singapore, Singapore
Full list of author information is available at the end of the article

expose patients with a potentially curable infection to unnecessary procedural risks.

The diagnostic yield of conventional (transbronchial biopsy) TBB for pulmonary TB has been reported to be 55–75.8 % [14, 15]. The current literature on radial EBUS is limited mostly to populations with high lung cancer prevalence and there is limited data on the role of radial EBUS guided bronchoscopic biopsy for PLLs in populations with a high incidence of pulmonary TB [9–11]. We aimed to evaluate the diagnostic yield of radial EBUS-guided sampling in PPLs for both malignant and benign lesions (including TB).

Methods

Study design and setting

This is a retrospective database review of an established database in Singapore General Hospital, a 1700-bedded university-affiliated tertiary hospital. A database of all adult consecutive patients at our hospital who consented for and underwent flexible bronchoscopy using radial EBUS was established in August 2008. This project was supported by government funding from the Ministry of Health, Singapore (under Health Services Development Project). As such, the project was closely audited by the funding agency and the Singapore General Hospital Quality Management Department. Therefore, completeness of data collection, diagnostic yield, technical details and complications were ensured. The study was approved by SingHealth Centralised Institutional Review Board (CIRB: 2008/458/B).

Study population

All consecutive patients who had PPLs and had undergone radial EBUS were considered for inclusion. Exclusion criteria were: 1) CT findings with any of the following: PPL < 1 cm diameter, endobronchial lesions, airway narrowing, pure 'ground-glass' appearance, or absence of CT bronchus sign, and 2) Presence of a submucosal lesion seen during flexible bronchoscopy. The study period was between August 2008 and December 2011 and data for included patients were reviewed retrospectively.

Study procedures

Bronchoscopy was performed under moderate sedation using a combination of midazolam and fentanyl. The pre-test probability of pulmonary TB was considered high if there was fever and sputum production clinically and if there was cavitation radiologically. All these patients had negative acid-fast bacilli smears prior to endoscopy.

During the procedure, the bronchoscope was maneuvered to the suspected sub-segmental airway and BAL was first performed. This was followed by insertion of a 20-MHz radial EBUS probe (UM-S20-20R; Olympus, Tokyo, Japan) with an external diameter of 2.2 mm via a guide-sheath through the 2.8 mm working channel of the flexible bronchoscope (Exera BF-1 T260; Olympus, Tokyo, Japan) with an outer diameter of 6.0 mm. The lesion was localized when the 'snow-storm' ultrasound appearance of aerated-normal lung was replaced with a soft tissue density on the processor monitor (EU-ME1; Olympus, Tokyo, Japan). The radial probe was adjusted until the probe was within the lesion. This was continued until all visible sub-segments were explored. Ultimately if the radial probe could not be placed within the lesion, the best CT-bronchoscopic correlation was used. Then, the probe was withdrawn leaving the guide-sheath in situ. Aliquots of 20 ml of normal saline solution were instilled and retrieved immediately with negative suction pressure that was adjusted to avoid airway collapse. A total of 100 to 200 ml of normal saline was instilled in each patient. Forceps biopsies were then taken under fluoroscopic guidance. Fluoroscopy served the dual purposes of ensuring that the guide-sheath was not dislodged and the forceps were closed at a safe distance from the pleura. Aliquots from the pooled BAL sample were sent for Gram stain, acid fast bacilli (AFB) smear, microbiologic (including tuberculous) culture and cytologic examination; forceps biopsies were sent for histopathology and tuberculous cultures.

Malignant PPLs was diagnosed based on histological evidence of malignancy obtained from bronchoscopic biopsies. A diagnosis of tuberculosis was derived based on the following outcomes: a) presence of positive cultures or b) demonstration of necrotizing granulomatous inflammation on histology with or without positive microbiology or c) clinical suspicion of TB and response to empirical anti-tuberculous treatment with radiological resolution of PPL [16]. All patients with non-diagnostic bronchoscopy were either subjected to an alternative biopsy (usually CT-guided or surgical biopsy) or followed up with a combination of radiology and clinical surveillance for a minimum of 12 months, depending on the managing physician's discretion. When an alternative diagnosis was established, these cases were designated as false negatives. If the patient showed both clinical and radiological stability, then the lesion was considered likely to be pulmonary scar tissue and designated as a true negative.

Statistical analysis

Statistical analysis was performed using a statistical package for social sciences software (Version 21.0). Confidence intervals of 95 % were reported, and all tests were 2-sided. Continuous variables were expressed as mean ± standard deviation, and comparisons were analysed with t-tests. Outcomes for categorical variables were analysed using chi-square test or Fisher's exact test. Sensitivity, specificity, predictive values and accuracy were calculated based on standard definitions. $p < 0.05$ was regarded as being statistically significant.

Results

Patient characteristics

Overall, 123 patients underwent bronchoscopy with radial EBUS guidance. 3 patients were excluded from analysis as the final diagnosis could not be determined due to death (2 patients) or loss to follow-up (1 patient) [Table 1]. The mean age of the patients was 62.6 ± 12.6 years and 60 % were males. The median number of forcep-biopsies performed was 5 (range 1–13). The median midazolam dose was 3.0 mg (range 0–10 mg) and the median fentanyl dose was 50.0 mcg (range 0–200 mcg). Patients diagnosed with malignant lesions were significantly older than those with benign lesions (mean age: 65.1 ± 10.3 vs. 58.2 ± 15.0 years, $p = 0.004$).

Diagnostic yield and outcomes

The final diagnosis was malignancy in 76 cases, giving an incidence of 62.5 %. Radial EBUS for malignant lesions had a sensitivity of 65.8 % (95 % CI: 53.9–76.0), positive predictive value of 100 % (95 % CI: 91.1–100), negative predictive value of 62.9 % (95 % CI: 50.4–73.9), and an overall diagnostic accuracy of 82.5 % [Table 2]. There was no difference for yield between malignant and non-malignant lesions ($p = 0.308$). 10 lesions were diagnosed to be pulmonary metastases; the bronchoscopic diagnostic yield for such lesions was only 20 %. 21 of 26 patients with non-diagnostic EBUS-guided sampling underwent further invasive investigations to confirm the diagnosis of malignancy [Table 3].

22 patients in our study group had a final diagnosis of pulmonary TB. Radial EBUS guided bronchoscopy successfully diagnosed pulmonary TB in 17 out of 22 cases, providing a diagnostic sensitivity of 77.3 % (95 % CI: 54.2–91.3), positive predictive value of 100 % (95 % CI: 77.1–100), negative predictive value of 95.1 % (95 % CI: 88.5–98.2) and a diagnostic accuracy of 95.8 % [Table 4]. Mycobacterial culture was positive in 15 of 17 (88.2 %) cases. These were obtained from BAL in all cases, whilst 6 cases yielded a positive culture from transbronchial biopsies as well. 10 of 22 patients demonstrated necrotizing granulomatous inflammation on their TBBs. In this subgroup with positive histology, all patients had negative AFB smears on bronchoscopic samples, and 2 patients had negative tuberculous cultures. In patients with negative histologic findings on biopsies, the main pathologic findings were chronic inflammatory changes without granulomatous inflammation (11 patients) or necrotic material (1 patient).

Data for ultrasound probe location was available for 105 patients. The probe was within the lesion in 78 patients (74.3 %), adjacent to the lesion in 22 patients (21.0 %), and outside of the lesion in 5 patients (4.7 %). Yield was significantly higher when the probe was positioned within the lesion (78.2 %) than when the probe was adjacent to or outside the lesion (44.4 %) ($p = 0.001$).

Mean lesion diameter was 25.6 ± 12.4 mm, with 71 patients (59.7 %) having lesions greater than 20 mm diameter. Mean lesion diameter was similar for malignant lesions (26 ± 12 mm) when compared to benign lesions (24 ± 13 mm) ($p = 0.357$). There was no significant difference in the yield for lesions greater than 20 mm diameter as compared to lesions ≤ 20 mm in diameter (67.6 % vs.70.8 %) ($p = 0.840$). Lobar location of the lesion also did not affect diagnostic outcome ($p = 0.590$). Mean lesion distance from pleura was 16.8 ± 13.5 mm.

Overall complication rate was 6.4 % [Table 5]. Seven patients (5.6 %) had bleeding that required cold saline or topical adrenaline for haemostasis and 1 patient (0.8 %) suffered a pneumothorax that was managed conservatively without requiring chest drainage. All complications were self-limited and no patient required escalation in the level of care.

Discussion

Although previous studies that investigated PLLs using bronchoscopy with radial EBUS guidance have demonstrated a high sensitivity for the detection of malignant lesions, it is worth noting that majority of the reports came from populations with high incidence of malignancy [17–20]. Lai et al. had a pulmonary TB incidence of 23.5 %, and reported a sensitivity of 55 % for tuberculous lesions diagnosed via conventional bronchoscopy and fluoroscopy [15]. In comparison, the incidence of pulmonary TB in our setting was 18.3 %. The addition of radial EBUS with guide-sheath increased the diagnostic sensitivity to 77.3 %, consistent with previous studies that highlighted an increased yield could be obtained when these 2 techniques are combined [5, 21, 22].

Another important finding from our study is that radial EBUS guided TBBs provided a more rapid diagnosis via histology in nearly half of patients with pulmonary TB, given their initial negative smear microscopy. Tuberculosis remains a global epidemic, and the ability to diagnose pulmonary TB early is important from a clinical and public health perspective. In 2011, there were an estimated 8.7 million new cases of TB and 1.4 million deaths from TB [23]. Around 3 million new cases of TB cases are diagnosed in South-East Asia each year, and this region accounts for 39 % of the global burden of TB [23]. Singapore, with an incidence of pulmonary tuberculosis of 50 per 100,000, is situated in a tuberculosis endemic region and offers a setting to further understand

Table 1 Demographics, clinical-radiological data and bronchoscopic results of malignant and benign peripheral lung lesions

	Malignant		Benign		*p*-value
Demographics					
Subjects (n)	76		44		
Age	65.1 ± 10.3		58.2 ± 15.0		0.004
Male gender (%)	60.5		70.5		0.326
Smoking (%)	44.6		33.3		0.247
Diabetes mellitus (%)	21.6		14.3		0.461
Presenting symptoms (n)					
Cough		27		14	0.841
Dyspnoea		14		1	0.037
Weight Loss		12		4	0.440
Hemoptysis		5		4	0.721
Fever		2		5	0.097
Asymptomatic		23		16	0.442
Size					
Mean (mm)	26 ± 12		24 ± 13		0.357
≤20 mm	28 (36.0)		21 (47.7)		
>20 mm	48 (64.0)		23 (52.3)		
Common radiologic characteristics					
Spiculation/Lobulation		44 (57.9)		10 (23.8)	<0.001
Cavitation		4 (5.3)		13 (31.0)	<0.001
Ground gass/Semisolid		4 (5.3)		3 (7.1)	0.698
Appearance					
Tree-in-bud changes		1 (1.3)		6 (13.6)	0.009
Distance of lesion from pleura (mm)	17 ± 13		16 ± 14		0.606
Lobar Position (n)					0.582
Right upper lobe	20		12		
Right middle lobe	6		5		
Right lower lobe	20		8		
Left upper lobe	28		14		
Left lower lobe	2		5		
Final diagnosis					
	Non-small cell lung cancer	63 (82.9)	Pulmonary tuberculosis	22 (50.0)	
			Pneumonia	15 (34.1)	
	Small cell lung cancer	2 (2.6)	Other diagnoses		
	Pulmonary metastases	10 (13.2)	Organising pneumonia	5 (11.4)	
	Bronchial carcinoid	1 (1.3)	Scarring	2 (4.6)	
Cases diagnosed by radial EBUS	Non-small cell lung cancer	45 (59.2)	Pulmonary tuberculosis	17 (38.6)	
			Pneumonia	12 (27.3)	
	Small cell lung cancer	2 (2.6)	Other diagnoses		
	Pulmonary metastases	2 (2.6)	Organising pneumonia	2 (4.5)	
	Bronchial carcinoid	1 (1.3)	Scarring	2 (4.5)	

Table 1 Demographics, clinical-radiological data and bronchoscopic results of malignant and benign peripheral lung lesions *(Continued)*

Yield based on known location of probe		
Within lesion	49 (71.6)	29 (78.9)
Adjacent to lesion	16 (23.9)	6 (15.8)
Outside lesion	3 (4.5)	2 (5.3)

Data presented as mean + SD and n (%), unless otherwise stated

EBUS diagnostic yields for both malignant and tuberculous diseases [24]. Early diagnosis and appropriate treatment of infectious patients with pulmonary TB are important steps to reduce transmission of *Mycobacterium Tuberculosis* and to achieve disease elimination [23]. Radial EBUS aided in obtaining histological diagnosis consistent with pulmonary TB infection in 58.8 % of our pulmonary TB patients thus enabling pulmonologists to diagnose the disease and start anti-tuberculous treatment earlier. However, histology does not replace mycobacterial cultures, which is the "gold standard" in diagnosis of pulmonary TB that gives additional important information on sensitivity to anti-tuberculous medications. Indeed, this is very important in the era of drug-resistant TB [23].

Our study demonstrated a low complication rate (6.4 %) comparable to previously reported safety data of radial EBUS (0–7.4 %) [9]. This is much lower compared to the generally quoted complication rate from percutaneous lung biopsy (15–25 %) [25, 26] with similar yield of 68.6 % for pulmonary TB [27]. The ability to diagnose pulmonary TB earlier with histology and low complication rate highlights the potential of radial EBUS as the preferred first step in an algorithm to evaluate PLLs when the pre-test probability of tuberculosis and malignancy are similarly high or for high risk patients who may not be able to tolerate the complication of pneumothorax (for example, patients with emphysema or chronic obstructive pulmonary disease). It is also noted that adding guide sheaths to the procedure does not worsen the safety profile and its use should be considered for sampling [28].

We postulate that our higher yield for benign lesions could be due to such lesions having surrounding inflammation with ill-defined borders - or in the case of pulmonary TB, associated consolidation, centrilobular nodules or tree-in-bud changes. In our group of pulmonary TB patients, the following associated radiologic characteristics were observed in addition to the PLLs: cavitation (9 lesions), scarring (3 lesions) and ground glass opacities (2 lesions). Another possible reason could be that benign lesions are less likely to cause airway distortion, in contrast to malignant lesions that have been recognized to directly compress and narrow the bronchus or indirectly narrow the proximal bronchial tree due to enlarged peribronchial or submucosal lymph nodes [29].

We report a sensitivity of 65.8 % for all malignant lesions, which is similar to yields obtained from previous

Table 2 Histologic and/or microbiologic results obtained from specimens derived from EBUS-guided sampling as compared to the final diagnosis of malignancy

	Final diagnosis of malignancy	Final diagnosis of benign lesion	Total
EBUS sampling positive for cancer	50	0	50
EBUS sampling negative for cancer	26	44	70
Total	76	44	120

Table 3 Evaluation of patients who had non-diagnostic radial-EBUS guided bronchoscopy

Malignant	n = 26
Final method of diagnosis	
Percutaneous lung biopsy	12
Surgical lung biopsy	9
Radiologic progression of pulmonary metastases	2
Transbronchial needle aspiration of associated lymph node metastases	1
Repeat bronchoscopic biopsy with radial EBUS guidance	1
Response to chemotherapy	1
Benign	n = 11
Tuberculosis	
Final method of diagnosis	
Responded to anti-tuberculous therapy	3
Percutaneous lung biopsy	1
Surgical lung biopsy	1
Infection	
Final method of diagnosis	
Responded to anti-microbial therapy	3
Organising pneumonia	
Final method of diagnosis	
Repeat bronchoscopic biopsy with radial EBUS	2
By different bronchoscopist	
Scarring	
Final method of diagnosis	
Interval stability on repeat imaging (up to 1 year)	1

Table 4 Histologic and/or microbiologic results obtained from specimens derived from EBUS-guided sampling as compared to the final diagnosis of tuberculosis

	Final diagnosis of tuberculosis	Not tuberculosis	Total
EBUS sampling positive for tuberculosis	17	0	17
EBUS sampling negative for tuberculosis	5	98	103
Total	22	98	120

radial EBUS studies [9]. However, our diagnostic yield for pulmonary metastases was much lower (20 %). This can be explained by spread of pulmonary metastases being haematogenous and not bronchial; hence visualization and diagnostic yield of such lesions by EBUS may be lower. This is supported by our observation that we could place our probe within the metastatic lesion in only 30 % of cases. Percutaneous lung biopsy might be more appropriate in such cases.

We identified several limitations in our study. Firstly, during the time of study, the use of nucleic acid amplification (NAA) tests as well as molecular tests to detect TB and mutations conferring rifampicin resistance (eg Xpert MTB/RIF) were not widely available for routine clinical use in our institution. The advantage of NAA is its ability to provide results within 24–48 h, compared to 3–5 days for histology and 2–6 weeks for TB cultures [30]. NAA testing has a high positive predictive value (>95 %) in AFB smear-positive sputum specimens (especially relevant in settings in which non-tuberculous mycobacteria are common). It can confirm the presence of Mycobacteria tuberculosis in 62.2–79.3 % of AFB smear-negative, culture-positive specimens [31, 32]. In our study group, all our pulmonary TB patients were sputum AFB smear negative. Given the low sensitivity of NAA in such patients and the fact that histology is necessary for the diagnosis of malignancy, these tests were unlikely to have made a huge impact in our clinical decision to perform bronchoscopy and radial EBUS. Secondly, being a retrospective analysis, selection bias could not be excluded. However, this was minimized by including all consecutive patients who received radial EBUS guidance in our institution. This meant that we could not apply clinical-radiologic models in predicting the probability of malignancy or infection prior to histologic investigation, which may subsequently influence the diagnostic yield of EBUS-TBB. We did not include a control group of patients with PPLs who underwent bronchoscopy with conventional fluoroscopic biopsy for comparison of diagnostic yields, as such patients should have been considered for an alternative procedure given the published data on low yields from conventional biopsies. Unlike previous reports where EBUS bronchoscopies were performed by selected few experts, radial EBUS bronchoscopies were performed by all 8 pulmonologists in our institution, hence variability in endoscopic competency may have affected the yield. Nevertheless, our hospital has a high bronchoscopic load with >1000 bronchoscopies performed every year and all pulmonologists were experienced bronchoscopists trained in EBUS at the same time. Therefore, endoscopic competency would not be a major factor in influencing the yield. Furthermore, this provides 'real-world' experience rather than procedures performed by selected specialized experts. It has been reported that performing trans-bronchial needle aspiration with radial EBUS guidance further improves the diagnostic yield [33]. This technique was not available to our center at the time of the study and could be evaluated in future studies. It was previously reported that EBUS-guided biopsies without the use of fluoroscopy had limited benefit for diagnosing smaller (≤20 mm) lesions [17]. For our study, we elected to combine both EBUS and fluoroscopy for optimal guidance of the forceps. Thus, the exact usefulness of EBUS may have been overestimated in our study especially for smaller lesions. This may also account for our similar diagnostic yields for smaller and larger lesions. Ideally, the gold standard for final diagnosis should be histologic or microbial confirmation of all PPLs. However, the risk-benefit ratio of multiple diagnostic procedures was considered and we included patients who we were confident of the final diagnosis based on appropriate observation or treatment.

Table 5 Complications arising from radial-EBUS guided sampling

	Malignant	Benign
Bleeding	5	2
Pneumothorax	0	1
Death	0	0

Limitations notwithstanding, the findings from our study have several clinical implications. Taking into account the high diagnostic accuracy for both malignant and benign lesions as well as the excellent safety profile of radial EBUS guided TBBs, we suggest using this as the first modality to investigate PLLs in which clinical characteristics and sputum studies remain inconclusive. This may in turn reduce morbidity and healthcare costs for patients who ultimately have benign lesions. Secondly, in cases where pre-test probability of pulmonary TB is high, whilst it is sufficient to obtain an eventual microbiologic diagnosis with BAL alone, the added benefit of a more rapid histologic diagnosis with radial EBUS guided TBB should be considered [34]. To validate these recommendations, prospective studies should be conducted in populations with a similar prevalence of pulmonary TB. This will allow for further analysis of the test performance of radial EBUS of pulmonary TB with the aim of creating a clear management algorithm of PLLs.

Conclusion

In our population with a high incidence of pulmonary TB, it is important to review the clinical and radiologic characteristics of PLLs before deciding on choice of investigation for histologic diagnosis. Where clinical suspicion of malignancy is indeterminate or when pulmonary tuberculosis is suspected following initial negative sputum studies, radial EBUS is to be considered as a viable first step in the evaluation of PLLs. The additional yield, faster time to diagnosis and favourable safety profile of radial EBUS are the positive factors contributing to our recommendation.

Abbreviations

AFB: Acid fast bacilli; BAL: Bronchoalveolar lavage; CT: Computed tomography; EBUS: Endobronchial ultrasound; NAA: Nucleic acid amplification; PLL: Peripheral lung lesion; TB: Tuberculosis; TBB: Transbronchial lung biopsies.

Competing interests

The authors declare that they have no competing interests.

Authors' contributions

MK was the Project Director of the Health Services Development Project for Radial Endobronchial Ultrasound. All authors designed the study and collected the data. AC analysed the data with input from all authors. AC drafted the article with critical input from all authors. All authors approved the final version. AC is the guarantor for the content of the manuscript, as well as the decision to publish.

Acknowledgements

The authors wish to thank Ms Ulina Santoso and the Singapore General Hospital's Department Of Quality Management for their assistance in auditing the radial EBUS service. The authors also appreciate the support of Duke-NUS/ SingHealth Academic Medicine Research Institute and the medical editing assistance of Taara Madhavan (Associate, Clinical Sciences, Duke-NUS Graduate Medical School).

Author details

[1]Department of Respiratory and Critical Care Medicine, Singapore General Hospital, Singapore, Singapore. [2]Duke- NUS Graduate Medical School, Singapore, Singapore.

References

1. Radke JR, Conway WA, Eyler WR, Kvale PA. Diagnostic accuracy in peripheral lung lesions. Factors predicting success with flexible fiberoptic bronchoscopy. Chest. 1979;76(2):176–9.
2. Shiner RJ, Rosenman J, Katz I, Reichart N, Hershko E, Yellin A. Bronchoscopic evaluation of peripheral lung tumours. Thorax. 1988;43(11):887–9.
3. Gasparini S, Ferretti M, Secchi EB, Baldelli S, Zuccatosta L, Gusella P. Integration of transbronchial and percutaneous approach in the diagnosis of peripheral pulmonary nodules or masses. Experience with 1,027 consecutive cases. Chest. 1995;108(1):131–7.
4. Baaklini WA, Reinoso MA, Gorin AB, Sharafkaneh A, Manian P. Diagnostic yield of fiberoptic bronchoscopy in evaluating solitary pulmonary nodules. Chest. 2000;117(4):1049–54.
5. Kurimoto N, Miyazawa T, Okimasa S, Maeda A, Oiwa H, Miyazu Y, et al. Endobronchial ultrasonography using a guide sheath increases the ability to diagnose peripheral pulmonary lesions endoscopically. Chest. 2004;126(3):959–65.
6. Kikuchi E, Yamazaki K, Sukoh N, Kikuchi J, Asahina H, Imura M, et al. Endobronchial ultrasonography with guide-sheath for peripheral pulmonary lesions. Eur Respir J. 2004;24(4):533–7.
7. Paone G, Nicastri E, Lucantoni G, Dello Iacono R, Battistoni P, D'Angeli AL, et al. Endobronchial ultrasound-driven biopsy in the diagnosis of peripheral lung lesions. Chest. 2005;128(5):3551–7.
8. Wang Memoli JS, Nietert PJ, Silvestri GA. Meta-analysis of guided bronchoscopy for the evaluation of the pulmonary nodule. Chest. 2012;142(2):385–93.
9. Steinfort DP, Khor YH, Manser RL, Irving LB. Radial probe endobronchial ultrasound for the diagnosis of peripheral lung cancer: systematic review and meta-analysis. Eur Respir J. 2011;37(4):902–10.
10. Fuso L, Varone F, Magnini D, Baldi F, Rindi G, Pagliari G, et al. Role of ultrasound-guided transbronchial biopsy in the diagnosis of peripheral pulmonary lesions. Lung Cancer. 2013;81(1):60–4.
11. Gould MK, Donington J, Lynch WR, Mazzone PJ, Midthun DE, Naidich DP, et al. Evaluation of individuals with pulmonary nodules: when is it lung cancer? Diagnosis and management of lung cancer, 3rd ed: American College of Chest Physicians evidence-based clinical practice guidelines. Chest. 2013;143(5 Suppl):e93S–120S.
12. Yew WW, Lange C, Leung CC. Treatment of tuberculosis: update 2010. Eur Respir J. 2011;37(2):441–62.
13. Seung KJ, Gelmanova IE, Peremitin GG, Golubchikova VT, Pavlova VE, Sirotkina OB, et al. The effect of initial drug resistance on treatment response and acquired drug resistance during standardized short-course chemotherapy for tuberculosis. Clin Infect Dis. 2004;39(9):1321–8.
14. Kohno S. Diagnostic value of bronchoscopy in diagnosis of pulmonary tuberculosis: bronchial aspirate, bronchial washing and transbronchial lung biopsy. Kekkaku. 1990;65(1):33–6.
15. Lai RS, Lee SS, Ting YM, Wang HC, Lin CC, Lu JY. Diagnostic value of transbronchial lung biopsy under fluoroscopic guidance in solitary pulmonary nodule in an endemic area of tuberculosis. Respir Med. 1996;90(3):139–43.
16. Blumberg HM, Burman WJ, Chaisson RE, Daley CL, Etkind SC, Friedman LN, et al. American Thoracic Society/Centers for Disease Control and Prevention/Infectious Diseases Society of America: treatment of tuberculosis. Am J Respir Crit Care Med. 2003;167(4):603–62.
17. Yoshikawa M, Sukoh N, Yamazaki K, Kanazawa K, Fukumoto S, Harada M, et al. Diagnostic value of endobronchial ultrasonography with a guide sheath for peripheral pulmonary lesions without X-ray fluoroscopy. Chest. 2007;131(6):1788–93.
18. Chung YH, Lie CH, Chao TY, Wang YH, Lin AS, Wang JL, et al. Endobronchial ultrasonography with distance for peripheral pulmonary lesions. Respir Med. 2007;101(4):738–45.
19. Chen A, Chenna P, Loiselle A, Massoni J, Mayse M, Misselhorn D. Radial probe endobronchial ultrasound for peripheral pulmonary lesions. A 5-year institutional experience. Ann Am Thorac Soc. 2014;11(4):578–82.
20. Herth FJ, Ernst A, Becker HD. Endobronchial ultrasound-guided transbronchial lung biopsy in solitary pulmonary nodules and peripheral lesions. Eur Respir J. 2002;20(4):972–4.
21. Ishida M, Suzuki M, Furumoto A, Tsuchihashi Y, Ariyoshi K, Morimoto K. Transbronchial biopsy using endobronchial ultrasonography with a guide sheath increased the diagnostic yield of peripheral pulmonary lesions. Intern Med. 2012;51(5):455–60.
22. Chavez C, Sasada S, Izumo T, Watanabe J, Katsurada M, Matsumoto Y, et al. Endobronchial ultrasound with a guide sheath for small malignant pulmonary nodules: a retrospective comparison between central and peripheral locations. J Thorac Dis. 2015;7(4):596–602.
23. WHO Global tuberculosis report 2014 World Health Organization, Geneva (2014) http://www.who.int/tb/publications/global_report/en/ (accessed 30 June 2015).
24. World Health Organisation Global Tuberculosis Report 2013: 270. www.who.int/iris/bitstream/10665/91355/1/9789241564656_eng.pdf (accessed: 11 July 2015).
25. Fielding DI, Chia C, Nguyen P, Bashirzadeh F, Hundloe J, Brown IG, et al. Prospective randomised trial of endobronchial ultrasound-guide sheath versus computed tomography-guided percutaneous core biopsies for peripheral lung lesions. Intern Med J. 2012;42(8):894–900.
26. Wiener RS, Wiener DC, Gould MK. Risks of transthoracic needle biopsy: How high? Clin Pulm Med. 2013;20(1):29–35.

27. Yew WW, Kwan SY, Wong PC, Fu KH. Percutaneous transthoracic needle biopsies in the rapid diagnosis of pulmonary tuberculosis. Lung. 1991;169(5):285–9.
28. Hayama M, Izumo T, Matsumoto Y, Chavez C, Tsuchida T, Sasada S. Complications with Endobronchial Ultrasound with a Guide Sheath for the Diagnosis of Peripheral Pulmonary Lesions. Respiration. 2015. [Epub ahead of print].
29. Tsuboi E, Ikeda S, Tajima M, Shimosato Y, Ishikawa S. Transbronchial biopsy smear for diagnosis of peripheral pulmonary carcinomas. Cancer. 1967;20(5):687–98.
30. Moore DF, Guzman JA, Mikhail LT. Reduction in turnaround time for laboratory diagnosis of pulmonary tuberculosis by routine use of a nucleic acid amplification test. Diagn Microbiol Infect Dis. 2005;52(3):247–54.
31. Guerra RL, Hooper NM, Baker JF, Alborz R, Armstrong DT, Maltas G, et al. Use of the amplified mycobacterium tuberculosis direct test in a public health laboratory: test performance and impact on clinical care. Chest. 2007;132(3):946–51.
32. Laraque F, Griggs A, Slopen M, Munsiff SS. Performance of nucleic acid amplification tests for diagnosis of tuberculosis in a large urban setting. Clin Infect Dis. 2009;49(1):46–54.
33. Chao TY, Chien MT, Lie CH, Chung YH, Wang JL, Lin MC. Endobronchial ultrasonography-guided transbronchial needle aspiration increases the diagnostic yield of peripheral pulmonary lesions: a randomized trial. Chest. 2009;136(1):229–36.
34. Du Rand IA, Blaikley J, Booton R, Chaudhuri N, Gupta V, Khalid S, et al. British Thoracic Society guideline for diagnostic flexible bronchoscopy in adults: accredited by NICE. Thorax. 2013;68 Suppl 1:i1–i44.

6

Isolated anterior mediastinal tuberculosis in an immunocompetent patient

S. Maguire[1*], S. H. Chotirmall[2], V. Parihar[1], L. Cormican[3], C. Ryan[4], C O'Keane[4], K. Redmond[5] and C. Smyth[1]

Abstract

Background: The differential diagnosis of a mediastinal mass is a common challenge in clinical practice, with a wide range of differential diagnosis to be considered. One of the rarer causes is tuberculosis. Atypical presentations of tuberculosis are well documented in immunocompromised patients, but should also be considered in the immunocompetent.

Case presentation: This case outlines a previously healthy 22 year-old immunocompetent male presenting with worsening chest pain, positional dyspnea, dry cough and dysphagia. Chest x-ray showed evidence of an isolated anterior mediastinal mass, which was confirmed on computed tomography. A mediastinoscopy was diagnostic as histology revealed necrotizing granulomatous inflammation and the presence of acid-fast bacilli, indicating mediastinal tuberculosis.

Conclusion: Typically the underlying presentation of mediastinal tuberculosis is mediastinal lymphadenitis. This case was unusual in that we detected an isolated large anterior mediastinal mass accompanied by a relatively small burden of mediastinal lymphadenitis. Cases similar to this have been documented in immunosuppressed patients however in our case no evidence of immunosuppression was found. This case report emphasizes the importance that a detailed and logical pathway of investigation is pursued when encountering a mediastinal mass.

Keywords: Tuberculosis, Atypical, Mycobacterium, Mass, Mediastinal

Background

Mediastinal masses are routinely encountered in clinical practice and a wide range of differential diagnoses must be considered. A less common cause is tuberculosis, a disease recognized for its atypical presentations attributed to its ability to affect almost any organ system. Tuberculosis has an incidence of 126 per 100,000 according to the latest report from the World Health Organization (WHO) [1]. *Mycobacterium tuberculosis* undergoes lympho-heamatogenous dissemination after entering the respiratory tract. Typically the mediastinal and hilar lymph nodes are the first lymphatic tissues *M. tuberculosis* will encounter [2] and it may then spread to other organ systems. Thirty percent of patients present with extra-pulmonary tuberculosis, an example of which is illustrated by this case [3].

* Correspondence: sineadmaguire@rcsi.ie
[1]Department of Gastroenterology, Connolly Hospital, Blanchardstown, Dublin Dublin 15, Ireland
Full list of author information is available at the end of the article

Case presentation

A 22-year-old Nigerian male presented to the accident and emergency department with a 2-week history of worsening chest pain associated with positional dyspnea, dry cough and dysphagia. He had no significant past history, was on no medication and denied any significant family history. The patient was resident in the Republic of Ireland since early childhood and had no recent travel abroad.

Chest radiography illustrated soft tissue enlargement within the right paratracheal stripe (Fig. 1a). Subsequent computed tomography of the thorax with contrast, revealed a large right-sided mediastinal mass with accompanying lymphadenopathy that encompassed the pre-tracheal, paratracheal, tracheobronchial, hilar and subcarinal regions superior to the right brachiocephalic vein, superior vena cava right pulmonary artery and superior right pulmonary vein (Fig. 1b).

Initial haematological testing revealed the following: C-reactive protein 62 (<5), ESR 102 (<20) and LDH 819 (208–378). Coagulation studies were also abnormal with a PT of 16.3 (11–13.5) and an INR of 1.4. Other laboratory

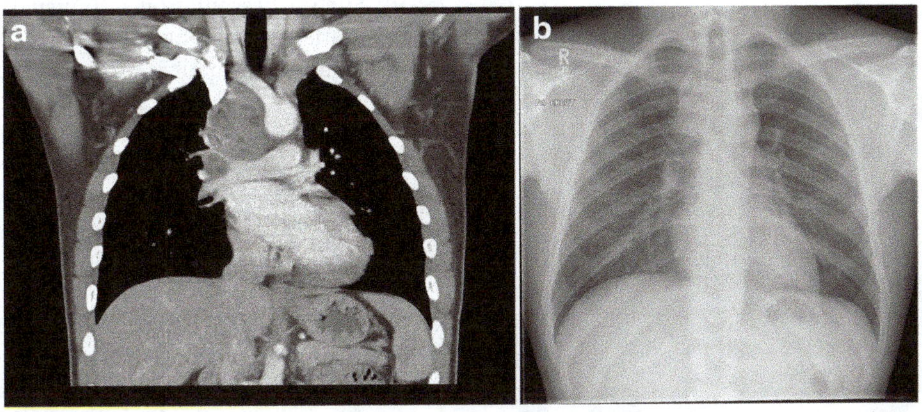

Fig. 1 **a** Initial chest x-ray demonstrates soft tissue enlargement within the right paratracheal stripe; **b** Contrast computed tomography of the thorax shows a large right-sided mediastinal mass with accompanying lymphadenopathy encompassing the pre-tracheal, para-tracheal, tracheobronchial, hilar and subcarinal regions. (The images have been placed in reverse order and so the caption does not match the image. The CXR should be Figure 1a and the CT image should be Figure 1b)

tests including full blood count, liver function test, troponin, electrolytes and glucose were normal as were the tumor markers beta human chorionic gonadotrophin (hCG) and alpha-fetoprotein. Computed tomography of the abdomen and pelvis was also concurrently done and found to be normal, with no evidence of other lymphadenopathy or masses.

Bronchoscopic evaluation illustrated 50 % external compression of the distal trachea with normal distal airways and no endobronchial mass visualized. Trans-bronchial biopsies showed no abnormality and bronchoalveolar lavage (BAL) showed pus cells but no organisms and tested negative for acid-fast bacilli. A full virology screen including HIV, hepatitis B and C were also negative. Whilst lymphoma was our primary working diagnosis due to the patient's age, mildly elevated LDH and the presence of a mass, tissue confirmation was pursued as initial bronchoscopic biopsies were not confirmatory.

A mediastinoscopy was subsequently performed and histology confirmed necrotizing granulomatous inflammation with the presence of acid fast bacilli (AFB) diagnostic of mediastinal tuberculosis (Fig. 2). The patient was commenced on a standard anti-tuberculosis regime for a total of 6 months and has since completed his course of treatment. His most recent chest x-ray (CXR) shows interval improvement (Fig. 3) and he has now been discharged from the respiratory service.

Conclusions

The differential diagnosis of a mediastinal mass is a common challenge in clinical practice (Table 1)[4]. Patients with these lesions are typically asymptomatic until they develop mass effects, such as chest pain, dyspnea or cough due to compression of local structures. Such symptoms prompted this patient's presentation. Investigation of such lesions must consider the wide range of differentials. As part of the initial evaluation, a detailed history and physical examination should be performed, looking specifically for lymphadenopathy, thyroid enlargement, testicular masses or evidence of immunosuppression. None of these features were present in this patient. A full haematological screen should be performed including relevant tumor markers including beta hCG and alpha-fetoprotein. Gene Xpert analysis is another well-recognized modality in rapid diagnosis of tuberculosis and should be considered in the work up of a mediastinal mass. Contrast computed tomography (CT) of the thorax is useful to further characterize a mediastinal mass. Radiographic findings suggestive of tuberculosis are a ghost like ring enhancement within a matted mass of nodes [5]. Importantly, tuberculosis has been shown to mimic malignancy both radiologically and

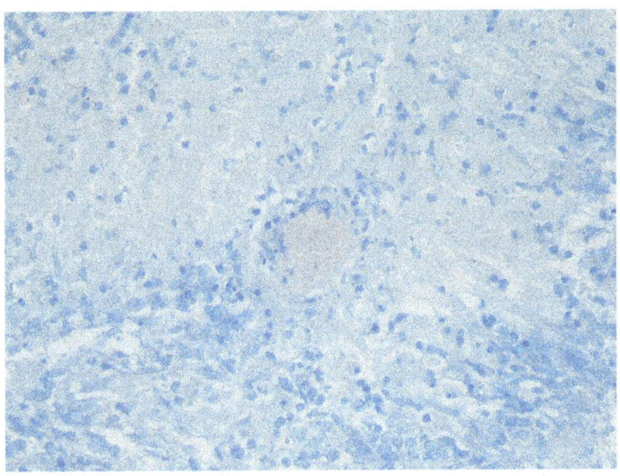

Fig. 2 Histology slide of a tissue specimen obtained via mediastinoscopy with Ziehl Neelsen staining shows a single acid-fast bacilli in center of necrosis

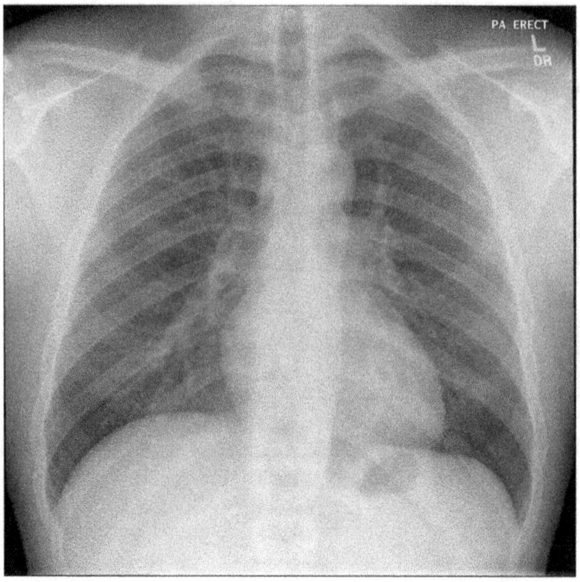

Fig. 3 Follow up chest x-ray shows considerable reduction in the soft tissue previously noted in relation to the right paratracheal stripe

clinically [6] hence diagnostic confirmation by histology is imperative prior to therapeutic intervention. This can be obtained by bronchoscopy or endoscopic bronchial ultrasound allowing for fine needle aspirate cytology or transbronchial needle aspirate to obtain a diagnostic pathological specimen.

There are several and varied presentations of mediastinal tuberculosis including lymph node calcification, oesophagomediastinal fistula, pericardial TB and fibrosing mediastinitis. The underlying cause of these lesions is mediastinal lymphadenitis, which extends to involve surrounding structures creating strictures and fistulation [7]. This case was unusual in that we detected an isolated large anterior mediastinal mass accompanied by a relatively small burden of mediastinal lymphadenitis. Prior cases similar to this have been noted to occur in immunosuppressed individuals such as those with seropositive HIV with a CD4 T lymphocyte count <200/mm^3 but are even more rarely found in HIV positive patients with a CD4 T lymphocyte count >200/mm^3 [8, 9]. Such a presentation is unusual in immunocompetent patients, although has been shown to occur more frequently in patients from countries where TB is endemic [10].

There are few documented cases of tuberculosis presenting as an isolated anterior mediastinal mass in an immunocompetent patient. Comprehensive review of the literature reveals ten similarly described cases with the majority occurring in the pediatric population aged 2 years or younger. Of the published cases on adults all three patients were male with age ranging from 32 to 76 years [11–14]. The masses varied in composition and behavior, with one case describing a cystic mass and another a mass infiltrating the right atrium. Similar to this case all three patients were treated with medical therapy. The limited published data on adult presentations of mediastinal tuberculosis in immunocompetent patients does reveal that presentation is usually associated with mass effect symptoms and that a diagnosis was only revealed following histological confirmation, both features observed in this case [15–20].

In summary, while the aetiology of a mediastinal mass can be difficult to establish because of the wide differential, it is imperative that a through and logical scheme of investigation including tissue diagnosis is pursued. This case aims to highlight the importance of considering tuberculosis in the differential even in immunocompetent patients presenting with an isolated mediastinal mass that cannot otherwise be explained.

Table 1 Differential diagnosis of a mediastinal mass

Lymphoma
Thymoma
Germ cell tumour
Thyroid enlargement
Vascular lesion
Lymphadenopathy
Cystic lesion (pleuropericardial or bronchogenic)
Tuberculosis

Ethics, consent & permissions

Written informed consent was obtained from the patient for publication of this case report and accompanying images. A copy of the written consent is available for review by the Editor of this journal. This project was carried out within an appropriate ethical framework. This manuscript conforms with the CARE guidelines published in 2013 (see Additional file 1).

Consent to publish

Written informed consent was obtained from the patient for publication of this case report and accompanying images. A copy of the written consent is available for review by the Editor of this journal.

Abbreviations

HIV: Human innunodeficiency virus; ESR: Erythrocyte sedimentation rate; LDH: Lactate dehydrogenase; INR: International normalized ratio; PT: Prothrombin time; Beta hCG: Human chorionic gonadotrophin;

CXR: Chest x-ray; ZN: Ziehl Neelsen; AFB: Acid fast bacilli; CT: Computed tomography.

Competing interests

None of the authors involved in this case report have any competing interest in accordance with BioMed Central's guidelines.

Authors' contributions

SM was the primary author and was responsible for gathering all relevant patient data, conducting a literature review and drafting the case report. SC was responsible for editing and formatting of the case report. VP also assisted with critical editing. LC provided advice on discussion points in the conclusion. CR and CO provided diagnostic evaluation of the tissue samples and supplied the histopathology images in this report. KR assisted in diagnostic investigations resulting in the diagnosis. CS was the primary consultant for this patient and also provided critical review of the case report. All authors read and approved the final manuscript.

Acknowledgements

N/A.

Funding

No funding was required for this case report or the research involved.

Author details

[1]Department of Gastroenterology, Connolly Hospital, Blanchardstown, Dublin Dublin 15, Ireland. [2]Lee Kong Chian School of Medicine, Nanyang Technological University, Singapore, Singapore. [3]Department of Respiratory Medicine, Connolly Hospital, Blanchardstown, Dublin Dublin 15, Ireland. [4]Department of Histopathology, Mater Misericordiae Hospital, Dublin Dublin 7, Ireland. [5]Department of Cardiothoracic Surgery, Mater Misericordiae Hospital, Dublin Dublin 7, Ireland.

References

1. World Health Organization. Global tuberculosis report 2014. Geneva: World Health Organization; 2014.
2. Rom WN, Garay SM. Tuberculosis. 2nd ed. New York: Little Brown and Company; 2000. p. 577.
3. CDC. Reported Tuberculosis in the United States, 2013. Atlanta: U.S. Department of Health and Human Services, CDC; 2014.
4. Strollo DC, Rosado de Christenson ML, Jett JR. Primary mediastinal tumors. Part 1: tumors of the anterior mediastinum. Chest. 1997;112(2):511–22.
5. Andronikou S, Joseph E, Lucas S, Brachmeyer S, Du Toit G, Zar H, et al. CT scanning for the detection of tuberculous mediastinal and hilar lymphadenopathy in children. Pediatr Radiol. 2004;34(3):232–6.
6. Tan CH, Kontoyiannis DP, Viswanathan C, Iyer RB. Tuberculosis: A benign imposter. AJR Am J Roentgenol. 2010;194(3):555–61.
7. Jeong YJ, Lee KS. Pulmonary Tuberculosis: Up-to-date imaging and management. AJR Am J Roentgenol. 2008;191(3):834–44.
8. Kim HY, Song KS, Goo JM, Lee JS, Lee KS, Lim TH. Thoracic sequelae and complications of tuberculosis. Radiographics. 2001;21(4):839–60.
9. Leung AN, Brauner MW, Gamsu G, Mlika-Cabanne N, Ben Romdhane H, Carrette MF, et al. Pulmonary tuberculosis: comparison of CT findings in HIV-seropositive and HIV-seronegative patients. Radiology. 1996;198(3):687–91.
10. Codecasa LR, Besozzi G, De Cristofaro L, Miradoli A, Sabolla L, Tagliaferri B. Epidemiological and clinical patterns of intrathoracic lymph node tuberculosis in 60 human immunodeficiency virus-negative adult patients. Monaldi Arch Chest Dis. 1998;53:277–80.
11. Vincken W, Vandenbrande P, Roels P, Pirngadi J, Welch W. Isolated paratracheal mass of tuberculosis origin in an adult patient. Eur J Respir Dis. 1983;64(8):630–5.
12. Jain N, Khilnani G, Hadda V, Iver V. Cystic mediastinal mass: A rare presentation of tuberculosis; Chest. 2013 Oct; 144:4 Meeting Abstract
13. Kumar N, Gera C, Philip N. Isolated mediastinal tuberculosis: a rare entity. J Assoc Physicians India. 2013;61(3):202–3.
14. Maeder M, Ammann P, Rickli H, Schoch OD. Fever and night sweats in a 22-year-old man with a mediastinal mass involving the heart. Chest. 2003;124(5):2006–9.
15. Gillies MJ, Farrugia MK, Lakhoo K. An unusual cause of a superior mediastinal mass in an infant. Pediatr Surg Int. 2008;24(4):485–6.
16. Ahmed A, Mirza S, Rothera MP. Mediastinal tuberculosis in a 10- month-old child. J Laryngol Otol. 2001;115(2):161–3.
17. Khilnani GC, Jain N, Hadda V, Arava SK. Anterior mediastinal mass: a rare presentation of tuberculosis. J Trop Med. 2011;2011:635385.
18. De Ugarte DA, Shapiro NL, Williams HL. Tuberculous mediastinal mass presenting with stridor in a 3-month-old child. J Pediatr Surg. 2003;38(4):624–5.
19. Thirithuvathas AJ, Ravikumar S, Gnanaseelan T. Huge prepericardial tuberculosis abscess in a 2-year-old child. J Pediatr Surg. 1989;24(11):1124.
20. Boussetta K, Tinsa F, Ghaffari H, Brini I, Aloui N, Jaubert F, et al. Mediastina Tuberculosis mass in a three-month-old boy. Tunis Med. 2010;88(8):602–4.

7

Later emergence of acquired drug resistance and its effect on treatment outcome in patients treated with Standard Short-Course Chemotherapy for tuberculosis

Jingtao Gao[1], Yan Ma[1], Jian Du[1], Guofeng Zhu[2], Shouyong Tan[3], Yanyong Fu[4], Liping Ma[5], Lianying Zhang[6], Feiying Liu[7], Daiyu Hu[8], Yanling Zhang[9], Xiangqun Li[10], Liang Li[1*] and Qi Li[1*]

Abstract

Backgrounds: The failure of current Standard Short-Course Chemotherapy (SCC) in new and previously treated cases with tuberculosis (TB) was mainly due to drug resistance development. But little is known on the characteristics of acquired drug resistant TB during SCC and its correlation with SCC failure. The objective of the study is to explore the traits of acquired drug resistant TB emergence and evaluate their impacts on treatment outcomes.

Methods: A prospective observational study was performed on newly admitted smear positive pulmonary TB (PTB) cases without drug resistance pretreatment treated with SCC under China's National TB Control Program (NTP) condition from 2008 to 2010. Enrolled cases were followed up through sputum smear, culture and drug susceptibility testing (DST) at the end of 1, 2, and 5 months after treatment initiation. The effect factors of early or late emergence of acquired drug resistant TB , such as acquired drug resistance patterns, the number of acquired resistant drugs and previous treatment history were investigated by multivariate logistic regression; and the impact of acquired drug resistant TB emergence on treatment failure were further evaluated.

Results: Among 1671 enrolled new and previously treated cases with SCC, 62 (3.7 %) acquired different patterns of drug resistant TB at early period within 2 months or later around 3–5 months of treatment. Previously treated cases were more likely to develop acquired multi-drug resistant TB (MDR-TB) (OR, 3.8; 95 %CI, 1.4–10.4; $P = 0.015$). Additionally, acquired MDR-TB cases were more likely to emerge at later period around 3-5 months after treatment starting than that of non-MDR-TB mainly appeared within 2 months (OR, 8.3; 95 %CI, 1.7–39.9; $P = 0.008$). Treatment failure was associated with late acquired drug resistant TB emergence (OR, 25.7; 95 %CI, 4.3–153.4; $P < 0.001$) with the reference of early acquired drug resistant TB emergence.

Conclusions: This study demonstrates that later development of acquired drug resistant TB during SCC is liable to suffer treatment failure and acquired MDR-TB pattern may be one of the possible causes.

Keywords: Tuberculosis, Multi-Drug Resistant Tuberculosis, Standard Short-Course Chemotherapy, Acquired drug resistant tuberculosis emergence

* Correspondence: liliang69@hotmail.com; lq703@hotmail.com
[1]Clinical Center on Tuberculosis, Beijing Chest Hospital, Capital Medical University, Beijing Tuberculosis and Thoracic Tumor Research Institute, Beijing, China
Full list of author information is available at the end of the article

Background

TB is a major global health problem with 8.6 million new cases and almost 1.3 million deaths attributed to the disease every year [1]. WHO recommended standardized first-line anti-TB drug regimen is a single 6-month or 8-month regimen composed of isoniazid (H), rifampicin (R), ethambutol (E), and streptomycin (S) with pyrazinamide (Z) [2]. This regimen is recommended for all new TB cases and previously treated cases in more than 90 countries. This strategy is designed and evaluated as the cost-effectiveness regimen used in resource-limited settings for decades for the consideration of convenient treatment management based on same number, dose, and types of medication. Though high cure rate was achieved of SCC for cases with drug-sensitive TB [3], the emergence of drug resistant TB, especially MDR-TB, and acquisition of additional drug resistance during treatment, brought much less efficacy of SCC both in trials [4–7] and under program conditions [8]. Few cohort studies, though the sample size was small, worked on the treatment of mono- or poly-resistant TB with SCC and presented poor results [9]. In most low- and middle-income countries, DST is not routinely performed for new cases nor for most previously treated cases [10, 11]; therefore, cases carrying drug-resistant strains of *Mycobacterium tuberculosis* (MTB) might be at greater risk for SCC failure and disseminating drug resistant strains [12]. China is one of the 27 countries with high MDR-TB burden, early detection and treatment could help prevent its transmission. Currently, China's NTP [13] provides new and previously treated cases with SCC under directly observed treatment (DOT) and monitors their response to SCC by sputum smear (SS) rather than sputum culture and DST due to limited resources. Sputum culture and DST are recommended to be performed for cases with initial treatment and retreatment failure, where possible, to develop appropriate chemotherapy regimens. Hence, little is known whether drug resistant TB occurs during treatment and few data available links acquired drug resistant TB to treatment failure with SCC. To address these issues, we conducted a prospective observational study tracing the emergence of acquired drug resistant TB at indicated time points among new and previously treated cases receiving first-line standard regimens to determine the characteristics and its effect on treatment failure.

Methods

Study settings and population

A prospective and observational cohort study was conducted in 8 provinces including Tianjin, Hebei, Henan, Shanghai, Chongqing, Yunnan, Guangxi, and Guangdong which are situated in northern, eastern, central-western, and southern China from October 2008 to September 2010. This study was embedded in the routine TB control program of each province. Case detection, smear microscopy, chemotherapy and treatment management were routine procedures under NTP; sputum culture and DST at varied time points were added. The sample size for new and previously treated cases of sputum smear-positive (SS+) TB was set at 1927 and 506 respectively which took into account a prevalence of overall resistance to first-line anti-TB drugs (H, R, E, S) of 18.6 % and 46.5 % respectively from a previous study [14], with desired precision of 1 %, a 95 % confidence level and a non-response rate of 10 %, assuming that 15 % of the culture samples would be lost due to failure to recover or due to growth of non-tuberculosis mycobacterium (NTM). Based on the requirements for sample size and the capacity to perform sputum culture and DST, the provincial TB Control and Prevention Centers in the above provinces were selected. The number of cases allocated to each province was based on the number of new SS+ cases reported by that province with the proportion to the total number of cases nationwide in 2007. Study subjects meeting all the following criteria were enrolled: 1. Aged ≥14 years; 2. Informed consent; 3. Newly registered confirmed PTB cases including cases with two positive direct smear microscopy results; or one positive direct smear microscopy result and lung imaging consistent with active PTB imaging manifestations [13]. 4. Not NTM strains infection; 5. Strains susceptible to all 4 first line anti-TB drugs (H, R, E, S) pretreatment (month 0). Demographic information and relevant medical history including age, gender, physical examinations, previous anti-TB treatment history and contact history with TB index cases were collected with a standard questionnaire given upon study entry. SS, culture, and DST results were examined at month 1, 2, and 5. Treatment outcomes were evaluated for both pan-susceptible cases all through SCC and acquired drug resistant TB cases during SCC.

Definitions

New cases of TB were defined as those who had never been treated for TB or had taken anti-TB drugs for less than one month. Previously treated cases were defined as those who had been previously treated for one month or more with anti-TB drugs [13]. In our study, according to the time of acquired drug resistant TB emergence for the first time, cases with any drug resistant TB emergence before the end of 2 months after treatment initiation were defined as early emergence of drug resistance while cases with drug resistant TB emergence after 2 months were defined as late emergence of drug resistance. Treatment outcomes were defined according to the WHO guidelines [2]. A patient who was initially SS+

and who was sputum smear-negative in the last month of treatment and on at least one previous occasion was defined as "Cured". A patient who completed treatment but did not meet the criteria for cure or failure was defined as "Completed treatment". A patient who died from any cause during treatment was defined as "Died". A patient who was initially SS+ and who remained SS+ at month 5 or later during treatment was defined as "Failed". A patient whose treatment was interrupted for two consecutive months or more was defined as "Defaulted". A patient whose treatment outcome was not known was defined as "Not evaluated". For analysis, a patient who was cured or who completed treatment was combined as "Successfully treated". In this study we mainly focus on cases with treatment success and failure of SCC.

Treatment regimen

All cases with pan-susceptible MTB strains prior treatment received SCC under qualified DOT. The initial standard regimen was $2H_3R_3Z_3E_3/4H_3R_3$, and the retreatment standard regimen was $2H_3R_3Z_3E_3S_3/6H_3R_3E_3$ [13]. For patients who could not use streptomycin for any reason, the intensive phase was extended for an additional month as $3H_3R_3Z_3E_3/6H_3R_3E_3$. The following regimen modifications were made after the second month SS examination: First, if a new SS+ TB patient was still tested SS+ at the end of the second month, the intensive phase was extended for an additional month, and the continuation phase remained unchanged. A smear microscopy was performed at the end of the third month. If the SS was negative at the end of the fifth month, the treatment regimen was $3H_3R_3Z_3E_3/4H_3R_3$. Second, if a retreatment SS + TB patient had a positive SS at the end of the second month, the intensive phase was extended for an additional month if the treatment regimen contained streptomycin and the continuation phase remained unchanged as $3H_3R_3Z_3E_3S_3/6H_3R_3E_3$, or the intensive phase was extended for another month, if the treatment regimen did not contain streptomycin, and the continuation phase remained unchanged as $4H_3R_3Z_3E_3/6H_3R_3E_3$. In both cases, a smear microscopy was performed at the end of the third month.

Bacteriologic examination

Three consecutive sputum samples (spot, night, and morning) were collected before the initiation of treatment (month 0) and 2 sputum samples were collected at months 1, 2, and 5 for each eligible patient. For isolation of the culture, each specimen was decontaminated, digested, and homogenized using the standard Petroff method [15]. An aliquot of 0.1 ml of the resulting specimen was inoculated into acidified Löwenstein–Jensen (LJ) slant tubes for primary isolation of the organism. Tubes were then incubated at 37 °C and inspected for growth of *Mycobacterium* for a period of 8 weeks. If no bacteria grew by week 8, the result was recorded as negative. Cultures with growing colonies were continued for identification and DST. Susceptibility testing of TB isolates to four first-line antimicrobial agents was performed by the indirect proportion method with LJ medium. The following drug concentrations were used to distinguish resistant isolates from susceptible isolates: isoniazid (H, 0.2 μg/mL), rifampicin (R, 40 μg/mL), ethambutol (E, 2 μg/mL), and streptomycin (S, 4 μg/mL). A strain was considered resistant when bacterial growth on a drug-containing medium was equal to or greater than 1 % of the colonies that grew on a drug-free medium. Quality-assured DST is critical to ensure accurate detection of drug resistance for subsequent treatment decisions and to avoid false diagnosis. All laboratories engaging in this study had external quality assessment coverage of DST. Internal control of sensitivity testing was assessed using a MTB sensitive strain (H37Rv).

Ethical considerations

This study was reviewed and approved by the Institutional Ethics Review Committee of Beijing Chest Hospital, Capital Medical University, Beijing Tuberculosis and Thoracic Tumor Research Institute, and selected 8 provincial TB Control and Prevention Centers. Written informed consent was obtained from all SS+ cases before enrollment in the study. In particular, for the minors enrolled in the study, written informed consent was obtained from themselves and their parents or guardians before enrollment. DST results were promptly reported back to the respective local health facilities the patients visited for further treatment management from above selected areas.

Statistics

The categorical variables were analyzed using Pearson's Chi-square test or Fisher's exact test as appropriate. To evaluate the effect factors of acquired drug resistant TB emergence, variables significant ($p < 0.05$) in the univariate analysis were subsequently analyzed by multiple logistic regression with a stepwise and forward method to identify the statistically significant factors to be maintained in the final model. For exploring the effect of acquired drug resistant TB emergence on treatment failure, we compared cases with late emergence to those with early emergence using univariate analysis by computing odds ratios (ORs) and their 95 % confidence intervals (CI). Data analysis was performed using SPSS version 18.0 (SPSS, Chicago). P value <0.05 was considered as criterion for statistical significance.

Results

Patient enrollment and demographic characteristics

During the study period, among 2142 confirmed pulmonary TB cases detected, 67 cases infected with NTM, 29 cases declined to participate the study, 321 cases with drug resistant TB and 54 cases with negative sputum culture results before treatment initiation. Therefore, according to the inclusion and exclusion criteria, the above cases were excluded and a total of 1671 pan-susceptible TB cases to all four first-line anti-TB drugs confirmed by pretreatment DST were enrolled and then received standardized anti-TB treatment (Fig. 1). Of these 1671 pan-susceptible cases pretreatment, 62 cases developed drug resistant TB during anti-TB therapy. Table 1 showed the analysis of univariate risk factors for acquired MDR-TB and Non-MDR-TB respectively. Non-MDR-TB refers to the cases with drug resistance other than MDR-TB. We found those aged 40–59 years (OR, 17.5; 95 %CI, 2.3–134.6; $P < 0.001$) was a significant factor for acquired MDR-TB development. Cases who had received previous TB treatment (OR, 3.8; 95 %CI, 1.4–10.4; $P = 0.015$) were more likely to develop acquired MDR-TB.

Acquired drug resistant TB emergence and its characteristics

Before starting treatment, 321 cases were resistant to at least one of the four first-line anti-TB drugs (H, R, E, and S), of which 251 were new and 70 were previously treated; 1671 cases were susceptible to all four drugs tested, of which 62 acquired drug resistant TB during SCC, composed of 49 new and 13 previously treated cases. The overall prevalence of drug resistance in our study was 17.6 % (300 of 1707) of new cases and 29.1 % (83 of 285) of previously treated cases. Furthermore, the prevalence of MDR-TB was 2.6 % (45 of 1707) of new cases and 14.0 % (40 of 285) of previously treated cases

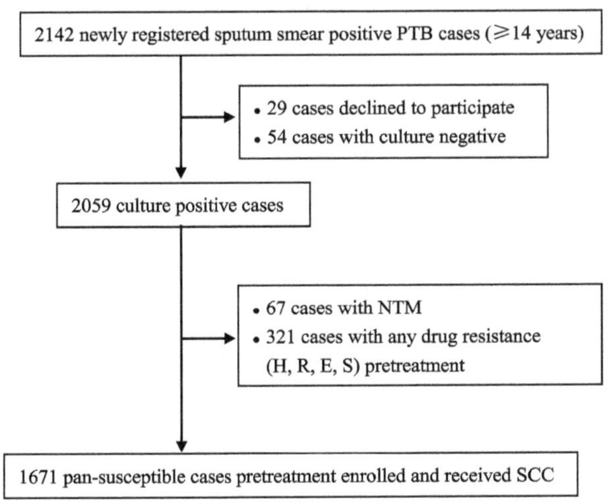

Fig. 1 Flow chart of TB subjects enrolled in the study

in the study (Additional file 1: Table S1). For the 62 acquired drug resistant TB cases, 89.8 % of new (44 of 49) and 61.5 % (8 of 13) of previously treated cases developed drug resistance within 2 months of SCC. In addition, 75.0 % newly acquired drug resistant TB (39 of 52) cases were resistant to 1 or 2 anti-TB drugs within first 2 months, while 70.0 % newly acquired drug resistant TB cases were resistant to 3 or 4 anti-TB drugs during 3–5 months after treatment starting. The acquired drug resistance patterns appeared within 2 months were mainly non-MDR-TB, accounted for 80.8 % (42 of 52) among patients with acquired drug resistance of same period, while 3–5 months after treatment starting, 70.0 % (7 of 10) newly acquired drug resistant TB cases were of MDR-TB pattern. In multivariate logistic regression analysis, late emergence of acquired drug resistant TB was associated with drug resistance patterns. Acquired MDR-TB cases were more likely to emerge at later period than that of acquired non-MDR-TB cases (OR, 8.3; 95 %CI, 1.7–39.9; $P = 0.008$) (Table 2).

Treatment outcomes of acquired drug resistant TB cases with standardized regimen

84.3 % of cases with pan-susceptible TB throughout were successfully treated and similar treatment success rate was achieved of cases with acquired drug resistant TB within 2 months of SCC, while only 20 % cases with late drug resistant TB emergence after 2 months were successfully treated (Table 3). The impact of time points of acquired drug resistant TB emergence on treatment outcomes evaluated indicated that treatment failure was significantly more likely among late emergence cases than among early emergence cases (OR, 25.7; 95 %CI, 4.3–153.4; $P < 0.001$) (Table 4). In addition, we analyzed the treatment outcomes of 62 acquired drug resistant cases during SCC based on drug resistance patterns. The treatment success rate of acquired MDR-TB cases was 52.9 %, much lower than that with non-MDR-TB pattern at 82.2 %.We further analyzed treatment success rate of 3 subgroups of non-MDR-TB. It is reported 92.3 % cases with any H resistance and 89.5 % cases with E/S resistance were successfully treated respectively. However, the treatment success rate of cases with any R resistance was 61.5 % (Additional file 1: Table S2).

Discussion

Up to date, this study is the first to evaluate traits of acquired drug resistant TB emergence and its impact on treatment failure of SCC under China's routine NTP condition. Majority of acquired drug resistant TB cases developed early within 2 months with SCC and late acquired drug resistant TB emergence after 2 months is more likely associated with the drug resistance pattern of MDR-TB. Furthermore, our results indicated a good

Table 1 Demographic characteristics and risk factors for patients with acquired drug resistant TB during SCC

Characteristics	Pan-susceptible TB throughout[a] n = 1609(%)	Any acquired drug resistant TB[b]		Acquired MDR-TB vs. Pan-susceptible TB throughout		Acquired Non- MDR-TB vs. Pan-susceptible TB throughout	
		MDR-TB[c] n = 17(%)	Non-MDR-TB[d] n = 45(%)	OR (95 % CI)[e]	*P* value	OR(95 % CI)	*P* value
Age(years)							
<40	756(47.0)	1(5.9)	19(42.2)	Reference		Reference	
40–59	560(34.8)	13(76.5)	20(44.5)	17.5(2.3–134.6)	<0.001	1.4(0.8–2.7)	0.278
≥60	293(18.2)	3(17.6)	6(13.3)	7.7(0.8–74.7)	0.079[g]	0.8(0.3–2.1)	0.665
Gender							
Male	1160(72.1)	14(82.4)	35(77.8)	Reference		Reference	
Female	449(27.9)	3(17.6)	10(22.2)	0.6(0.2–1.9)	0.427[g]	0.7 (0.4–1.5)	0.401
BMI[f] (Kg/m^2)							
BMI < 18.5	620(38.5)	3(17.6)	18(40.0)	Reference		Reference	
BMI ≥ 18.5	989(61.5)	14(82.4)	27(60.0)	2.9(0.8–10.2)	0.078	0.9(0.5–1.7)	0.842
Treatment history							
New	1407(87.4)	11(64.7)	38(84.4)	Reference		Reference	
Previously treated	202(12.6)	6(35.3)	7(15.6)	3.8(1.4–10.4)	0.015[g]	1.3(0.6–2.9)	0.550

[a]Pan-susceptible TB throughout in our study was defined as cases with TB strains susceptible to all four first-line anti-TB drugs including soniazid(H), rifampicin(R), ethambutol(E), and streptomycin(S) both pretreatment and throughout therapy
[b]Any acquired drug resistant TB in our study was defined as cases with TB strains that were susceptible to all four first-line anti-TB drugs pretreatment, but developed resistance to at least one of the four drugs during SCC
[c] MDR-TB was defined as TB that was at least resistant to both isoniazid and rifampicin
[d]Non-MDR-TB in our study was defined as TB cases with any drug resistance pattern except MDR-TB
[e]OR, odds ratio. CI, confidence interval
[f]BMI, body mass index, calculated as the weight in kilograms divided by the square of the height in meters
[g]*P* value was determined by Fisher's Exact Test. Not indicated was determined by Pearson's Chi-Square Test

response to SCC in cases with pan-susceptible strains throughout therapy which reconfirmed the SCC effectiveness for cases with susceptible strains [8, 16]. However, our findings presented poor response of SCC in cases with acquired drug resistant TB, especially with late drug resistant TB. It is shown that late acquired drug resistant TB emergence after 2 months is 25.7 times higher to result in treatment failure than that within 2 months.

In our study, the data from 8 provinces in China indicating a overall drug resistant TB prevalence of 17.6 % in new cases and 29.1 % in previously treated cases and a MDR-TB prevalence of 2.6 % and 14.0 % in new and

Table 2 Frequency and effect factors of acquired drug resistant TB emergence at varied time points during SCC

Variable	Month1(1) n = 35 (%)	Month2(2) n = 17 (%)	Month3-5(3) n = 10 (%)	Univariate analysis (3) vs (1 + 2)	Multivariate logistic regression (3) vs (1 + 2)	
				P value	OR(95 % CI)	*P* value
Treatment history				0.027*		
New	32 (91.4)	12 (70.6)	5 (50.0)			
Previously treated	3 (8.6)	5 (29.4)	5 (50.0)			
No. of drugs to which isolate is resistant				0.015*		
1	21(60)	6(35.3)	2(20.0)			
2	9(25.7)	3(17.6)	1(10.0)			
3	4(11.4)	5(29.5)	5(50.0)			
4	1(2.9)	3(17.6)	2(20.0)			
Drug resistance patterns				0.003*		
Non-MDR-TB	30 (85.7)	12 (70.6)	3 (30.0)		Reference	
MDR-TB	5 (14.3)	5 (29.4)	7 (70.0)		8.3(1.7–39.9)	0.008

**P* value was determined by Fisher's Exact Test

Table 3 Treatment outcomes of both pan-susceptible TB cases throughout SCC and those acquired drug resistant TB during treatment

Treatment outcomes n(%)	Pan-susceptible TB throughout[a] N = 1609	Acquired drug resistant TB N = 62		
		≦2 months	3–5 months	Total
Successfully treated	1357(84.3)	44(84.6)	2(20.0)	46(74.1)
Failed	102(6.3)	6(11.5)	7(70.0)	13(21.0)
Died	36(2.2)	0(0.0)	1(10.0)	1(1.6)
Defaulted	39(2.4)	1(1.9)	0(0.0)	1(1.6)
Not evaluated	75(4.7)	1(1.9)	0(0.0)	1(1.6)

[a]Pan-susceptible TB throughout in our study was defined as cases with TB strains susceptible to all four first-line anti-TB drugs including isoniazid(H), rifampicin (R), ethambutol (E), and streptomycin (S) both pretreatment and throughout the therapy

previously treated cases respectively are lower than that from China's national drug resistance survey in 2007 [17]. The reduction of drug resistant TB and MDR-TB prevalence in our study could be explained by two possible reasons. Firstly, given the prevalence of TB and MDR-TB not balanced which was highest in western China, 2 provinces from 4 main areas in the study may not be representative of the overall situation in China. Secondly, the drug resistant TB cases in the study were from TB Control and Prevention Centers system not TB specialized hospitals system where more previously treated cases tend to access for further second line anti-TB drugs due to MDR-TB pretreatment [18].

It is well known that previous TB treatment is a strong determinant of drug resistance [17, 19–22]. Current data suggests that previously treated cases are more likely to develop acquired drug resistance, especially MDR-TB, during therapy than that of new cases. However, it is impossible for us to determine the identified reason of acquired drug resistant TB during SCC without DNA fingerprinting analysis of resistant strains compared to that of original strains pretreatment. This represents a limitation of the study. Two reasons might contribute to the acquired drug resistant TB emergence under qualified DOT and quality-assured drug apply under China's NTP. First, the selection of resistant mutants in mixed bacterial population infected pretreatment due to killing of susceptible strains by anti-TB drugs of SCC. Second, infection of new drug resistant strains may be another explanation for the acquired drug resistant TB emergence during SCC [23].

Several researchers have reported that amplification of resistance to additional anti-TB drugs while receiving WHO recommended SCC [24]. Few data was reported on the traits of acquired drug resistant TB emergence receiving SCC with susceptible strains pretreatment. However, it is important to identify drug-resistant cases in time with standard treatment and prevent its dissemination. We found the time point of acquired drug resistant TB emergence was associated with drug resistance patterns. Cases with MDR-TB development were 8.3 times more likely to be late emergence compared to the non-MDR-TB pattern. Moreover, the cases with late emergence of acquired drug resistance are of high risk to contribute to SCC failure. In line with other studies, anti-TB drug resistance especially MDR-TB has a negative impact on treatment outcome of SCC [8, 12, 16, 25–29]. Treatment success rate of MDR-TB cases was 58 % in Peru and 60 % in Hongkong with SCC [8]. One study in rural counties of eastern China indicated that the cure rate of MDR-TB and other drug resistant TB were 58.3 % and 91.0 % of SCC [30]. Different from these studies, we excluded the drug resistant TB cases pretreatment to target on the characteristics of drug resistant TB emergence during SCC and further explore its impact on treatment outcome. Treatment success rate of cases with acquired MDR-TB was 52.9 % while 82.2 % with non-MDR-TB, a little lower than that in Peru, Hongkong and eastern China. We also analyzed treatment success rate of 3 subgroups of non-MDR-TB indicating that cases with any H resistance and E/S resistance have higher treatment success rate around 90 % while much lower treatment success rate of 61.5 % with any R resistance with SCC. Some discordant impacts of drug susceptibility patterns on treatment success are reported in the literature [25, 31, 32]. This could be explained by the different target population in our study. The greatest finding of this study is that the time point of acquired drug resistant TB emergence significantly impacted treatment outcomes with SCC. Cases with acquired drug resistant TB at 3–5 months were 25.7 times higher (OR, 25.7; 95 %CI, 4.3–153.4; $P < 0.001$) than that of cases with acquired drug resistant TB within 2 months of SCC to experience treatment failure.

Table 4 Effect of acquired drug resistant TB emergence during SCC on treatment failure

Time of acquired drug resistance emergence	Total	Treatment success n(%)	Treatment failure n(%)	Univariate analysis	
				OR(95 % CI)	*P* value
≦2 months	52	44(84.6)	6(11.5)	Reference	<0.001*
3–5 months	10	2(20.0)	7(70.0)	25.7(4.3–153.4)	

**P value was determined by Fisher's Exact Test*

Besides drug resistant TB emergence time point, many other factors including low BMI, smoking, and some behaviors such as alcohol consumption and drug abuse are also associated with poor treatment outcomes [33–36]. Diabetes and baseline disease severity of TB also have been shown to be independent risk factors for poor treatment outcomes in previous studies [18, 26, 37–39].

As reported, the use of standard first-line anti- TB treatment on cases with drug resistant TB pretreatment have greater likelihood to get relapse, treatment failure and acquired drug resistance [12, 40–42]. Therefore, pretreatment DST were carried out for individual patients and those with any drug resistance were excluded from our study and transferred to a DOTS-Plus program with the consideration of providing a more tailored regimen for optimal treatment outcomes. Without doubt, DST performed before and during SCC could provide information to recognize drug resistant TB, particularly MDR-TB. Our studies suggested DST should be taken before treatment starting and subsequent DST should be checked regarding patients who remain bacteriological positive at the month 2 or 3 and it is better to provide accordingly effective regimen rather than keeping using SCC in the setting with drug resistant TB emergence later after 2 months as these cases are more likely to fail with SCC. The pressing need to prevent MDR-TB warrants this recommendation and this approach will help decrease its transmission.

Our study has several limitations. First, we did not provide longer follow-up information to evaluate recurrence rates and correlated risk factors for long-term prognosis among successfully treated acquired drug-resistant TB cases. Second, this study was limited by the relatively small number of acquired drug resistant TB cases during SCC. A larger sample could better present the association of treatment failure and its impact factors. Hence, larger scale cohort studies are still needed to further verify the findings of our study. Third, we were not able to measure certain factors possibly related to treatment failure, for example, comorbidities including diabetes, chronic obstructive pulmonary disease, chronic hepatitis, and bacterial load. Fourth, our study is lack of DNA fingerprinting examination to differentiate the origin of acquired drug resistant TB.

Despite these limitations, to date, this might be the first study to evaluate the characteristics of acquired drug resistant TB and its effect on treatment failure with SCC. This study demonstrated later emergence of acquired drug resistant TB during SCC is the prognostic risk factor for treatment failure. Our findings may help relevant policy makers to take more consideration of treatment management on TB cases with potential failed outcomes. Early detection of treatment failure will decrease transmission and decrease likelihood of additional drug resistance acquisition, providing more probability to choose effective regimen. Administration of effective regimen may optimize cure rates and drug resistance acquisition may be avoided. Rapid, feasible and economical culture and molecular biology methods such as GeneXpert are imperative to be applied for identifying drug resistant TB in time pretreatment or during SCC. Effective and comprehensive TB control strategies with adapted DOT is needed to prevent drug resistance especially MDR-TB development. More strict infection control and health education measures should be taken to minimize the transmission of TB and drug resistant TB bacilli in public and ensure patients adherence to treatment preventing drug resistance development. In addition, we expect more robust predictors developed which could evaluate factors that could affect underlying pathological process of the disease being treated and measure the effects of interventions on clinical outcomes in multiple aspects [43].

Conclusion

Later emergence of acquired drug resistant TB during SCC is prognostic risk factor for treatment failure. Early detection of treatment failure will decrease transmission and decrease likelihood of additional drug resistance acquisition, providing more probability to choose effective regimen.

Abbreviations

DOT: directly observed treatment; DST: drug susceptibility testing; E: ethambutol; H: isoniazid; LJ: Löwenstein–Jensen; MDR-TB: multi-drug resistant TB; MTB: mycobacterium tuberculosis; NTM: non-tuberculosis mycobacterium; NTP: national TB control program; OR: odds ratios; PTB: pulmonary TB; R: rifampicin; S: streptomycin; SCC: standard short-course chemotherapy; SS: sputum smear; SS+: sputum smear-positive; TB: tuberculosis; Z: pyrazinamide.

Competing interests

The authors declared that they have no competing interests.

Authors' contributions

LL and GFZ conceived and designed the study. JTG, YM, JD, GFZ, SYT, YYF, LPM, LYZ, FYL, DYH, YLZ and LL performed the study. JTG, LL and QL analyzed the data. JTG prepared the final version of the manuscript. All authors read and approved the final manuscript.

Acknowledgments

The authors are grateful to the physicians and microbiologists of the network in all settings for their active and ongoing participation, without which this study would not have been possible.

Author details

[1]Clinical Center on Tuberculosis, Beijing Chest Hospital, Capital Medical University, Beijing Tuberculosis and Thoracic Tumor Research Institute,

Beijing, China. [2]State Key Laboratory for Molecular Virology and Genetic Engineering, Institute of Pathogen Biology, Chinese Academy of Medical Sciences & Peking Union Medical College, Beijing, China. [3]Department of TB Control, Guangzhou Chest Hospital, Guangzhou, Guangdong, China. [4]Department of TB Control, Tianjin Centers for Disease Control and Prevention, Tianjin, China. [5]Department of TB Control, Henan Center for Disease Control and Prevention, Zhengzhou, Henan, China. [6]Department of TB Control, Hebei Center for Disease Control and Prevention, Shijiazhuang, Hebei, China. [7]Department of TB Control, Guangxi Center for Disease Control and Prevention, Nanning, Guangxi, China. [8]Department of TB Control, Chongqing Anti-tuberculosis Institute, Chongqing, China. [9]Department of TB Control, Yunnan Center for Disease Control and Prevention, Kunming, Yunnan, China. [10]Department of TB Control, Shanghai Municipal Center for Disease Control and Prevention, Shanghai, China.

References

1. World Health Organization. Global tuberculosis report 2013. Geneva: WHO; 2013. WHO/HTM/TB/ 2013. 11.
2. World Health Organization. Treatment of tuberculosis guidelines. 4th ed. Geneva: WHO; 2010. WHO/HTM/STB/2009.420.
3. Fox W, Ellard GA, Mitchison DA. Studies on the treatment of tuberculosis undertaken by the British Medical Research Council tuberculosis units, 1946–1986, with relevant subsequent publications. Int J Tuberc Lung Dis. 1999;3(10):S231–79.
4. Hong Kong Chest Service; British Medical Research Council. Controlled trial of 4 three-times-weekly regimens and a daily regimen all given for 6 months for pulmonary tuberculosis. Second report: the results up to 24 months. Tubercle. 1982;63(2):89–98.
5. Service HKC, Council BMR. Controlled trial of 2, 4, and 6 months of pyrazinamide in 6-month, three-times-weekly regimens for smear-positive pulmonary of isoniazid, rifampicin, and pyrazinamide: results at 30 months. Am Rev Respir Dis. 1991;143(4):700–6.
6. Service ST, Council BMR. Clinical trial of three 6-month regimens of chemotherapy given intermittently in the continuation phase in the treatment of pulmonary tuberculosis. Am Rev Respir Dis. 1985;132(2): 374–8.
7. Council K-Z-BMR. Controlled clinical trial of levamisole in short-course chemotherapy of pulmonary tuberculosis. Am Rev Respir Dis. 1989;140(4): 990–5.
8. Espinal MA, Kim SJ, Suarez PG, Kam KM, Khomenko AG, Migiori GB, et al. Standard short-course chemotherapy for drug-resistant tuberculosis: treatment outcomes in 6 countries. JAMA. 2000;283(19):2537–45.
9. World Health Organization. Companion handbook to the WHO guidelines for the programmatic management of drug-resistant tuberculosis. Geneva: WHO; 2014. WHO/ HTM/ TB/ 2014. 11.
10. World Health Organization. Treatment of tuberculosis: guidelines for national programmes. Geneva: WHO; 2003. WHO/CDS/TB/2003.313.
11. Enarson DA, Rieder HL, Arnadottir T, Trebucq A. Management of tuberculosis: a guide for low income countries. 5th ed. Paris: International Union Against Tuberculosis and Lung Disease; 2000.
12. Mak A, Thomas A, Del Granado M, Zaleskis R, Mouzafarova N, Menzies D. Influence of multidrug resistance on tuberculosis treatment outcomes with standardized regimens. Am J Respir Crit Care Med. 2008;178(3): 306–12.
13. Ministry of Health. Guidelines for implementing the national tuberculosis control program in China. Beijing: Peking Union Medical College Press; 2008.
14. Liu Y, Jiang G, Zhao L, Fu Y, Li Y, Bi Z, et al. Drug resistance of mycobacterium tuberculosis in a nationwide epidemiological survey in China in the year of 2000. Zhonghua Jie He He Hu Xi Za Zazhi. 2002;25(4):224–7.
15. Kent P, Kubica G. Public health mycobacteriology: a guide for the level III laboratory. Atlanta: Centers for Disease Control; 1985.
16. Han T. Effectiveness of standard short-course chemotherapy for treating tuberculosis and the impact of drug resistance on its outcome. Int J Evid Based Healthc. 2006;4(2):101–17.
17. Zhao Y, Xu S, Wang L, Chin DP, Wang S, Jiang G, et al. National survey of drug-resistant tuberculosis in China. N Engl J Med. 2012;366(23):2161–70.
18. Tang S, Tan S, Yao L, Li F, Li L, Guo X, et al. Risk factors for poor treatment outcomes in patients with MDR-TB and XDR-TB in China: retrospective multi-center investigation. PLoS ONE. 2013;8(12):e82943.
19. Liu Q, Zhu L, Shao Y, Song H, Li G, Zhou Y, et al. Rates and risk factors for drug resistance tuberculosis in Northeastern China. BMC Public Health. 2013;13:1171–7.
20. Rifat M, Milton AH, Hall J, Oldmeadow C, Islam MA, Husain A, et al. Development of multidrug resistant tuberculosis in Bangladesh: a case-control study on risk factors. PLoS ONE. 2014;9(8):e105214.
21. Zhao P, Li XJ, Zhang SF, Wang XS, Liu CY. Social behaviour risk factors for drug resistant tuberculosis in mainland China: a meta-analysis. J Int Med Res. 2012;40(2):436–45.
22. Espinal MA, Laserson K, Camacho M, Fusheng Z, Kim SJ, Tlali RE, et al. Determinants of drug-resistant tuberculosis: analysis of 11 countries. Int J Tuberc Lung Dis. 2001;5(10):887–93.
23. Matthys F, Rigouts L, Sizaire V, Vezhnina N, Lecoq M, Golubeva V, et al. Outcomes after chemotherapy with WHO category Ilregimen in a population with high prevalence of drug resistant tuberculosis. PLoS ONE. 2009;4(11):e7954.
24. Seung KJ, Gelmanova IE, Perementin GG, Golubchikova VT, Pavlova VE, Sirotkina OB, et al. The effect of initial drug resistance on treatment response and acquired drug resistance during standardized short-course chemotherapy for tuberculosis. Clin Infect Dis. 2004;39(9):1321–8.
25. Anuwatnonthakate A, Whitehead SJ, Varma JK, Silachamroon U, Kasetjaroen Y, Moolphate S, et al. Effect of mycobacterial drug resistance patterns on patient' survival: a cohort study in Thailand. Glob J Health Sci. 2013;5(6):60–72.
26. Choi H, Lee M, Chen RY, Kim Y, Yoon S, Joh JS, et al. Predictors of pulmonary tuberculosis treatment outcomes in South Korea: a prospective cohort study, 2005–2012. BMC Infect Dis. 2014;14:360.
27. Chang KC, Leung CC, Yew WW, Ho SC, Tam CM. A nested case-control study on treatment-related risk factor for early relapse of tuberculosis. Am J Respir Crit Care Med. 2004;170(10):1124–30.
28. Seyoum B, Demissie M, Worku A, Bekele S, Aseffa A. Prevalence and drug resistance patterns of mycobacterium tuberculosis among new smear positive pulmonary tuberculosis patients in eastern Ethiopia. Tuberc Res Treat. 2014;2014:753492.
29. Jordan TS, Davies PD. Clinical tuberculosis and treatment outcomes. Int J Tuberc Lung Dis. 2009;14(6):683–8.
30. Hu Y, Jiang WL, Wang WB, Xu B. A-cohort study on the standard short-course chemotherapy program for drug resistant tuberculosis in the rural counties in Eastern China. Zhonghua Liu Xing Bing Xue Za Zhi. 2008;29(6): 540–4.
31. Bang D, Andersen PH, Andersen AB, Thomsen V. Isoniazid-resistant tuberculosis in Denmark: mutations, transmission and treatment outcome. J Infect. 2010;60(6):452–7.
32. Jacobson KR, Theron D, Victor TC, Streicher EM, Warren RM, Murray MB. Treatment outcomes of isoniazid-resistant tuberculosis patients, Western Cape Province, South Africa. Clin Infect Dis. 2011;53(4):369–72.
33. Reed GW, Choi H, Lee SY, Lee M, Kim Y, Park H, et al. Impact of diabetes and smoking on mortality in tuberculosis. PLoS ONE. 2013;8(2):e58044.
34. Kolappan C, Gopi PG. Tobacco smoking and pulmonary tuberculosis. Thorax. 2002;57(11):964–6.
35. Maciel EL, Brioschi AP, Peres RL, Guidoni LM, Ribeiro FK, Hadad DJ, et al. Smoking and 2-month culture conversion during anti-tuberculosis treatment. Int J Tuberc Lung Dis. 2013;17(2):225–8.
36. Franke MF, Appleton SC, Bayona J, Arteaga F, Palacios E, Llaro K, et al. Risk factors and mortality associated with default from multidrug-resistant tuberculosis treatment. Clin Infect Dis. 2008;46(12):1844–51.
37. Faustini A, Hall A, Perucci C. Risk factors for multidrug resistant tuberculosis in Europe: a systematic review. Thorax. 2006;61(2):158.
38. Kim HR, Hwang SS, Kim HJ, Lee SM, Yoo CG, Kim YW, et al. Impact of extensive drug resistance on treatment outcomes in Non-HIV-infected patients with multidrug-resistant tuberculosis. Clin Infect Dis. 2007;45(10):1290–5.
39. Dalton T, Cegielski P, Akksilp S, Asencios L, Campos Caoili J, Cho SN, et al. Prevalence of and risk factors for resistance to second-line drugs in people with multidrug-resistant tuberculosis in eight countries: a prospective cohort study. Lancet. 2012;380(9851):1406–17.
40. Lew W, Pai M, Oxlade O, Martin D, Menzies D. Initial drug resistance and tuberculosis treatment outcomes: systematic review and meta-analysis. Ann Intern Med. 2008;149(2):123–34.

41. Menzies D, Benedetti A, Paydar A, Royce S, Madhukar P, Burman W, et al. Standardized treatment of active tuberculosis in patients with previous treatment and /or with mono-resistance to isoniazid: a systematic review and meta-analysis. PLoS Med. 2009;6(9), e1000150.
42. Yoshiyama T, Yanai H, Rhiengtong D, Palittapongarnpim P, Nampaisan O, Supawitkul S, et al. Development of acquired drug resistance in recurrent tuberculosis patients with various previous treatment outcomes. Int J Tuberc Lung Dis. 2004;8(1):31–8.
43. Wallis RS, Kim P, Cole S, Hanna D, Andrade BB, Maeurer M, et al. Tuberculosis biomarkers discovery: developments, needs, and challenges. Lancet Infect Dis. 2013;13(4):362–72.

Treatment of multiple-level tracheobronchial stenosis secondary to endobronchial tuberculosis using bronchoscopic balloon dilatation with topical mitomycin-C

Mohamed Faisal[1*], Hafaruzi Harun[2], Tidi M. Hassan[1], Andrea Y. L. Ban[1], Sanjay H. Chotirmall[3] and Jamalul Azizi Abdul Rahaman[2]

Abstract

Background: Tracheobronchial stenosis is a known complication of endobronchial tuberculosis. Despite antituberculous and steroid therapy, the development of bronchial stenosis is usually irreversible and requires airway patency to be restored by either bronchoscopic or surgical interventions. We report the use of balloon dilatation and topical mitomycin-C to successful restore airway patency.

Case presentation: We present a 24-year old lady with previous pulmonary tuberculosis and laryngeal tuberculosis in 2007 and 2013 respectively who presented with worsening dyspnoea and stridor. She had total left lung collapse with stenosis of both the upper trachea and left main bronchus. She underwent successful bronchoscopic balloon and manual rigid tube dilatation with topical mitomycin-C application over the stenotic tracheal segment. A second bronchoscopic intervention was performed after 20 weeks for the left main bronchus stenosis with serial balloon dilatation and topical mitomycin-C application. These interventions led to significant clinical and radiographic improvements.

Conclusion: This case highlights that balloon dilatation and topical mitomycin-C application should be considered in selected patients with tracheobronchial stenosis following endobronchial tuberculosis, avoiding airway stenting and invasive surgical intervention.

Keywords: Case report, Endobronchial tuberculosis, Bronchoscopic intervention, Mitomycin-C

Background

Endobronchial tuberculosis (EBTB) is a consequence of pulmonary TB (PTB) extending into the endobronchial or endotracheal wall, and its incidence has been reported to range from 6 to 50 % of cases [1–3]. EBTB can affect any region of the tracheobronchial tree, with higher rates of central EBTB (proximal to lobar bronchi) compared to segmental bronchi [3]. The true incidence and complications of EBTB are unknown as routine bronchoscopy is not performed in all patients with PTB.

The clinical presentation of EBTB can be non-specific with cough, dyspnoea and stridor; however patients may also be asymptomatic. Generally, stridor occurs when the proximal airway diameter in an adult diminishes to approximately 6 mm [4]. Bronchial stenosis and strictures are sequelae of EBTB and may develop in up to 95 % of cases despite adequate antituberculous therapy [5, 6]. Eradication of the tubercle bacilli is the primary goal of treatment for EBTB, similar to standard first line treatment approaches Corticosteroids have improved clinical outcomes when used as an adjunct therapy in

* Correspondence: arabinose@hotmail.com
[1]Department of Medicine, Respiratory Unit, Universiti Kebangsaan Malaysia Medical Centre, Jalan Yaacob Latiff, Bandar Tun Razak, 56000 Cheras, Kuala Lumpur, Malaysia
Full list of author information is available at the end of the article

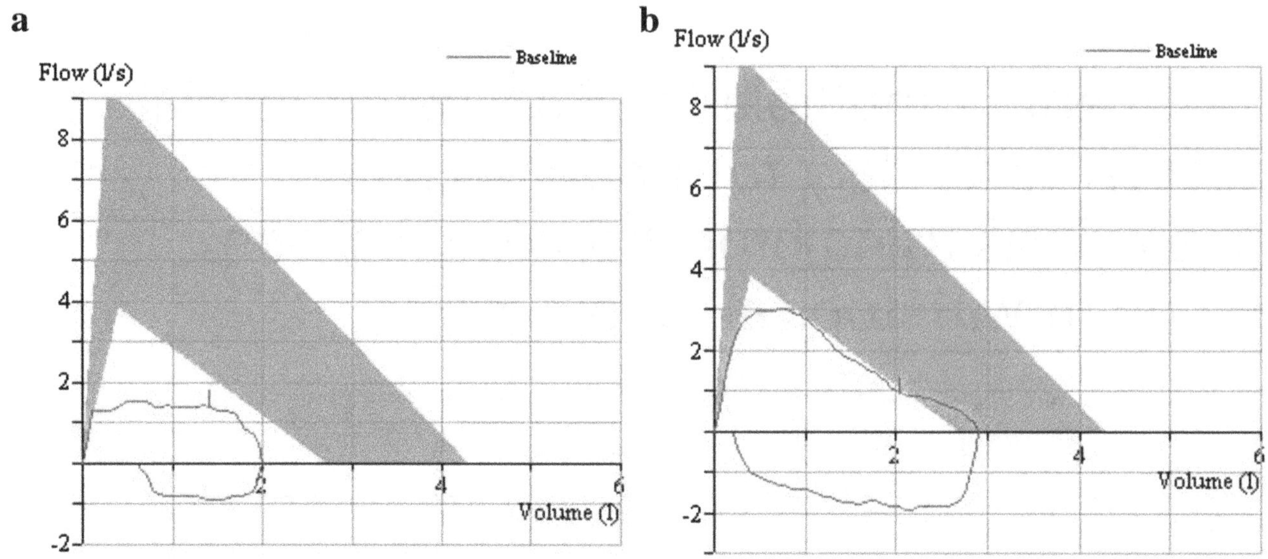

Fig. 1 FV loop pre- and post-intervention. **a** FV loop showing flattening of inspiratory and expiratory limbs indicating fixed upper airway obstruction. **b** FV loop at 36 weeks following intervention showed improvement of both the inspiratory and expiratory limbs

children, however this has not been shown to prevent bronchostenosis in adults and clinical concerns about its immunosuppressive effects in this setting persist [7].

Despite antituberculous and steroid therapy, the development of bronchial stenosis or strictures is usually irreversible and therefore requires airway patency to be restored by either bronchoscopic or surgical interventions [8]. There are various bronchoscopic techniques including laser, balloon dilatation and stent insertion [9–11]. We report a female patient who had two previous episodes of tuberculosis complicated by multi-level fibrostenotic EBTB involving the left main bronchus and the trachea. The left lung was successfully expanded following serial endoscopic treatment with subsequent use of mitomycin-C preventing the need for an airway stent.

Case presentation

A 24-year-old female presented with a 3-month history of worsening dyspnoea and stridor. She was unable to climb one flight of stairs or walk more than 50 meters on a flat surface, requiring domiciliary oxygen therapy. She also had significant loss of appetite and loss of weight. Her past medical history included acid-fast bacilli (AFB) smear-positive PTB in 2007 and laryngeal TB in 2013 for which she completed 6 months of standard anti-tuberculous (anti-TB) regimen on both occasions.

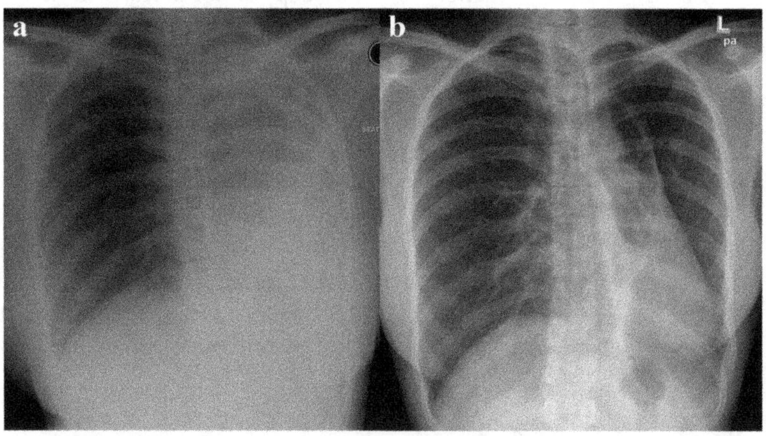

Fig. 2 Chest radiograph pre- and post-intervention. **a** Chest radiograph showed total left lung collapse. **b** Chest radiograph at 36 weeks following intervention illustrating re-expansion of the left lung field

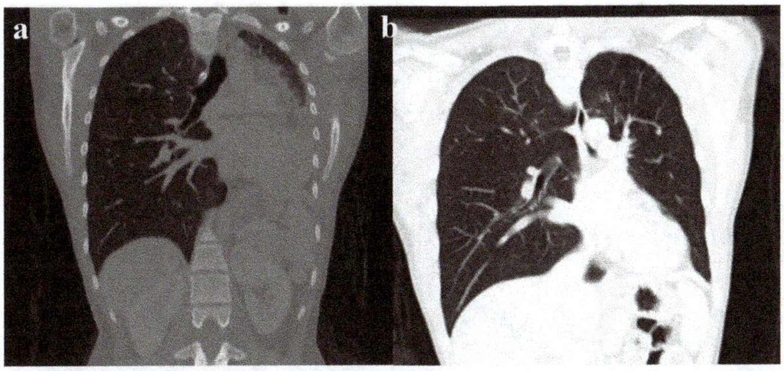

Fig. 3 CT Thorax pre- and post-intervention. **a** Coronal view CT Thorax showed total left lung collapse. **b** Coronal view CT Thorax at 36 weeks following intervention showing re-expansion of the left lung

Respiratory examination revealed tracheal deviation to the left, decreased chest expansion, reduced vocal fremitus and dullness to percussion of the left lung. Oxygen saturation on room air was 95 %.

On this presentation, sputum smear examination for AFB was negative. Flow volume (FV) loop was consistent with fixed airway obstruction (Fig. 1a) with her best functional vital capacity (FVC) of 2.03 litres (58 % predicted). Chest radiograph (Fig. 2a) and computed tomography (CT) scan of thorax (Fig. 3a) showed total left lung collapse. The CT thorax also revealed 1-cm segment of tracheal stenosis (Fig. 4a) and left main bronchus (LMB) stenosis (Fig. 5a) with mediastinal shift to the left (Fig. 6a).

Flexible bronchoscopy revealed a web-like 90 % tracheal stenosis and the visualisation of airways distally from this point was not possible. A clinical judgement of PTB reactivation was made based on the bronchoscopic appearance and the presence of constitutional symptoms. The standard four anti-TB regimen was therefore commenced. Patient was then referred to an interventional pulmonology centre for bronchoscopic intervention.

The first intervention performed was sequential tracheal dilatation to 10 mm via controlled radial expansion CRE® balloon (Boston Scientifics, USA) and mechanical dilatation with rigid bronchoscopy followed by mitomycin-C application (0.4 mg/ml) with a total contact time of 8 min. The first intervention was successful, as bronchoscopic surveillance performed at 3, 8 and 16 weeks (Fig. 7a) showed no recurrence of tracheal stenosis with a tracheal diameter of 10 mm. The airway distal to the tracheal stenosis became accessible which subsequently revealed the LMB stenosis with a pinpoint opening as previously reported in the CT thorax. We then proceeded with dilatation of the LMB.

The second intervention was performed at 20 weeks and the stenosed LMB was dilated using a CRE® balloon at 8, 9 and 10 mm. At 26 weeks, the balloon dilatation

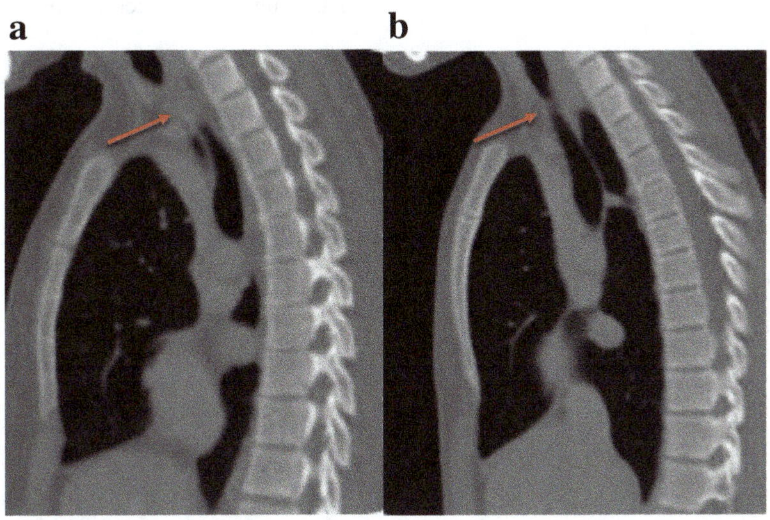

Fig. 4 CT Thorax pre- and post-intervention. **a** Lateral view of a CT Thorax showing 1 cm of total stenosis at the upper one third of trachea. **b** Lateral view CT Thorax at 36 weeks following successful intervention

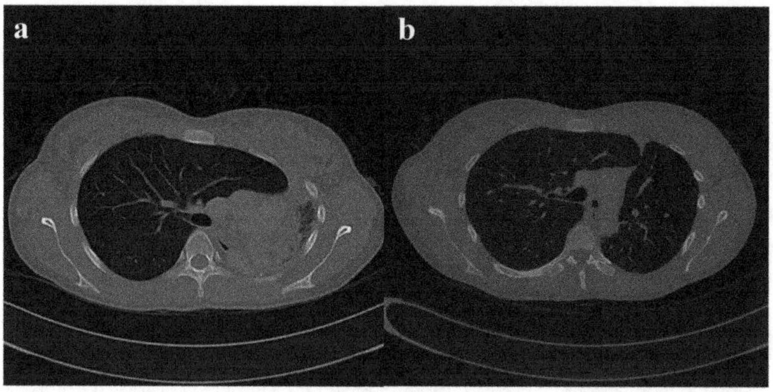

Fig. 5 Axial view of a CT Thorax at the main carina level pre- and post-intervention. **a** CT Thorax showed left main bronchus stenosis with collapsed left lung. **b** CT Thorax at 36 weeks following intervention with residual left main bronchus stenosis and re-expansion of the left lung

was repeated with the adjuvant treatment of topical mitomycin-C application (0.4 mg/mls) with the same contact time of 8 min. These procedures were repeated again at 36 weeks to re-examine further the LMB stenosis. There were no immediate complications.

Following these interventions, the patient showed significant and sustained improvement. The FV loop (Fig. 1b) illustrated improvement in both inspiratory and expiratory limbs and the FVC increased to 2.91 litres (83 % predicted). Chest radiograph (Fig. 2b) and CT thorax showed re-expansion of the left lung (Fig. 3b), tracheal patency (Fig. 4b) and the mediastinum back to its original position (Fig. 6b).

The patient is currently able to climb more than four flights of stairs and walk more than 1 kilometre without dyspnoea. She had completed a total 9 months of anti-TB therapy. She no longer requires oxygen and is back to her usual daily activities.

Discussion

We report a rare case of multiple level tracheobronchial stenoses secondary to endobronchial tuberculosis. The risk factors present include female gender, symptom duration of more than 4 weeks and multiple previous episodes of PTB; these are significant predictors of EBTB [4]. Our patient had a unique presentation in which bronchoscopy revealed tracheal fibrostenosis as well as LMB involvement. These are both rare sites for EBTB as current literature reports that the right upper lobe and right main bronchus are the most common sites [5, 6, 12].

Although presentation of EBTB varies, patients are more commonly reported to present with cough and wheezing [13]. Localised rhonchi on respiratory examination should prompt the clinician to assess for the presence of an endobronchial lesion in which correlation of loop spirometry, CT findings and bronchoscopy may aid the diagnosis. The

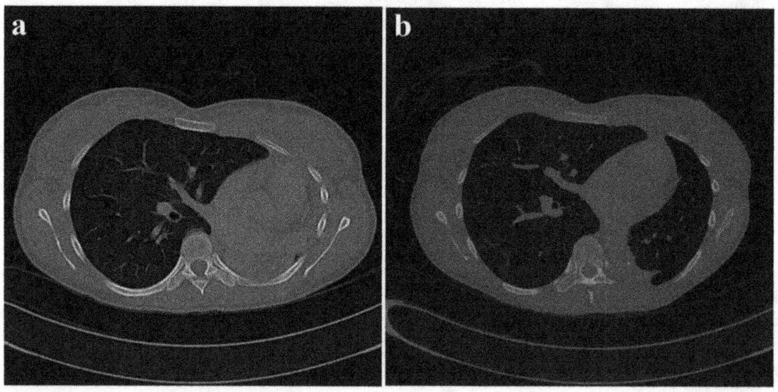

Fig. 6 Axial view CT Thorax pre- and post-intervention. **a** CT Thorax showed mediastinal shift to the left. **b** CT Thorax at 36 weeks following intervention showed normal location of the mediastinum

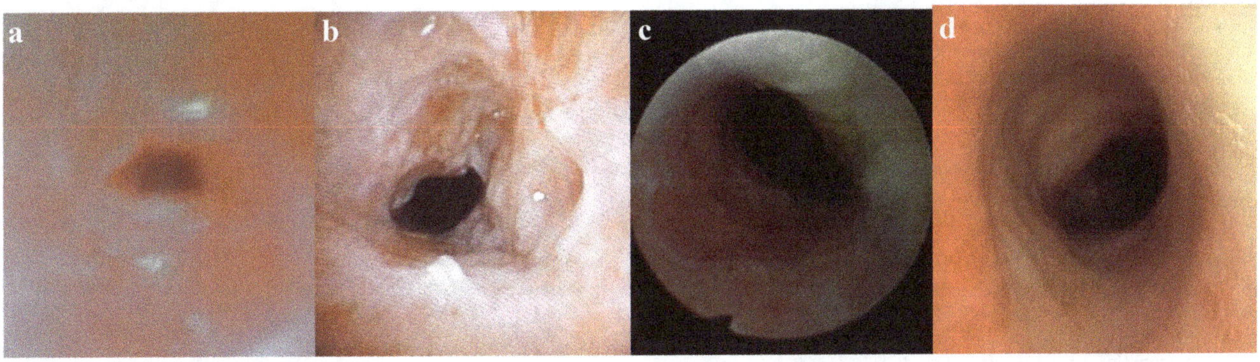

Fig. 7 Bronchoscopic findings (**a**) during presentation showing stenotic upper tracheal segment. **b** 3 weeks **c** 8 weeks and **d** 16 weeks post-intervention

involvement of the trachea was the reason for the patient's rare presentation of dyspnea and stridor.

Simple tracheal stenosis can be treated endoscopically while complex stenosis should be evaluated for surgery [8]. Various bronchoscopic techniques include laser, cryosurgery, controlled heat application, balloon dilatation and stent insertion are available [9–11]. Persistent airway stenosis following balloon dilatation has been described especially if active inflammation, calcification and malacia are evident. Patients who require more than one session of balloon dilatation may need more definitive treatment such as stenting or ablative procedures [10].

As there was no bronchomalacia evident in our patient, an airway stent was not inserted into the LMB to avoid long-term complications associated with this foreign device. This option would be considered however, if the LMB stenosis re-occurred following topical mitomycin-C application.

The use of mitomycin-C as an adjunct therapy to bronchoscopic procedures in our case was influenced by reports of successful treatment in patients with tracheal stenosis secondary to intubation [14, 15]. There are no controlled studies and very few case reports in the literature describing the utility of mitomycin-C for tracheabronchial stenosis secondary to EBTB. Two previous reports had shown the success of topical mitomycin-C for obstructive granuloma and a 90 % occlusion of the upper trachea secondary to EBTB [16, 17]. Mitomycin-C is an antineoplastic antibiotic agent that inhibits fibroblast proliferation and modulates wound healing and scarring. Due to its teratogenic effects, use in a women of childbearing age woman should be coupled with contraceptive use.

This patient was successfully managed with clinical (symptoms and FV loop) and radiological improvements at short-term follow-up, despite having residual LMB stenosis. As there was no bronchomalacia, an airway stent was not inserted to the LMB.

Conclusion

This case report contributes to the current literature and evidence base that balloon dilatation and topical mitomycin-C application should be considered in selected patients with tracheobronchial stenosis post EBTB. Importantly, this technique might obviate the need for airway stenting and further invasive surgical intervention.

Consent

Written informed consent was obtained from the patient for publication of this case report.

Abbreviations

EBTB: endobronchial tuberculosis; PTB: pulmonary tuberculosis; LMB: left main bronchus; AFB: acid fast bacilli; FV: flow volume; FVC: functional vital capacity; CT: computed tomography.

Competing interests

The authors declare that they have no competing interests.

Authors' contributions

MFAH is the main author and corresponding author for this article. HH was involved in literature review. TMH, AYLB SHC and JAR edited and approved the final version of the case report. All authors approved the final manuscript as submitted.

Acknowledgements

We would like to acknowledge Prof Dato Dr. Raymond Azman Ali, Dean of the Medical Faculty and the Director of the Universiti Kebangsaan Malaysia Medical Centre.

Author details

[1]Department of Medicine, Respiratory Unit, Universiti Kebangsaan Malaysia Medical Centre, Jalan Yaacob Latiff, Bandar Tun Razak, 56000 Cheras, Kuala Lumpur, Malaysia. [2]Respiratory Unit, Serdang Hospital, Jalan Puchong, 43000 Kajang, Selangor Darul Ehsan, Malaysia. [3]Lee Kong Chian School of Medicine, Nanyang Technological University, Singapore, Singapore.

References

1. An JY, Lee JE, Park HW, Lee JH, Yang SA, Jung SS, et al. Clinical and bronchoscopic features in endobronchial tuberculosis. Tuberc Respir Dis. 2006;60:532–9.
2. Kurasawa T, Kuze F, Kawai M, Amitani R, Murayama T, Tanaka E, et al. Diagnosis and management of endobronchial tuberculosis. Intern Med. 1992;31:593–8.
3. Kashyap S, Solanki A. Challenges in endobronchial tuberculosis: from diagnosis to management. Pulm Med. 2014;2014:594806.
4. Jung S-S, Park H-S, Kim J-O, Kim S-Y. Incidence and clinical predictors of endobronchial tuberculosis in patients with pulmonary tuberculosis. Respirology (Carlton, Vic). 2015;20(3):488–95. doi:10.1111/resp.12474.
5. Puchalski J, Musani AI. Tracheobronchial Stenosis : causes and advances in medicine. Clin Chest Med. 2013;34(3):557–67.
6. Lee JH, Park SS, Lee DH, et al. Endobronchial tuberculosis: clinical and bronchoscopic feature in 121 cases. Chest. 1992;102(4):990–3.
7. Park IW, Choi BW, Hue SH. Prospective study of corticosteroid as an adjunct in the treatment of endobronchial tuberculosis in adults. Respirology. 1997; 2(4):275–81.
8. Galluccio G, Lucantoni G, Battistoni P, Paone G, Batzella S, Lucifora V, et al. Interventional endoscopy in the management of benign tracheal stenoses: definitive treatment at long-term follow-up. Eur J Cardiothorac Surg. 2009; 35(3):429–34.
9. Puchalski J, Musani AI. Tracheobronchial stenosis: causes and advances in management. Clin Chest Med. 2013;34(3):557–67.
10. Shitrit D, Kuchuk M, Zismanov V, Rahman NA, Amital A, Kramer MR. Bronchoscopic balloon dilatation of tracheobronchial stenosis: long-term follow-up. Eur J Cardiothorac Surg. 2010;38(2):198–202.
11. Bolliger CT, Sutedja TG, Strausz J, Freitag L. Therapeutic bronchoscopy with immediate effect: laser, electrocautery, argon plasma coagulation and stents. Eur Respir J. 2006;27(6):1258–71.
12. Aneja A, Krishnaswamy UM, Thyagaraj V, et al. Endobronchial Tuberculosis: Two Case Reports and Review of the the literature. Case Reports Pulmonol. 2014;2014:283972. http://www.ncbi.nlm.nih.gov/pubmed/?term=Aneja+A%2C+Krishnaswamy+UM%2C+Thyagaraj+V%2C+et+al.+Endobronchial+Tuberculosis%3A+Two+Case+Reports+and+Review+of+the+the+literature.+Case+Reports+Pulmonol.+2014%3B2014
13. Cordovilla R, Jiménez-Massa A. Endobronchial tuberculosis: a case report and review of the literature. J Bronchology Interv Pulmonol. 2009;16(2):121–3. doi:10.1097/LBR.0b013e3181a13768.
14. Viveiros F, Gomes J, Oliveira A, Neves S, Almeida J, Moura e Sá J. Topical application of mitomycin-C as an adjuvant treatment to bronchoscopic procedures in post-intubation tracheal stenosis. Rev Port Pneumol. 2013; 19(6):276–80.
15. Wong JL, Tie ST, Samril B, Lum CL, Rahman MRA, Rahman JAA. Successful treatment of tracheal stenosis by rigid bronchoscopy and topical mitomycin C: a case report. Cases J. 2010;3:2. doi:10.1186/1757-1626-3-2.
16. Penafiel A, Lee P, Hsu A, Eng P. Topical mitomycin-C for obstructing endobronchial granuloma. Ann Thorac Surg. 2006;82(3):e22–3.
17. Cary C, Jhaji M, Cinicola J, Evans R, Cheriyath P, Gorrepati VS. A rare case of fibrostenotic endobronchial tuberculosis of trachea. Ann Med Surg(Lond). 2015;4(4):479–82.

Lung functions among patients with pulmonary tuberculosis in Dar es Salaam

Mohamed Manji[1*], Grace Shayo[1], Simon Mamuya[2], Rose Mpembeni[3], Ahmed Jusabani[4] and Ferdinand Mugusi[1]

Abstract

Background: Approximately 40–60 % of patients remain sufferers of sequela of obstructive, restrictive or mixed patterns of lung disease despite treatment for pulmonary tuberculosis (PTB). The prevalence of these abnormalities in Tanzania remains unknown.

Methods: A descriptive cross-sectional study was carried out among 501 patients with PTB who had completed at least 20 weeks of treatment. These underwent spirometry and their lung functions were classified as normal or abnormal (obstructive, restrictive or mixed). Logistic regression models were used to explore factors associated with abnormal lung functions.

Results: Abnormal lung functions were present in 371 (74 %) patients. There were 210 (42 %) patients with obstructive, 65 (13 %) patients with restrictive and 96 (19 %) patients with mixed patterns respectively. Significant factors associated with abnormal lung functions included recurrent PTB (Adj OR 2.8, CI 1.274 - 6.106), Human Immunodeficiency Virus (HIV) negative status (Adj OR 1.7, CI 1.055 - 2.583), age more than 40 years (Adj OR 1.7, CI 1.080 - 2.804) and male sex (Adj OR 1.7, CI 1.123 - 2.614).

Conclusion: The prevalence of abnormal lung functions is high and it is associated with male sex, age older than 40 years, recurrent PTB and HIV negative status.

Keywords: Spirometry, TB sequlae, Obstruction, Restriction

Background

Tuberculosis (TB) is among the top infectious causes of death worldwide [1]. Patients with treated TB may remain lifelong sufferers of disabling sequelae of the disease which subsequently impair their quality of life [2]. Many studies have shown that partially treated pulmonary tuberculosis can result in airflow obstruction [3–7]. Studies with longer follow-up have revealed that a large percentage of patients with treated pulmonary tuberculosis show signs of permanent airflow obstruction or restrictive impairment [8–11]. Post tuberculosis pulmonary impairment, therefore has emerged as a distinct clinical entity [12].

With 170,000 reported TB cases in the year 2014, Tanzania ranked the 18th among the 22 WHO high TB burdened countries in the world [13]. The prevalence of bacteriologically confirmed TB in Tanzania was 295 per 100,000 adults in the year 2010 [14]. Despite this high burden of TB, there is no formal evidence of post tuberculous pulmonary abnormalities from Tanzania. Factors associated with these complications or factors that may predict long term residual abnormalities in such patients has also been poorly addressed. This study was aimed at determining the prevalence and the factors associated with these abnormalities.

Methods

Study design and population

We conducted a health facility-based descriptive cross sectional study between July and December 2014 in Temeke municipality, the largest of three municipalities

* Correspondence: mohd_manji@hotmail.com
[1]Department of Internal Medicine, Muhimbili University of Health and Allied Sciences (MUHAS), P.O. Box 65001, Dar es Salaam, Tanzania
Full list of author information is available at the end of the article

in Dar es Salaam city. Two busy TB clinics in this municipality, the Temeke municipal hospital and the Mbagala rangi tatu health centre, were chosen. The target population was patients with pulmonary tuberculosis (PTB), both sputum smear positive and smear negative TB regardless of their HIV status. Eligible patients were aged 18 years or older, had attended the clinic and completed at least 20 of the 24 weeks of anti TB treatment. Prior research has shown that peak lung function loss in patients with TB occurs within 6 months of diagnosis [8]. We enrolled patients who had completed 20 of the 24 weeks of anti TB treatment (i.e. 5 months), since most of these subjects would have achieved a microbiological cure, and that such timing would enable identification of sequel of disease without considering active disease. This timing was also reasonable in allowing data collection for a maximal number of subjects given that patients are discharged from the clinic at 6 months after which it would be difficult to access them. Participants were enrolled in a consecutive manner. The exclusion criteria were participants who had preexisting asthma or COPD, paraplegia, heart failure, stroke, extra pulmonary tuberculosis, contraindications to spirometry (e.g. recent surgery, myocardial infarction, vertigo, vomiting), spine deformities (kyphosis, scoliosis), chest deformities, and pregnancy.

A total of 501 participants were enrolled in the study (Fig. 1). All participants gave consent for participation. Ethical clearance for conducting the study was obtained from the Muhimbili University of Health and Allied Sciences (MUHAS) institutional review board.

Data collection

Evaluations were incorporated into routine TB clinic visits. A clinical record form (CRF) was used for data collection. A thorough history and physical examination was performed for each participant and recorded on the CRF. The modified Medical research council dyspnea scale was used to assess their functional status [15]. The patients TB02 treatment card was used to obtain other relevant information including duration on anti TB treatment, serostatus for HIV and whether the PTB was smear negative or positive for acid fast bacilli (AFB) at diagnosis. This information was filled in the CRF. A digital weighing scale (OMRON) was used to measure body weight in kilograms (kg). Weight was measured in erect position wearing only light clothing and without shoes. Height was measured in centimeters using meter rods. Waist circumference was measured using a tape measure midway between the lower rib cage margin and the anterior superior iliac spine. Mid upper arm circumference (MUAC) was measured with a tape measure midway between the tip of the shoulder (the acromion) and the tip of the elbow (olecranon process).

This was followed by spirometry by means of the ndd EasyOne™ spirometer (manufactured by ndd Medizintechnik (Switzerland)). The EasyOne™ spirometer complies with the 2005 ATS/ERS spirometry standards. The spirometer

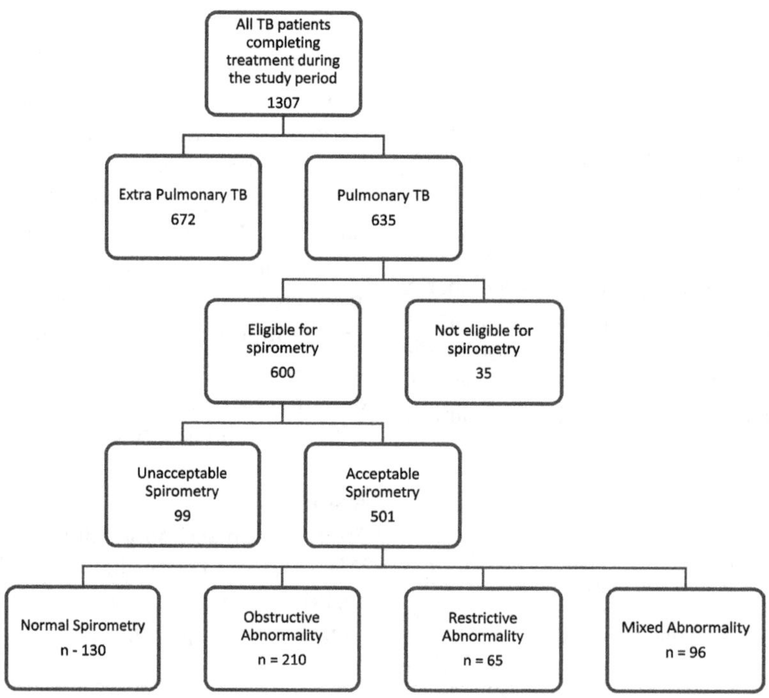

Fig. 1 Flow diagram for recruitment into the study

does not need daily calibration [16–18]. It has been used in several studies before both locally and internationally [19–22]. Thus pre testing of the tool was not performed. The device is portable and not affected by environmental conditions. Precautionary measures in using the spirometer included the use of disposable mouthpiece (spirette) per participant to avoid cross contamination. Spirometry was performed in a vacant area with open sunlight and face masks and gloves were used to protect the investigator/assistants.

The forced expiratory maneuvers, the within and between maneuver evaluation for acceptability as well as test result selection were in accordance with the ATS/ERS guidelines [23]. Spirometry was performed in the standing position. The forced expiratory maneuvers were explained in local language by trained assistants (3 doctors and 1 nurse) to the participants before they underwent spirometry. Spirometry was performed without a nose clip owing to the results of a pilot study among 25 patients prior to this research that observed that patients were uncomfortable when nose clips were used during spirometry. Furthermore, a nose clip is recommended, but not a compulsory requirement for spirometry [23] and other studies have not shown significant differences in results among users and non-users of nose clips [24, 25]. Disposable mouthpieces (spirettes) were discarded after individual use. Parameters measured included forced expiratory volume in one second (FEV1) and the forced vital capacity (FVC). The highest FEV1 and FVC from three acceptable maneuvers were used for further comparison and analysis. The FEV1: FVC% was then calculated from these.

Data analysis

The lung functions were categorized into normal, obstruction, restriction and mixed patterns of lung disease according to the algorithm from the National Lung Health Education Program (NLHEP) [26].

The predicted values were derived from regression equations for healthy Tanzanian adults [22]. To compare the observed and predicted lung functions, we used the percentage of predicted values (the ratio of observed to predicted values times 100) for FVC (FVC %) and FEV1 (FEV1%). Severity for obstruction and restriction were graded according to Global Initiative for Chronic Obstructive Lung Disease (GOLD) [27] and the American Thoracic Society/European Respiratory Society (ATS/ERS) task force recommendations [28] respectively.

Data was analyzed using SPSS (version 15.0) statistical software. Means ± standard deviation (SD) and proportions were calculated for continuous and categorical data respectively. Median and interquartile range (IQR) was used for non-normally distributed numerical data. The Chi square test and t-test were used to determine associations between variables. If more than 20 % of the cells had an expected frequency of <5, Fischer's exact test was used instead.

Logistic regression was done to determine predictors of abnormal lung function. The dependent variable was lung function which was reported as normal or abnormal. The independent variables that were run in multivariate models were those that had a p value of < 0.2 in univariate analysis. These included age, sex, level of education, Modified Medical Research Council Dyspnea Score (MMRC Score), smoking status, sputum smear status at diagnosis (positive or negative), TB episode number (first episode or recurrent), duration from symptoms to diagnosis of TB, HIV serostatus (positive or negative) and CD4 counts. Statistically significance was achieved when $p < 0.05$.

Results

Study population

There were a total of 501 participants in the study (Fig. 1). Males constituted 60.5 % (303/501) of the study participants. More than 60 % (326/501) of participants were aged 40 years or younger. Majority were married or cohabiting (52.5 %) (263/501), had attained primary level education (65.9 %) (330/501) and were domestic workers (34.1 %) (171/501). Approximately 29.3 % (147/501) were ever smokers with a median of 2.5 pack years. With respect to their clinical characteristics, approximately 54.3 % (272/501) had smear positive pulmonary TB and 90.1 % (245/272) of these had converted to smear negative at 2 months of treatment. Majority (85 %) (426/501) of the patients had presented with a first episode of TB. The median time from first symptom presentation to TB diagnosis was 30 days. Approximately 30 % (152/501) of the population was HIV co-infected. Approximately 46 % (70/152) of the patients had CD4+ cell count <200cells/μL. Majority (81 %) (407/501) had good functional scores (1 to 2) for dyspnea as reported by the MMRC score (Table 1). The mean FEV1, FVC and FEV1: FVC% were 1.83 ± 0.75, 2.95 ± 1.11 and 63.02 ± 17.99 respectively.

Prevalence and severity of abnormal lung functions

The overall prevalence of lung function abnormalities was 74 % (371/501). Majority was due to obstruction (42 %) (210/501) followed by mixed (19 %) (96/501) and restrictive (13 %) (65/501) abnormalities. Approximately 73 % (48/65) of patients with restrictive dysfunction has mild to moderate severity. Approximately 79 % (166/210) of patients with obstructive dysfunction had mild to moderate severity (Fig. 2).

Factors associated with abnormal lung functions

Patients who were aged 40 years or younger were less likely to present with abnormal lung functions (69.9 %)

Table 1 Sociodemographic and clinical characteristics of participants

Characteristics (N = 501)	Frequency	Percent (%)
Age Groups (years)		
18–30	166	33.1
31–40	160	31.9
41–50	96	19.2
51–60	42	8.4
>60	37	7.4
Sex		
Male	303	60.5
Female	198	39.5
Marital Status		
Single	169	33.7
Married/Cohabiting	263	52.5
Divorced/Widowed	69	13.8
Education		
No Formal	62	12.4
Primary	330	65.9
Secondary	84	16.8
Post-Secondary	25	5.0
Occupation		
Agriculture	19	3.8
Domestic	171	34.1
Industrial	64	12.8
Office	119	23.8
Other	128	25.5
MMRC score		
1–2	407	81.2
3–5	94	18.8
Cigarette smoking		
Never smokers	354	70.7
Ever Smokers	147	29.3
Smoking Pack Years (Median (IQR))	2.5 (5.3)	
Smear for Acid Fast Bacilli		
Positive	272	54.3
Negative	229	45.7
Time to Negative Sputum Conversion (months)(n=272)		
Smear Negative at 2 Months	245	90.1
Smear Positive at 2 Months	27	9.9
TB Episode		
First	426	85.0
Recurrent	75	15.0

Table 1 Sociodemographic and clinical characteristics of participants *(Continued)*

Duration to TB diagnosis (months)		
≤1 Month	275	54.9
>1 Month	226	45.1
HIV Status		
Positive	152	30.3
Negative	349	69.7
CD4 count (n = 152)		
<200	70	46.2
200–350	50	33.0
>350	32	20.9

MMRC Score Modified Medical Research Council Dyspnea Score, *BMI* Body Mass Index, *IQR* Interquartile range

compared to those older than 40 years (81.7 %), $p = 0.004$. Abnormal lung function was more prevalent among males (78.9 %) than among females (66.7 %) ($p = 0.002$). However more males developed restrictive ($p = 0.034$) and mixed ($p < 0.001$) abnormalities while more females developed obstruction ($p < 0.001$) (Table 2). As far as clinical characteristics are concerned, higher MMRC scores were significantly associated with any abnormality (84 % for scores 3–5 vs 71.7 % for score 1–2) ($p = 0.013$). A similar finding was seen for mixed abnormalities ($p = 0.009$). However lower scores were significantly more associated with obstruction ($p = 0.04$). Patients who had more than 5 pack years of smoking had significantly higher obstructive abnormalities than those who had smoked for less than 5 pack years (73.3 % vs. 41.9 %) ($p = 0.005$). Patients with recurrent TB were also more likely to have abnormal lung functions compared to those with a first episode of TB (89.3 % vs 71.4 %) ($p = 0.001$). Also HIV negative patients constituted significantly greater percentage of individuals with abnormal lung functions (77.1 %) compared to HIV infected patients (67.1 %) ($p = 0.019$). This relationship was also true for mixed lung disease ($p = 0.012$). However obstructive dysfunction was more common in HIV infected (66.7 %) than in HIV negative patients (52.4 %) ($p = 0.014$) (Table 3).

In multivariate analysis significant predictors for any abnormality were age > 40 years (Adj OR 1.740, CI 1.080 - 2.804), male sex (Adj OR 1.713, CI 1.123 - 2.614), TB recurence (Adj OR 2.789, CI 1.274 - 6.106) and HIV negative status (Adj OR 1.651, CI 1.055 - 2.583) (Table 4).

Discussion

The prevalence of abnormal lung functions of any type in this study was 74 % and the prevalence of individual patterns of impairment was 42, 13 and 19 % for obstructive, restrictive and mixed patterns of lung disease respectively. These findings indicate a huge burden of

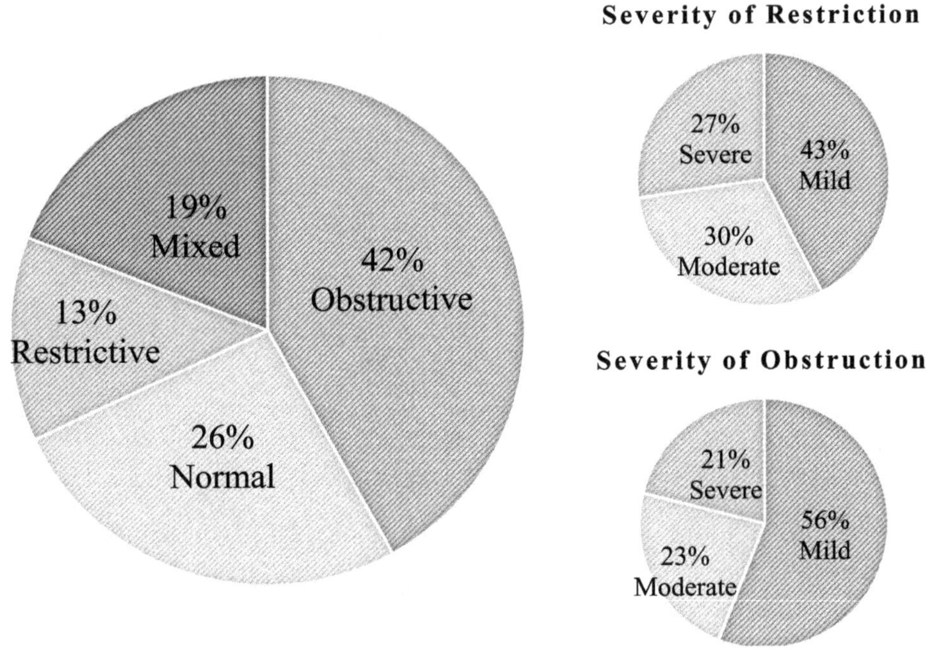

Fig. 2 Prevalence and severity of abnormal lung functions. Pie charts showing the prevalence of the different types of lung function abnormalities (large pie chart, $N = 501$). The smaller pie charts show the severity of patients who had restrictive (small upper, $n = 65$) and obstructive abnormalities (small lower, $n = 210$)

Table 2 Sociodemographic factors associated with abnormal lung functions

Characteristics	Total	Any Abnormality		*P*	Obstructive		*P*	Restrictive		*P*	Mixed		*P*
Age groups (number, %)													
≤40 years	326	228	69.9 %	0.004*	121	53.1 %	0.132*	46	20.2 %	0.163*	61	26.8 %	0.715*
>40 years	175	143	81.7 %		88	61.5 %		20	14.0 %		35	24.5 %	
Sex (number, %)													
Males	303	239	78.9 %	0.003*	112	46.9 %	<0.001*	50	20.9 %	0.034*	77	32.2 %	<0.001*
Female	198	132	66.7 %		97	73.5 %		16	12.1 %		19	14.4 %	
Marital Status (number, %)													
Single	169	120	71.0 %	0.432	64	53.3 %	0.679	23	19.2 %	0.723	33	27.5 %	0.874
Married/Cohabiting	263	201	76.4 %		115	57.2 %		36	17.9 %		50	24.9 %	
Divorced/W idowed	69	50	72.5 %		30	60.0 %		7	14.0 %		13	26.0 %	
Education (number, %)													
No Formal Education	62	47	75.8 %	0.080	29	61.7 %	0.063	7	14.9 %	0.912	11	23.4 %	0.036
Primary Education	330	249	75.5 %		148	59.4 %		45	18.1 %		56	22.5 %	
Secondary Education	84	62	73.8 %		26	41.9 %		11	17.7 %		25	40.3 %	
Post-Secondary Education	25	13	52.0 %		6	46.2 %		3	23.1 %		4	30.8 %	
Occupation (number, %)													
Agriculture	19	18	94.7 %	0.05	11	61.1 %	0.005	1	5.6 %	0.236	6	33.3 %	0.013
Domestic	171	119	69.6 %		81	68.1 %		19	16.0 %		19	16.0 %	
Industrial	64	44	68.8 %		16	36.4 %		10	22.7 %		18	40.9 %	
Office	119	96	80.7 %		53	55.2 %		14	14.6 %		29	30.2 %	
Other	128	94	73.4 %		48	51.1 %		22	23.4 %		24	25.5 %	

* fishers exact

Table 3 Clinical factors associated with abnormal lung functions

Characteristics	Total	Any Abnormality		*P*	Obstructive		*P*	Restrictive		*P*	Mixed		*P*
MMRC score (number, %)													
1–2	407	292	71.7 %	0.013*	173	59.2 %	0.04*	53	18.2 %	0.868*	66	22.6 %	0.00
3–5	94	79	84 %		36	45.6 %		13	16.5 %		30	38.0 %	9*
Cigarette smoking (number, %)													
Never smokers	354	255	72.0 %	0.118*	151	59.2 %	0.114*	49	19.2 %	0.309*	55	21.6 %	0.00
Ever Smokers	147	116	78.9 %		58	50.0 %		17	14.7 %		41	35.3 %	7*
Smoking Pack Years (number, %) (n=147)													
≤5	107	86	80.4 %	0.5*	36	41.9 %	0.005*	16	18.6 %	0.068*	34	39.5 %	0.12
>5	40	30	75.0 %		22	73.3 %		1	3.3 %		7	23.3 %	6*
Smear for Acid Fast Bacilli (number, %)													
Smear Positive	272	198	72.8 %	0.54*	110	55.6 %	0.754*	31	15.7 %	0.278*	57	28.8 %	0.19
Smear Negative	229	173	75.5 %		99	57.2 %		35	20.2 %		39	22.5 %	2*
Time to Negative Sputum Conversion (number, %)													
Smear Positive at 2 Months	27	19	70.4 %	0.82*	11	57.9 %	1.0*	3	15.8 %	1.0*		26.3 %	1.0*
Smear Negative at 2 Months	245	179	73.1 %		99	55.3 %		28	15.6 %			29.1 %	
TB Episode Number (number, %)													
First	426	304	71.4 %	0.001*	171	56.3 %	1.0*	59	19.4 %	0.111*	74	24.3 %	0.16
Recurrent	75	67	89.3 %		38	56.7 %		7	10.4 %		22	32.8 %	6*
Duration to TB diagnosis (mo) (number, %)													
≤1 Month	275	207	75.3	0.539*	117	56.5 %	1.0*	40	19.3 %	0.414*	50	24.2 %	0.40
>1 Month	226	164	72.6		92	56.1 %		26	15.9 %		46	28.0 %	6*
HIV Status (number, %)													
HIV Positive	152	102	67.1 %	0.026*	68	66.7 %	0.014*	17	16.7 %	0.764*	17	16.7 %	0.01
HIV Negative	349	269	77.1 %		141	52.4 %		49	18.2 %		79	29.4 %	2*
CD4 count (Median (IQR))		202.50 (210)				192.5 (225)			200 (156)			260(167)	

* fishers exact, *MMRC score* Modified Medical Research Council Dyspnea score, *BMI* Body Mass Index, *IQR* Interquartile range

Table 4 Logistic regression analysis of sociodemographic and clinical parameters

Characteristic (n = 501)	Comparison	OR	95 % CI	*P*	Adj OR	95 % CI	*P*
Age >40 years	≤40 years	1.921	1.224–3.014	0.005	1.740	1.080–2.804	0.023
Male	Female	1.867	1.24 -2.797	0.002	1.713	1.123–2.614	0.013
Any Formal Education	No Formal	0.899	0.944–8.087	0.736	-	-	-
MMRC score 3–5	MMRC ≤2	2.074	1.147 -3.752	0.016	1.786	0.962–3.316	0.066
Ever Smoker	Never smoker	1.453	0.918–2.300	0.111	-	-	-
Smear Positive TB	Smear Negative	0.866	0.579–1.296	0.484	-	-	-
Smear Positive at 2 months	Smear negative at 2 months	0.876	.366–2.096	0.766	-	-	-
TB recurrence (Any recurrence)	1st episode	3.361	1.568–7.206	0.002	2.789	1.274–6.106	0.010
Duration to Diagnosis >1 month	≤1 months	0.869	0.582–1.297	0.492	-	-	-
HIV Negative	HIV Positive	1.648	1.082–2.510	0.020	1.651	1.055–2.583	0.028
CD4 count >350	<350	0.362	0.124–1.059	0.064	-	-	-

MMRC Score Modified Medical Research Council Dyspnea Score, *Adj* Adjusted

post treatment pulmonary function abnormalities in patients with pulmonary tuberculosis. It was also found that majority of patients with obstructive and restrictive abnormalities had mild to moderate severity. The findings of the present study are similar to those done elsewhere. For instance, in a study by Pasipanodya et al. (2007) in the USA, the prevalence of abnormal lung function of any type was 59 % and the prevalence of individual subtypes of impairment for obstructive, restrictive and mixed were 15, 31 and 13 % respectively [29]. While the prevalence of pulmonary impairment was higher in our study, it suffices to note that pulmonary functions are abnormal in the majority of patients upon completion of chemotherapy. This has been a consistent finding in studies done in other parts of the world [6, 9, 30].

A striking difference can be observed in the proportion of obstructive lung disease between the Pasipanodya study and the present study. The present study revealed a markedly higher proportion of patients who had obstructive lung disease (42 % vs 15 %). In some studies pulmonary infections (like childhood pneumonias, pneumocystis jirovecii, pertussis and measles) contribute up to a third of cases of obstructive airway disease [31–36]. Childhood pneumonias and measles are common in Tanzania. Other studies have found that the odds of developing obstructive disease may be even higher with TB than with smoking [19, 37, 38]. Poor socioeconomic status [39] and low birth weights [40] have also been linked with the development of obstructive impairments both of which are applicable to the Tanzanian setup. For example, 9.7 % of the Tanzanian population are below the food and poverty line [41] and 13 % of Tanzanian newborns are low birth weight [42]. Therefore, a predominance of obstructive sequelae after TB may not be so surprising in this part of the world.

We have shown that patients who presented with recurrent tuberculosis had a 2.8 fold higher likelihood of developing abnormal lung functions at the end of treatment than those with a first episode of TB. Considering that Tanzania is among the high burden countries, the burden of recurrent TB is also high. Studies in other parts of the world have also shown recurrent tuberculosis to be associated with adverse spirometric outcomes. In a population wide Korean study, Lee and colleagues showed that previous TB predicted almost 3 fold higher chance of developing obstructive lung disease [43]. Another South African study of approximately 27,000 miners showed incremental rise in lung function abnormalities with the number of TB episodes (18, 27 and 35 % among first, second and third time sufferers of TB respectively) [8].

In the present study, it was found that HIV negative individuals had a 1.7 fold more likelihood of presenting with any form of lung impairment than were HIV infected patients. These findings can be explained by the fact that the mechanisms by which tuberculosis damages the lung depend extensively on cell mediated immune processes [44]. Many typical tuberculous changes may not be found in individuals who are HIV infected due to defects in their cell mediated immunity. These have been shown in studies comparing radiographic presentations of TB among HIV positive and negative individuals [45]. For example, HIV infected patients may not have typical upper lobe involvement or form typical cavities which confer significant structural alteration to the lung morphology [45]. As a result, it is likely that HIV positive patients end up with less spirometric abnormalities for lack of gross functional alteration due to relatively preserved lung parenchyma unlike their HIV negative counterparts.

The findings of this study warrant an active search among TB patients for these abnormalities. According to these results, practitioners in TB clinics can predict patients who may be at a higher risk for these impairments. Patients with recurrent tuberculosis, patients who are HIV negative, male patients and patients older than 40 years run the highest risk of these abnormalities. The tools to detect such abnormalities are fairly simple, rapid and not overly costly and there should not be a reason to miss this population who may require assistance beyond standard anti tuberculous therapy.

One may argue that these results actually make a case for an even more intensified and rapid detection of TB patients such that earlier treatment may offset the development of these sequelae. While this concept looks plausible in theory, the findings of the present study suggest otherwise. In a subgroup analysis of duration of symptoms to TB diagnosis and lung function, there was no significant difference among patients who were diagnosed and started treatment within 1 month against those who were diagnosed and started treatment later (Table 3). This relationship was also non-significant for obstructive, restrictive and mixed disease suggesting that simply having tuberculosis imparts a risk irrespective of how soon treatment is started.

The prevalence of these abnormalities among patients completing anti TB is alarmingly high. The morbidity and impairment in quality of life conferred by these sequelae is likely to be similarly high. While such data on long term morbidity is missing in Tanzania, literature from other parts of the world suggests that these sequelae confer a significant impact on everyday functioning and quality of life [2, 46–48]. In fact, some studies suggest greater morbidities from the sequelae rather than from the disease itself [2, 48]. These non-communicable post tuberculous sequelae bring to light the often overlooked processes by which TB impacts quality of life. Tuberculosis therefore imposes an infectious and non-infectious burden to the healthcare infrastructure. While the infectious and microbiologic domain has received much attention in TB treatment, a lot is still left to be desired in the non-infectious sequela.

Conclusions

The magnitude of residual lung function abnormalities among patient with tuberculosis is high despite successful administration of anti TB medications. Important factors associated with abnormal lung functions include recurrent TB, HIV negative status, age more than 40 years and male sex. The findings of this study warrant an active search of these impairments among TB patients. Studies that look at the quality of life and socioeconomic impact of residual lung function abnormalities, screening strategies and treatment need to be conducted to supplement the findings of this study.

Consent for publication

Not applicable.

Abbreviations

Adj: adjusted; ATS: American Thoracic Society; CI: confidence interval; COPD: chronic obstructive pulmonary disease; CRF: clinical record form; DALYS: disability adjusted life years; ERS: European Respiratory Society; FEV1: forced expiratory volume in 1st second; FVC: forced vital capacity; HIV: human immunodeficiency virus; IQR: interquartile range; MMRC: modified medical research council dyspnea score; MUAC: mid upper arm circumference; MUHAS: Muhimbili University of Health and Allied Sciences; OR: odd's ratio; PFT: pulmonary function test; PTB: pulmonary tuberculosis; SPSS: statistical package for social sciences; TB: tuberculosis.

Competing interests

The authors declare that they have no competing interests.

Authors' contributions

MM, GS and FM were involved in designing the methodology, data analysis and discussion of the paper. MM, GS, FM, SM and AJ were involved in planning and technical aspects of data collection. MM, GS and RM conducted the data analysis. MM, GS and FM wrote the manuscript. All authors read and approved the final manuscript.

Acknowledgements

We extend our gratitude to the International Clinical, Operational and Health Services Research and Training Award (ICOHRTA) for their support. The authors would like to thank all the participants and their families for their cooperation and support. We would like to extend our appreciation to Ahmad Walji, Jaffer Lalji, Alihussein Molloo and Aliabbas Molloo who worked tirelessly during data collection. We would also like to thank Vasudev Uttamsingh and Sanjoy Basak for supplying the mouthpieces for this study. We would like to thank the staff of the Temeke Municipal Hospital and the Mbagala Rangi Tatu health centre TB clinics where the study was conducted.

Author details

[1]Department of Internal Medicine, Muhimbili University of Health and Allied Sciences (MUHAS), P.O. Box 65001, Dar es Salaam, Tanzania. [2]Department of Environmental Occupational Health, Muhimbili University of Health and Allied Sciences (MUHAS), P.O. Box 65001, Dar es Salaam, Tanzania. [3]Department of Epidemiology and Biostatistics, Muhimbili University of Health and Allied Sciences (MUHAS), P.O. Box 65001, Dar es Salaam, Tanzania. [4]Department of Radiology, The Aga Khan Hospital, P.O Box 2289, Dar es Salaam, Tanzania.

References

1. WHO. The Global Burden of Disease 2004 Update. WHO. 2008.
2. Miller TL, McNabb SJN, Hilsenrath P, Pasipanodya J, Weis SE. Personal and societal health quality lost to tuberculosis. PLoS One. 2009;4:e5080.
3. Snider G, Doctor L, Demas T, Shaw A. Obstructive airway disease in patients with treated pulmonary tuberculosis. Am Rev Respir Dis. 1971;103(5):625–40.
4. Birath G, Caro J, Malmberg R, Simonsson BG. Airways obstruction in pulmonary tuberculosis. Scand J Respir Dis. 1966;47:27–36.
5. Lancaster JF, Tomashefski JF. Tuberculosis–a cause of emphysema. Am Rev Respir Dis. 1963;87:435–7.
6. Plit ML, Anderson R, Van Rensburg CE, Page-Shipp L, Blott JA, Fresen JL, Feldman C. Influence of antimicrobial chemotherapy on spirometric parameters and pro-inflammatory indices in severe pulmonary tuberculosis. Eur Respir J. 1998;12:351–6.
7. Simpson DG, Uschner M, Mcclement J. Respiratory function in pulmonary tuberculosis. Am Rev Respir Dis. 1963;87:1–16.
8. Hnizdo E, Singh T, Churchyard G. Chronic pulmonary function impairment caused by initial and recurrent pulmonary tuberculosis following treatment. Thorax. 2000;55:32–8.
9. Willcox PA, Ferguson AD. Chronic obstructive airways disease following treated pulmonary tuberculosis. Respir Med. 1989;83:195–8.
10. Krishna K, Bond S, Artvinli M, Reid KDG, McHardy GJR, Crofton JW. Pulmonary function in treated tuberculosis; a long-term follow-up. Am Rev Respir Dis. 1977;115:402–4.
11. Vargha G. Fifteen year follow-up of lung function in obstructive and non-obstructive pulmonary tuberculosis. Acta Med Hung. 1983;40:271–6.
12. Seaton A, LA Seaton D. Crofton and Douglass's Respiratory Disease. United Kingdom: Blackwell Science; 2002.
13. WHO. Global Tuberculosis Report 2015. 2015.
14. The First National Tuberculosis Prevalence Survey in the United Republic of Tanzania Final Report. 2013.
15. Stenton C. The MRC breathlessness scale. Occup Med (Lond). 2008;58:226–7.
16. Walters JAE, Wood-baker R, Walls J, Johns DP. Stability of the EasyOne ultrasonic spirometer for use in general practice. 2006. p. 306–10.
17. Skloot GS, Edwards NT, Enright PL. Four-Year Calibration Stability of the EasyOne Portable Spirometer. Respir Care. 2010;55:873–7.
18. Barr RG, Stemple KJ, Mesia-vela S, Basner C, Derk S, Henneberger P, Milton DK, Taveras B. Reproducibility and Validity of a Handheld Spirometer. Respir Care. 2008;53:433–41.
19. Hallal PC, Muin A, Lopez MV, Valdivia G, Talamo C, Pertuze J. Tuberculosis and airflow obstruction: evidence from the PLATINO study in Latin America ". Eur Respir J. 2007;30:1180–5.
20. Carlsen HK, Gislason T, Benediktsdottir B, Kolbeinsson TB, Hauksdottir A, Thorsteinsson T, Briem H. A survey of early health effects of the Eyjafjallajökull 2010 eruption in Iceland : a population-based study. 2012.
21. Schirnhofer L, Firlei N. Using Targeted Spirometry to Reduce Non-Diagnosed Chronic Obstructive Pulmonary Disease. Respiration. 2011;81:476–82.
22. Knudsen TM, Mørkve ODD, Mfinanga S, Hardie JONA. Predictive equations for spirometric reference values in a healthy adult suburban population in Tanzania. Tanzan J Health Res. 2011;13:1–10.
23. Miller MR, Hankinson J, Brusasco V, Burgos F, Casaburi R, Coates A, Crapo R, Enright P, van der Grinten CPM, Gustafsson P, Jensen R, Johnson DC, MacIntyre N, McKay R, Navajas D, Pedersen OF, Pellegrino R, Viegi G, Wanger J. Standardisation of spirometry. Eur Respir J. 2005;26:319–38.
24. Chavasse R, Johnson P, Francis J, Balfour-Lynn I, Rosenthal M, Bush A. To clip or not to clip? Noseclips for spirometry. Eur Respir J. 2003;21:876–8.
25. Newall C, McCauley T, Shakespeare J, Cooper B. Is it necessary to use a noseclip in the performance of spirometry using a wedge bellows device? Chron Respir Dis. 2007;4:53–7.
26. Ferguson G, Enright P, Buist A. Office spirometry for lung health assessment in adults: a consensus statement from the National Lung Health Education Program. Chest. 2000;117:1146–61.
27. Pauwels RA, Buist AS, Calverley PM, Jenkins CR, Hurd SS. Global strategy for the diagnosis, management, and prevention of chronic obstructive

pulmonary disease. NHLBI/WHO Global Initiative for Chronic Obstructive Lung Disease (GOLD) Workshop summary. Am J Respir Crit Care Med. 2001; 163:1256–76.

28. Pellegrino R, Viegi G, Brusasco V, Crapo RO, Burgos F, Casaburi R, Coates A, Van Der Grinten CPM , Gustafsson P, Hankinson J, Jensen R, Johnson DC, Macintyre N, Mckay R, Miller MR, Navajas D, Pedersen OF, Wanger J. Interpretative strategies for lung function tests. Eur Respir J. 2005;26:948–968.
29. Pasipanodya JG, Miller TL, Vecino M, Munguia G, Garmon R, Bae S, Drewyer G, Weis SE. Pulmonary impairment after tuberculosis. Chest. 2007;131:1817–24.
30. Lee JH, Chang JH. Lung function in patients with chronic airflow obstruction due to tuberculous destroyed lung. Respir Med. 2003;97:1237–42.
31. Shoemark A, Ozerovitch L, Wilson R. Aetiology in adult patients with bronchiectasis. Respir Med. 2007;101:1163–70.
32. Konietzko NF, Carton RW, Leroy EP. Causes of death in patients with bronchiectasis. Am Rev Respir Dis. 1969;100:852–8.
33. Pasteur MC, Helliwell SM, Houghton SJ, Webb SC, Foweraker JE, Coulden RA, Flower CD, Bilton D, Keogan MT. An investigation into causative factors in patients with bronchiectasis. Am J Respir Crit Care Med. 2000;162(4 Pt 1): 1277–84.
34. Nicotra MB, Rivera M, Dale AM, Shepherd R, Carter R. Clinical, pathophysiologic, and microbiologic characterization of bronchiectasis in an aging cohort. Chest. 1995;108:955–61.
35. Escombe AR, Moore DAJ, Gilman RH, Pan W, Navincopa M, Ticona E, Martínez C, Caviedes L, Sheen P, Gonzalez A, Noakes CJ, Friedland JS, Evans CA. The infectiousness of tuberculosis patients coinfected with HIV. PLoS Med. 2008;5:e188.
36. Calderon EJ, Rivero L, Respaldiza N, Morilla R, Montes-Cano MA, Friaza V, Munoz-Lobato F, Varela JM, Medrano FJ, de la Horra C. Systemic Inflammation in Patients with Chronic Obstructive Pulmonary Disease Who Are Colonized with Pneumocystis jiroveci. Clin Infect Dis. 2007;45:e17–9.
37. Ehrlich RI, White N, Norman R, Laubscher R, Steyn K, Lombard C, Bradshaw D. Predictors of chronic bronchitis in South African adults. Int J Tuberc Lung Dis. 2004;8:369–76.
38. Caballero A, Torres-Duque CA, Jaramillo C, Bolívar F, Sanabria F, Osorio P, Orduz C Guevara DP, Maldonado D. Prevalence of COPD in five Colombian cities situated at low, medium, and high altitude (PREPOCOL study). Chest. 2008;133:343–9.
39. Prescott E, Lange P, Vestbo J. Socioeconomic status, lung function and admission to hospital for COPD: results from the Copenhagen City Heart Study. Eur Respir J. 1999;13:1109.
40. Rona RJ, Gulliford MC, Chinn S. Effects of prematurity and intrauterine growth on respiratory health and lung function in childhood. BMJ. 1993;306:817–20.
41. National Bureau of Statistics: Tanzania in Figure 2014. Dar es Salaam. 2015.
42. UNICEF. Children and Women in Tanzania. 2010.
43. Lee SW, Kim YS, Kim D-S, Oh Y-M, Lee S-D. The risk of obstructive lung disease by previous pulmonary tuberculosis in a country with intermediate burden of tuberculosis. J Korean Med Sci. 2011;26:268–73.
44. Cooper AM. Cell mediated immune responses in Tuberculosis. Annu Rev Immunol. 2009;27:393–422.
45. Swaminathan S, Narendran G, Menon PA, Padmapriyadarsini C, Arunkumar N, Sudharshanam NM, Kumar SR, Chandrasekhar S, Swaminathan S. Impact of HIV Infection on Radiographic Features in Patients with Pulmonary Tuberculosis. Indian J Chest Dis Allied Sci. 2007;49:133–6.
46. Weis SE, Miller TL, Hilsenrath PE, Moonan PK. Comprehensive cost description of tuberculosis care. Int J Tuberc Lung Dis. 2005;9:467.
47. Miller TL, Reading JA, Hilsenrath P, Weis SE. What are the costs of suspected but not reported tuberculosis? Ann Epidemiol. 2006;16:777–81.
48. Pasipanodya JG, McNabb SJ, Hilsenrath P, Bae S, Lykens K, Vecino E, Munguia G, Miller TL, Drewyer G, Weis SE. Pulmonary impairment after tuberculosis and its contribution to TB burden. BMC Public Health. 2010;10:259.

Ultrathin bronchoscopy for solitary pulmonary lesions in a region endemic for tuberculosis

Daniel Franzen[1], Andreas H. Diacon[2], Lutz Freitag[1], Pawel T. Schubert[3,4], Colleen A. Wright[3,4] and Macé M. Schuurmans[1,2*]

Abstract

Background: The evaluation of solitary pulmonary lesions (SPL) requires a balance between procedure-related morbidity and diagnostic yield, particularly in areas where tuberculosis (TB) is endemic. Data on ultrathin bronchoscopy (UB) for this purpose is limited. To evaluate feasibility and safety of UB compared to SB for diagnosis of SPL in a TB endemic region.

Methods: In this prospective randomised trial we compared diagnostic yield and adverse events of UB with standard-size bronchoscopy (SB), both combined with fluoroscopy, in a cohort of patients with SPL located beyond the visible range of SB.

Results: We included 40 patients (mean age 55.2 years, 45 % male) with malignant SPL ($n = 16$; 40 %), tuberculous SPL ($n = 11$; 27.5 %) and other benign SPL ($n = 13$; 32.5 %). Mean procedure time in UB and SB was 30.6 and 26.0 min, respectively ($p = 0.15$). By trend, adverse events were recorded more often with UB than with SB (30.0 vs. 5.0 %, $p = 0.091$), including extensive coughing ($n = 2$), blocked working channel ($n = 2$), and arterial hypertension requiring therapeutic intervention ($n = 1$), all with UB. The overall diagnostic yield of UB compared to SB was 55.0 % vs. 80.0 %, respectively ($p = 0.18$). Sensitivity for the diagnosis of malignancy of UB and SB was 50.0 % and 62.5 %, respectively ($p = 0.95$).

Conclusion: UB is not superior to SB for the evaluation of SPL in a region endemic with tuberculosis, when combined with fluoroscopic guidance only.

Keywords: Solitary pulmonary nodule, Ultrathin bronchoscopy, Lung cancer, Diagnostic yield, Histology

Background

Solitary pulmonary lesions (SPL) are frequently detected in computed tomography (CT) scans of the chest. A fourth of the patients who underwent a low-dose chest CT scan in the U.S. National Lung Screening Trial (NSLT) had a positive screening result; mostly presenting as one or more SPL or a pulmonary mass suspicious for lung cancer [1]. Thus, by following a lung cancer screening program with low-dose chest CT, an increasing number of SPL for evaluation is to be expected. However, more than 95 % of SPL detected by low-dose CT screening show false positive findings due to a non-malignant final diagnosis [1]. In a tuberculosis (TB) endemic area, the prevalence of benign SPL may be even higher [2], and therefore efforts have been undertaken to establish diagnostic modalities to distinguish between malignant and benign lesions without excess perioperative mortality [3]. According to guidelines for the diagnosis of SPL, there are three possibilities to manage these patients depending on the probability of an underlying malignancy: serial CT scans, tissue biopsy, or direct surgical resection [4]. Direct surgical resection is not

* Correspondence: mace.schuurmans@usz.ch
[1]Division of Pulmonology, University Hospital Zurich, University of Zurich, Raemistrasse 100, Zurich 8091, Switzerland
[2]Department of Internal Medicine, Lung Unit, Tygerberg Academic Hospital, University of Stellenbosch, Cape Town, South Africa
Full list of author information is available at the end of the article

justified in the majority of cases given the high rate of false positive findings in the context of SPL in a high TB burden environment. The goal is to diagnose malignant SPL promptly, to permit timely surgical resection, while avoiding invasive testing or surgery in patients with benign SPL [5]. The sensitivity of traditional transbronchial biopsy (TBB) with flexible bronchoscopy ranges between 14 % and 63 %, depending on size and location of the SPL [6]. Recently, new navigational bronchoscopy techniques have emerged which guide the bronchoscopist to the SPL using various image-processing modalities. These technologies including electromagnetic navigation bronchoscopy (ENB), virtual bronchoscopy (VB), and radial endobronchial ultrasound (R-EBUS) have shown to have a better diagnostic yield than traditional TBB [5]. In countries with limited resources, these technologies may not be available due to financial constraints.

Data on the utility of ultrathin bronchoscopy (UB) for the diagnosis of SPL is limited [7]. The smaller outer diameter of the instrument might improve access to SPL not visible by standard-size bronchoscopy (SB) and thus improve the diagnostic yield compared to TBB using SB. Based on the considerably smaller outer diameter of the UB it may be possible to visualise endoscopically more peripheral lesions and thus increase the yield of sampling in the area of interest. We undertook this prospective randomised trial to compare the overall diagnostic yield and adverse event rate of UB with that of SB for the diagnosis of SPL in lesions that were not visible on SB in a TB endemic region.

Methods

Study design and patient selection

The present prospective single-centre randomised pilot study was performed at Tygerberg Academic Hospital, a tertiary university hospital in Cape Town, South Africa, with a referral drainage area of 1.5 million people and TB notification rate of up to 1'000/100'000 persons per year when the study was performed. Between November 2000 and November 2003 all patients referred to the lung unit with single pulmonary lesion ≤ 6 cm in diameter on chest CT were considered. SPL was defined as a single and circumscribed pulmonary lesion with a diameter ≤ 6.0 cm, surrounded by aerated lung tissue, without evidence of satellite lesions, adenopathy or characteristic signs of malignant or benign lesions [3]. Location and maximal diameter of all indeterminate SPLs were recorded from the chest CT prior to enrolment of patients. Inclusion criteria were a previous cytological and microbiological negative sputum examination, absence of enlarged mediastinal or hilar lymph nodes on chest CT scan, and informed consent obtained before start of the procedure. Exclusion criteria were SPL with lesion size unchanged over two years, inability to undergo bronchoscopy or thoracotomy, and pregnancy. The study flow diagram is displayed in Fig. 1. Participants with consent for participation in the study in whom the lesion was found to be visible on SB were then not randomised and not considered part of the study population. Written informed consent was obtained from all patients before inclusion in the study, which was approved by the Committee for Human Research of Stellenbosch University (Cape Town, South Africa) with the reference number 2000/C094. The study is registered at ClinicalTrials.gov (Identifier: NCT02490059).

Randomisation during bronchoscopic procedure

All procedures were started using SB with an external diameter of 5.0–6.0 mm with a biopsy channel of 2.2–

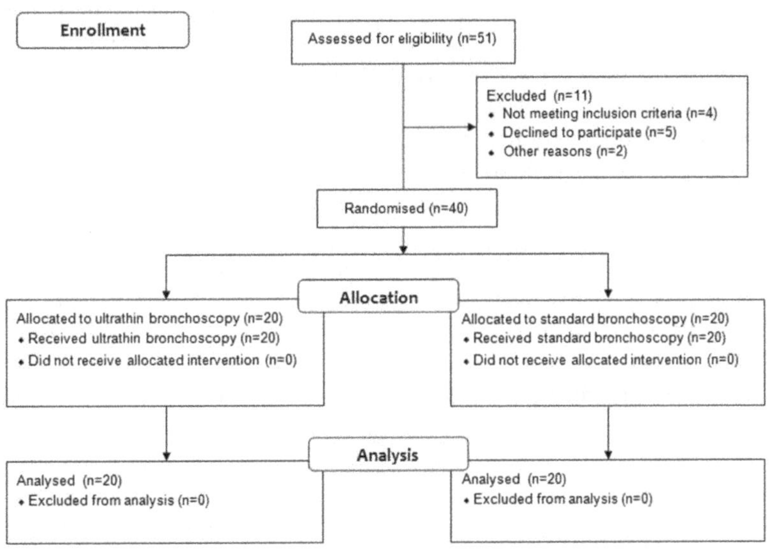

Fig. 1 Study flow diagram (CONSORT flow chart)

2.8 mm (models Olympus BF-30 and BF-1 T160, Olympus, Tokyo, Japan). If during SB the lesion was endoscopically visible the bronchoscopy was continued as standard diagnostic procedure and the patients were excluded from the analysis. Only if no tumour was visible during complete inspection of the bronchial tree using the SB, a participant was randomised by opening a numbered sealed opaque envelope. Randomisation was performed using sequentially numbered (1–40) sealed opaque envelopes (block randomisation: block size 4). For subjects allocated to the SB group, the examination was immediately continued with the same SB bronchoscope. For subjects randomised to UB, the instrument was changed immediately to an Olympus BF-XP 40 ultrathin bronchoscope with an outer diameter of 2.8 mm and a working channel 1.2 mm during the same bronchoscopy session.

Procedural details

Five experienced operators performed all procedures under topical anaesthesia (1 % lidocaine) and conscious sedation (intravenous midazolam). Sampling of SPL was performed with brush and forceps biopsies under fluoroscopic guidance, and with bronchial washing as deemed appropriate by the bronchoscopist. Using all modalities was encouraged by the protocol. Three or more samples were taken using the biopsy forceps and at least 2 samples using the brush. A study-specific case report form including a checklist on the bronchoscopic procedures and findings was completed by the bronchoscopist directly after the procedure. The lesion was considered "reached" if the biopsy forceps and/or brush were placed within the lesion, and it was considered "moved" when push and pull manoeuvers with the biopsy forceps and/or brush were transferrable to the lesion, both as assessed by two-dimensional fluoroscopic visualisation. Procedure duration time was measured from insertion of bronchoscope to extraction and in the case of randomisation to UB included the change over time from SB to UB. All laboratory staff was blinded to study group allocation. Biopsy specimens obtained by bronchoscopy were compared with the diagnosis made by surgical resection or CT-guided trans-thoracic needle aspiration if applicable. Efforts were made to obtain confirmatory histological diagnosis for all patients. Alternatively, when invasive diagnosis was not feasible or appropriate (as assessed by a multidisciplinary tumour board) radiological follow-up examinations were performed over two years.

Outcomes

The primary outcome was to determine and compare the overall diagnostic yield and the sensitivity for the diagnosis of malignancy of UB versus SB. The diagnostic yield was calculated by identifying cases for which a definitive histological or cytological diagnosis could be made or follow-up examinations after two years suggested a benign disease. The following formula was used to compute the overall diagnostic yield: diagnostic yield (%) = 100 × cases diagnosed by UB or SB/total number of patients with completed procedures. The sensitivity was calculated as previously described [8], and is related to the diagnosis of malignancy. The secondary outcome was to compare the adverse event rate and procedure duration of UB versus SB.

Adverse events

The intensity levels of the adverse events (AEs) were graded according to a standard three-grade scale [9]. Grade 1, or mild AE, was defined as "no effect on bronchoscopic procedure"; Grade 2, or moderate AE, was considered when "some interference with bronchoscopic procedure" occurred; and Grade 3, or severe AE, was present if "early termination of bronchoscopy was required". For purpose of this study only grade 2 and 3 AEs were recorded.

Statistical analysis

All statistical analyses were performed using IBM SPSS Statistics for Windows, version 22 (IBM corporation, Armonk NY, USA). Data are reported as median (interquartile range, IQR), or mean ± standard deviation (SD), or percentages as appropriate. Distribution of normality was tested with the one-sample Kolmogorov-Smirnov test. The difference between patients between the groups was calculated using the Fisher's exact test (for 2 × 2 tables) or χ^2 test for categorical data, and Mann–Whitney *U*-test or student's *t*-test for continuous data. Both overall diagnostic yield and sensitivity between the groups were compared using the χ^2 test. *P*-values of all outcomes were two-sided; a value less than 0.05 was considered to indicate statistical significance. There was no sample size calculation as the study was designed as a pilot trial to test feasibility.

Results

Forty patients were included in the study (see Additional file 1). Baseline characteristics and the final diagnoses are displayed in Table 1. Neither localization of SPL in the upper lobes ($p = 0.33$), nor lesion size > 3 cm was associated with active TB ($p = 0.21$). Although none of the lesions were visible by SB (inclusion criterion), two of the 20 lesions (10 %) were visualized endoscopically by UB. The mean procedure time for UB and SB allocated patients was 30.6 and 26.0 min, respectively ($p = 0.15$). By trend, AEs were significantly more frequent in the UB compared to the SB group (30.0 vs. 5.0 %, $p = 0.091$). AEs in the UB group included extensive coughing ($n = 2$), blocked

Table 1 Baseline characteristics of patients in the study

	Ultrathin bronchoscopy ($n = 20$)	Standard size bronchoscopy ($n = 20$)	*P* value
Age, mean (SD), y	54.8 (12.4)	55.7 (12.7)	0.72
Male gender, No. (%)	10 (50.0)	8 (40.0)	0.75
Previous tuberculosis, No. (%)	4 (20.0)	4 (20.0)	0.99
Lobar localisation			0.65
Upper lobe, No. (%)	12 (60.0)	11 (55.0)	
Middle lobe, No. (%)	2 (10.0)	1 (5.0)	
Lower lobe, No. (%)	6 (30.0)	8 (40.0)	
Lesion size, median (IQR), cm	2.7 (1.7–3.5)	2.4 (1.8–3.9)	0.40
Lesion size ≥ 2 cm, No. (%)	14 (70.0)	14 (70.0)	0.99
NSCLC, No. (%)	8 (40.0)	8 (40.0)	
Benign final diagnosis, No. (%)	12 (60.0)	12 (60.0)	0.66
Tuberculosis	5 (25.0)	6 (30.0)	
Otherwise benign lesion[a]	7 (35.0)	6 (30.0)	
Confirmation of final diagnosis			0.62
Surgery	11 (55.0)	8 (40.0)	
Radiological follow-up (no histological confirmation)	8 (40.0)	11 (55.0)	
Loss of follow-up (no histological confirmation)	1 (5.0)	1 (5.0)	

[a]scar ($n = 1$), bacterial infection ($n = 2$), silicosis ($n = 1$), hamartoma ($n = 1$), unknown ($n = 8$)
SD standard deviation, *IQR* interquartile range, *NSCLC* non-small cell lung cancer

working channel or weak suctioning ($n = 3$), and hypertensive urgency requiring therapeutic intervention ($n = 1$). No grade 3 AEs were documented. In the SB group, there was one case of extensive bleeding, which was stopped by topical application of adrenaline through the working channel of the bronchoscope. Procedural details were equally distributed within the groups (Table 2). The overall diagnostic yield of fluoroscopic guided UB compared to SB was 55.0 % vs. 80.0 %, respectively ($p = 0.18$). Sensitivity for the diagnosis of malignancy of UB and SB was 50.0 % and 62.5 %, respectively (Table 3). Rates of true positives, true negatives and false negatives in UB compared to SB were 20 % vs. 25 %, 60 % vs. 60 %, and 20 % vs. 15 %, respectively. The diagnostic yield of lesions that were fluoroscopically moved was 90.9 % compared to 88.0 % in lesions that were fluoroscopically reached. However, only a "reached" SPL was a significant predictor of the diagnostic yield ($p <$ 0.001), whereas a "moveable" SPL was not significant ($p = 0.052$). The size of the lesion was not significantly associated with increased diagnostic yield ($p = 0.40$).

Discussion

This randomised trial investigating endoscopically nonvisible SPL up to 6 cm diameter by SB showed no diagnostic benefit of switching to UB for the diagnostic bronchoscopic sampling when compared to the procedure

Table 2 Procedural details

	Ultrathin bronchoscopy ($n = 20$)	Standard size bronchoscopy ($n = 20$)	P value
Biopsy method, No. (%)			
Forceps	14 (70.0)	10 (50.0)	0.33
Brushing	14 (70.0)	18 (90.0)	0.23
Washing	20 (100)	19 (95.0)	0.99
Combination of all three methods	12 (60.0)	7 (35.0)	1
Combination of two methods	4 (20.0)	12 (60.0)	0.99
Washing only	4 (20.0)	1 (5.0)	1
Lesion reached, No. (%)[a]	12 (60.0)	13 (65.0)	0.99
Lesion moved, No. (%)[a]	4 (20.0)	7 (35.0)	0.48

[a]fluoroscopically determined

Table 3 Overall diagnostic yield and sensitivity for the diagnosis of malignancy of ultrathin versus standard size bronchoscopy

	Ultrathin bronchoscopy (*n* = 20)	Standard size bronchoscopy (*n* = 20)	*P*-value
Overall diagnostic yield	55.0	80.0	0.18
Sensitivity	50.0 (16.0–84.0)	62.5 (24.7–91.0)	0.95

Data in the table are mean values, displayed in % (95 % CI)

performed with the SB alone, when used under fluoroscopic guidance. There is only limited evidence from randomised controlled trials comparing the diagnostic yield of UB with that of SB. We found that UB had no diagnostic advantage compared to SB but was more cumbersome for operators. Moreover, the procedure time was nearly five minutes longer with UB, although the difference was not statistically significant. The clinical relevance of four minutes time difference can maybe neglected, since the change from the standard to the ultrathin bronchoscope is omitted in daily routine but was part of procedure time here. Although the classical definition of SPLs considers lesions ≤ 3 cm, we have chosen to investigate lesions ≤ 6 cm, since tuberculomas of nearly double that size have been reported [10].

Data concerning the diagnostic yield of fluoroscopic guided UB compared to SB in the literature is scarce, especially for the evaluation of SPL. Considering the existing evidence in this field, the diagnostic yield of fluoroscopic guided UB in our study (55.0 %) was within the published range from 30.0 to 69.0 % reported by others [11–13], although these studies used different sampling methods and were in different populations. In a small prospective, single-arm study published by Rooney et al. on 17 patients, the diagnostic yield of UB was only 30.0 %, perhaps because only a small biopsy brush was used for the ultrathin bronchoscope [11]. The combined use of histological and cytological biopsy techniques has led to an improved diagnostic yield obtained with UB of 60.0 % [12]. Using a slightly thicker bronchoscope (outer diameter 3.5 mm) in a prospective study on 102 patients, Oki et al. reported a diagnostic yield of 69.0 % for the thin bronchoscopy irrespective of lesion size. This result was obtained without using a brush; only forceps biopsy and bronchial washing were performed [13]. We used forceps, brushing, and bronchial washings under fluoroscopic guidance as sampling methods. We did not investigate the diagnostic utility of the combined use of UB and SB in this context as sampling was only performed with the allocated bronchoscope (UB or SB). The diagnostic yield in our study may have been influenced by the prevalence of TB in our cohort (27.5 %), which is clearly higher than in the three other studies ranging from 5.9 to 12.5 %.

Technological advances in recent years have led to the availability of newer modalities helping to navigate to SPLs [14]. The weighted diagnostic yield of ENB, VB, and R-EBUS for the work-up of SPLs without the use of UB is in the range of 67–74 % which is comparable with conventional methods mentioned above [5, 15]. However, in the context of the new navigational bronchoscopic techniques the utility of UB needs to be reinvestigated. The usefulness of UB may play an important role when it is used with other new modalities such as CT-fluoroscopy or virtual bronchoscopic navigation. The combination of UB and CT-fluoroscopy is reported to have a similar diagnostic yield of 78 % in one study [16]. Data regarding VB combined with UB are conflicting. In the randomised study by Asano et al, there was no significant difference of the diagnostic yield between the VB-assisted group (67 %) and the non-VB-assisted group (60 %) [17]. However, under the combined use of EBUS, fluoroscopy, and virtual bronchoscopic navigation guidance, a recent randomised study published by Oki et al. could show that the diagnostic yield for malignant lesions was significantly higher with a 3.0-mm ultrathin bronchoscope (74 %) compared to a 4.0-mm thin bronchoscope (59 %) [18]. The authors concluded that the combination of UB with navigational technology and endobronchial ultrasound (EBUS) seems to combine the best two modalities for evaluating peripheral pulmonary lesions [18]. Interestingly, the diagnostic yield of UB was markedly higher in the study by Oki et al. (74 %) compared to our study (55 %). In contrast, the yield of SB was higher in our study (80 %) compared to 59 % by Oki et al., although a slightly thinner bronchoscope was used in their study [18]. On one hand, this underlines the conclusion that advanced navigational technologies improve the diagnostic yield of UB. On the other hand, these differences raise the issue of the operator's experience and a possible influence by the higher TB prevalence in our cohort. An additional aspect to consider is that VB- or ENB-guided biopsy techniques increase average costs, which is not feasible in many parts of the world [19]. Compared to video-assisted thoracoscopic surgery (VATS) or (18)F-fluoro-deoxyglucose positron emission tomography (FDG-PET), ENB is more cost-effective to diagnose lung cancer in moderate-to high-risk patients [20]. Another issue, which should be considered, is training. The recommended training requirement for R-EBUS is at least 50 supervised procedures [21]. Issues of costs and training need to be considered before acquisition and introduction of such modalities. Some of these diagnostic modalities may not be feasible in less affluent settings. In addition, the benefit of these highly sophisticated diagnostic tools in an area with high incidence of TB remains questionable.

The limitations of this study are its small sample size, since it was originally designed as pilot trial, and that not all bronchoscopic results were confirmed by surgical sampling. Interestingly, none of the individuals in whom observation was considered the appropriate strategy by the clinical board had a malignant lesion. Furthermore, a new ultrathin bronchoscope with a larger working channel has been introduced which most probably leads to higher yields [13]. All of the UB procedures were done with a fiberscope, which might have influenced diagnostic yield and could have caused a bias. We did not evaluate the distance of SPL from hilum or presence of bronchus sign as possible predictors of the diagnostic yield. Lastly, the bronchoscopies were performed by five different operators, which may have introduce a certain bias. However, three of the five operators had a documented track record from a previous study, and at least one of them was present in the bronchoscopy suite for all study related procedures [22].

Conclusions

We conclude that the inspection and sampling with UB in endoscopically non-visible SPL showed no advantage over sampling with SB in the evaluation of undiagnosed SPL in a TB-endemic area, when combined with fluoroscopic guidance only. It seems that for the diagnostic work-up of SPL, tumour visibility is less important than getting higher volumes of material. Sample material volume consisting of tumour cells and fluid markers is determined by the diameter of the bronchoscope.

Abbreviations

AE: adverse event; CT: computed tomography; ENB: electromagnetic navigation bronchoscopy; IQR: interquartile range; R-EBUS: radial endobronchial ultrasound; SB: standard size bronchoscopy; SD: standard deviation; SPL: solitary pulmonary lesion; TB: tuberculosis; TBB: transbronchial biopsy; UB: ultrathin bronchoscopy.

Competing interests

The authors declare that they have no competing interests.

Authors' contributions

DF, LF and MMS drafted the manuscript and analysed the data. MMS, AHD, PTS, and CAW designed the study and were involved in acquisition of the data. All authors approved the final version of the manuscript.

Acknowledgements

Chris T Bolliger was the initiator and promoter of this pilot study. He passed away on November 2, 2012.

Funding

There is no funding source of this study.

Author details

[1]Division of Pulmonology, University Hospital Zurich, University of Zurich, Raemistrasse 100, Zurich 8091, Switzerland. [2]Department of Internal Medicine, Lung Unit, Tygerberg Academic Hospital, University of Stellenbosch, Cape Town, South Africa. [3]Division of Anatomical Pathology, Tygerberg Academic Hospital, University of Stellenbosch, Cape Town, South Africa. [4]NHLS, Port Elizabeth and Tygerberg Hospital, Cape Town, South Africa.

References

1. Aberle DR, Adams AM, Berg CD, Black WC, Clapp JD, Fagerstrom RM, Gareen IF, Gatsonis C, Marcus PM, Sicks JD. Reduced lung-cancer mortality with low-dose computed tomographic screening. N Engl J Med. 2011;365(5):395–409.
2. Lai RS, Lee SS, Ting YM, Wang HC, Lin CC, Lu JY. Diagnostic value of transbronchial lung biopsy under fluoroscopic guidance in solitary pulmonary nodule in an endemic area of tuberculosis. Respir Med. 1996;90(3):139–43.
3. Schuurmans MM, Ellmann A, Bouma H, Diacon AH, Dyckmans K, Bolliger CT. Solitary pulmonary nodule evaluation with 99mTc-methoxy isobutyl isonitrile in a tuberculosis-endemic area. Eur Respir J. 2007;30(6):1090–5.
4. Gould MK, Fletcher J, Iannettoni MD, Lynch WR, Midthun DE, Naidich DP, Ost DE. Evaluation of patients with pulmonary nodules: when is it lung cancer?: ACCP evidence-based clinical practice guidelines (2nd edition). Chest. 2007;132(3 Supp):108s–30.
5. Wang Memoli JS, Nietert PJ, Silvestri GA. Meta-analysis of guided bronchoscopy for the evaluation of the pulmonary nodule. Chest. 2012; 142(2):385–93.
6. Baaklini WA, Reinoso MA, Gorin AB, Sharafkaneh A, Manian P. Diagnostic yield of fiberoptic bronchoscopy in evaluating solitary pulmonary nodules. Chest. 2000;117(4):1049–54.
7. Schoenfeld NTT, Fisseler-Eckhoff A, et al. Ultrathin bronchoscopy as a new tool in the diagnosis of peripheral lung lesions: preliminary results of a prospective evaluation. In: Yoshimura H, Niimi S, Kida A, Kaneko M, Arai T, Kitahara S, editors. Bronchology and bronchoesophagology: state of the art 2001. Amsterdam: Elsevier; 2001. p. 785–7.
8. Linnet K, Bossuyt PM, Moons KG, Reitsma JB. Quantifying the accuracy of a diagnostic test or marker. Clin Chem. 2012;58(9):1292–301.
9. Common Terminology Criteria for Adverse Events v4.O2 (CTCAE), May 28 waoC–Q, Reference_5x7.pdf.
10. Palmer PE. Pulmonary tuberculosis–usual and unusual radiographic presentations. Semin Roentgenol. 1979;14(3):204–43.
11. Rooney CP, Wolf K, McLennan G. Ultrathin bronchoscopy as an adjunct to standard bronchoscopy in the diagnosis of peripheral lung lesions. A preliminary report. Respiration. 2002;69(1):63–8.
12. Yamamoto S, Ueno K, Imamura F, Matsuoka H, Nagatomo I, Omiya Y, Yoshimura M, Kusunoki Y. Usefulness of ultrathin bronchoscopy in diagnosis of lung cancer. Lung Cancer. 2004;46(1):43–8.
13. Oki M, Saka H, Kitagawa C, Tanaka S, Shimokata T, Mori K, Kajikawa S. Novel thin bronchoscope with a 1.7-mm working channel for peripheral pulmonary lesions. Eur Respir J. 2008;32(2):465–71.
14. Narula T, Machuzak MS, Mehta AC. Newer modalities in the work-up of peripheral pulmonary nodules. Clin Chest Med. 2013;34(3):395–415.
15. Gex G, Pralong JA, Combescure C, Seijo L, Rochat T, Soccal PM. Diagnostic yield and safety of electromagnetic navigation bronchoscopy for lung nodules: a systematic review and meta-analysis. Respiration. 2014;87(2):165–76.
16. Matsuno Y, Asano F, Shindoh J, Abe T, Shiraki A, Ando M, Suzuki T, Seko A, Moriwaki H. CT-guided ultrathin bronchoscopy: bioptic approach and factors in predicting diagnosis. Intern Med. 2011;50(19):2143–8.

17. Asano F, Shinagawa N, Ishida T, Shindoh J, Anzai M, Tsuzuku A, Morita S. Virtual bronchoscopic navigation combined with ultrathin bronchoscopy. A randomized clinical trial. Am J Respir Crit Care Med. 2013;188(3):327–33.
18. Oki M, Saka H, Ando M, Asano F, Kurimoto N, Morita K, Kitagawa C, Kogure Y, Miyazawa T. Ultrathin bronchoscopy with multimodal devices for peripheral pulmonary lesions. A randomized trial. Am J Respir Crit Care Med. 2015;192(4):468–76.
19. Dale CR, Madtes DK, Fan VS, Gorden JA, Veenstra DL. Navigational bronchoscopy with biopsy versus computed tomography-guided biopsy for the diagnosis of a solitary pulmonary nodule: a cost-consequences analysis. J Bronchology Interv Pulmonol. 2012;19(4):294–303.
20. Deppen SA, Davis WT, Green EA, Rickman O, Aldrich MC, Fletcher S, Putnam JB, Jr., Grogan EL. Cost-effectiveness of initial diagnostic strategies for pulmonary nodules presenting to thoracic surgeons. Ann Thorac Surg. 2014;98(4):1214–22.
21. Ernst A, Silvestri GA, Johnstone D. Interventional pulmonary procedures: Guidelines from the American College of Chest Physicians. Chest. 2003;123(5):1693–717.
22. Schuurmans MM, Michaud GC, Diacon AH, Bolliger CT. Use of an ultrathin bronchoscope in the assessment of central airway obstruction. Chest. 2003;124(2):735–9.

11

Vitamin D deficiency associates with susceptibility to tuberculosis in Pakistan, but polymorphisms in *VDR*, *DBP* and *CYP2R1*

Kashaf Junaid[1*], Abdul Rehman[1], David A. Jolliffe[2], Tahir Saeed[3], Kristie Wood[4] and Adrian R. Martineau[2]

Abstract

Background: Single nucleotide polymorphisms (SNPs) in the genes encoding the vitamin D receptor (*VDR*) and the vitamin D binding protein (*DBP*) have been reported to modify the influence of vitamin D deficiency on susceptibility to active tuberculosis (TB) in the UK, but this phenomenon has not been investigated in settings with a high TB burden. SNPs in *CYP2R1*, which encodes a vitamin D 25-hydroxylase enzyme, are known to influence vitamin D status, but their potential role in determining susceptibility to TB has not previously been investigated in any setting.

Method: We conducted a case–control study in 260 pulmonary TB patients and 112 controls recruited in Lahore, Pakistan. Analyses were conducted to test for main effects of vitamin D status and SNPs in *VDR* (rs731236, rs2228570 and rs1544410), *DBP* (rs7041 and rs4588) and *CYP2R1* (rs2060793, rs10500804 and rs10766197) on susceptibility to TB, and to investigate whether these SNPs modify the association between vitamin D status and disease susceptibility.

Results: Profound vitamin D deficiency (serum 25-hydroxyvitamin D concentration ≤ 20 nmol/L) was common among TB patients (118/260, 45 %), and was independently associated with susceptibility to TB (adjusted odds ratio 1.87, 95 % CI 1.15 to 3.04, $P = 0.01$). However, none of the SNPs investigated associated with susceptibility to TB, either in main effects analysis, or in interaction with vitamin D status.

Conclusion: Profound vitamin D deficiency was common among TB patients in this high-burden setting, and was independently associated with disease susceptibility. However, no statistically significant associations between SNPs in the vitamin D pathway and disease susceptibility was demonstrated.

Keywords: Tuberculosis, Vitamin D, Vitamin D Receptor, Hypovitaminosis D, Vitamin D binding protein, Vitamin D 25-hydroxylase

Background

Tuberculosis (TB) is a leading global cause of morbidity and mortality, responsible for an estimated 1.5 million deaths in 2014 [1]. The identification of factors which increase disease susceptibility has potential to inform control strategies. Case control studies have previously reported independent associations between vitamin D deficiency and susceptibility to active TB [2]. However, interpretation of such studies is limited by their cross-sectional nature, as they cannot determine whether vitamin D deficiency is a cause or a consequence of active TB. The case for vitamin D deficiency playing a causal role in enhancing disease susceptibility is supported by findings of genetic studies reporting that polymorphisms in the vitamin D receptor (VDR) and the vitamin D binding protein (DBP) genes modify the influence of vitamin D status on susceptibility to active disease in the UK [3, 4]. Only one study is present who have investigated such gene-environment interactions; analogous investigations in high TB burden countries are therefore needed [5]. Moreover, no study has previously investigated whether polymorphisms in the gene encoding the

* Correspondence: kashaf_junaid@hotmail.com
[1]Department of Microbiology and Molecular Genetics, University of the Punjab, Quaid-e-Azam Campus, Lahore 5400, Pakistan
Full list of author information is available at the end of the article

vitamin D hydroxylase enzyme, *CYP2R1,* are associated with susceptibility to TB, either as a main effect, or as a modifier of the effects of vitamin D status. This gene is a plausible candidate for effect modification, as 25-hydroxylation of 'parent' vitamin D_3 (cholecaciferol, synthesized in the skin on exposure to ultra-violet B radiation) to form the major circulating vitamin D metabolite 25-hydroxyvitamin D (25[OH]D) is a key determinant of circulating 25(OH)D concentrations [6].

We therefore conducted a case–control study to determine the influence of vitamin D status and single nucleotide polymorphisms (SNPs) in *VDR*, *DBP* and *CYP2R1* on susceptibility to active TB in Pakistan, a high-burden setting where TB incidence in 2014 was estimated at 270 cases per 100,000 population per year [1]. Having demonstrated an independent association between vitamin D deficiency and susceptibility to active TB in the study population, we proceeded to investigate whether this was modified by SNPs in the vitamin D pathway.

Methods

Study design

We conducted a case control study. Cases were patients aged 14–60 years with newly-diagnosed smear-positive pulmonary TB, recruited from the Gulab Devi Chest hospital, Lahore. Patients with any of the following conditions documented in the hospital record were excluded: diabetes mellitus, ischemic heart disease, chronic renal failure, jaundice or seropositivity for hepatitis B surface antigen, Hepatitis C Virus or Human Immunodeficiency Virus. Controls were healthy relatives of TB patients or hospital staff working at the same hospital with no history of previous tuberculosis but exposed to TB cases. Participants who fulfilled eligibility criteria were asked to complete a questionnaire detailing their age, gender and monthly income. Informed consent was taken from all participants before sample collection. The study was approved from the ethical committee of the University of Punjab (Ref No: SBS 873–12) and also from Gulab Devi Chest Hospital, Lahore.

Five mL of blood were drawn from a median cubital vein; 2 mL were transferred into vials containing EDTA and frozen at −20 °C for subsequent DNA extraction, and 3 mL were added to serum vials and sent to the laboratory within two hours of collection, where serum was isolated from clotted blood by centrifugation and stored at −20 °C for subsequent determination of 25(OH)D concentration.

Serum 25 (OH)D assay

Serum 25(OH)D concentration was determined by ELISA (Immunodiagnostic Systems, Boldon,UK). Calibrators and controls provided with kits were run in duplicate. For the purpose of this study, a patient with 25(OH) vitamin D level equal or less than 20 nmol/L was considered to be vitamin D deficient. Inter-assay CV for serum 25(OH)D assay for our samples was 12.5 %.

Genotyping

Genomic DNA was extracted from whole blood and quantified using a nanodrop spectrophotometer as previously described [7]. TaqMan allelic probe assays (Applied Biosystems, Foster City, CA, USA) were used to genotype polymorphisms in genes encoding the vitamin D receptor *VDR* [(rs731236 Taq I), (rs2228570 Bsm I); (rs1544410 Fok I)]; the vitamin D 25-hydroxylase *CYP2R1* [(rs2060793, rs10500804, rs10766197)] and the vitamin D binding protein *DBP* [(rs7041) and (rs4588)]. All primers were commercially prepared. Details of primers used in this study has been provided in Additional file 1. The PCR reaction mixture contained 7.5 μL of TaqMan Genotyping master mixture, 0.75 μL of TaqMan SNP (probes), 1 μL of genomic DNA (1–10 ng), and 5.75 μL nuclease free water. Thermal conditions were as follows: initial denaturation at 95 °C for 10 min, 40 cycles were run at 95 °C for 15 seconds (denaturing) followed by 60 °C for 1 min (annealing/extension). PCR plates were read by 7900HT seq detection system ABI prism.

Sample size and statistical analysis

Sample size was calculated using OpenEpi sample calculator [8] assuming an expected frequency of 57 % vitamin D deficiency in cases and 33 % in controls [9]. Statistical analyses were done with SPSS version 20. Chi square tests were used for univariate analyses exploring potential determinants of vitamin D status and susceptibility to active TB, and binary logistic regression analysis was used for corresponding multivariate analyses. Sub-group analyses were performed to determine whether genetic variation in the vitamin D pathway modified effects of vitamin D status on susceptibility to active TB by repeating primary efficacy analyses with the inclusion of a term for an interaction between vitamin D status and genotype. Odds ratios are presented with 95 % confidence intervals and *P*-values.

Results

Participant characteristics

A total of 260 cases with smear-positive pulmonary TB and 112 controls were recruited to the study between August 2012 and September 2013. The mean age of cases and controls was 31.6 years (s.d. 10.5 years, range 14–55 years) vs. 30.6 years (s.d. 9.3, range 15–56 years) respectively. Fifty-four percent of cases and 48 % of controls were female. Forty-five percent of cases and

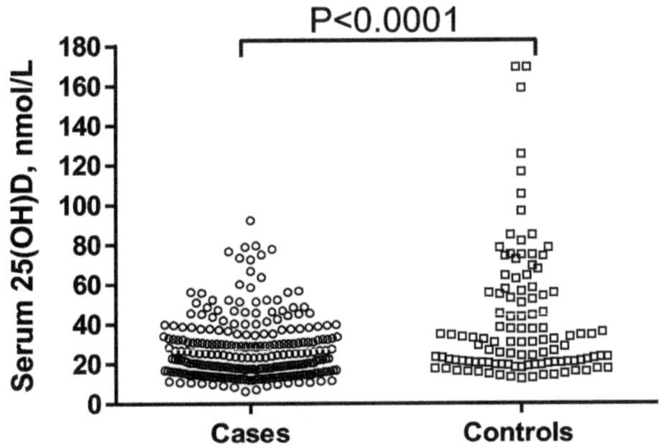

Fig. 1 Serum 25-hydroxyvitamin D (25[OH]D) concentrations in TB cases ($n = 260$) and healthy controls ($n = 112$). *P* value from unpaired *t* test comparison of means

30 % of controls had profound vitamin D deficiency (serum 25[OH]D ≤20 nmol/L), and mean serum 25(OH)D concentration was lower in cases vs. controls (27.3 vs. 43.3 nmol/L respectively, 95 % CI for difference 11.5–22.8, $P < 0.0001$; Fig. 1).

Determinants of vitamin D status in cases and controls

Table 1 presents determinants of vitamin D status in cases and controls. Vitamin D deficiency was independently associated with female vs. male gender (aOR 2.31, 95 % CI 1.33 to 4.01, $P = 0.003$; aOR 3.67, 95 % CI 1.38 to 9.70, $P = 0.01$) and sampling in October-March vs. April-September (aOR 1.89, 95 % CI 1.14 to 3.16, $P = 0.01$; aOR 2.55, 95 % CI 1.03 to 6.31, $P = 0.04$) in both case and control populations, respectively (Table 1).

Association between phenotypic features and susceptibility to active tuberculosis

Table 2 presents results of univariate and multivariate analyses testing for associations between participants' phenotypic features and susceptibility to active TB. Active TB was independently associated with lower monthly income (aOR 1.68, 95 % CI 1.06 to 2.66, $P = 0.02$) and presence of profound vitamin D deficiency (aOR 1.87, 95 % CI 1.15 to 3.04, $P = 0.01$). The following phenotypic features were not found to associate with susceptibility to active TB: age, sex, marital status or season of recruitment.

Association between vitamin D pathway genotype and susceptibility to active tuberculosis

Table 3 presents results of analyses testing for associations between genetic variation in *VDR, CYP2R1* and *DBP* and susceptibility to active TB, adjusting for monthly income and vitamin D status. No statistically significant association was observed between susceptibility to active TB and any polymorphism investigated.

Association between vitamin D deficiency and host genotype, stratified by vitamin D status

We next proceeded to investigate whether genetic variation in *VDR, DBP* or *CYP2R1* modified the association between vitamin D deficiency and susceptibility reported above. Results of the pertinent sub-group and interaction analyses are presented in Table 4: these revealed no evidence to support the hypothesis that polymorphisms in the vitamin D pathway modify the effect of vitamin D deficiency on risk of active TB.

Discussion

We report that vitamin D deficiency is very common among TB patients in Pakistan, and that it associates

Table 1 Determinants of vitamin D status in TB cases and controls

		TB cases			Control		
Characteristics		25 (OH) D ≤20 nmol/l	aOR(95 % CI)[a]	P	25(OH) D ≤20 nmol/l	aOR(95 % CI)[a]	P
Age	>30 years	56/124 (45 %)	Ref		17/50 (34 %)	Ref	
	≤30 years	62/136 (46 %)	1.26(0.71-2.32)	0.44	17/62 (27 %)	1.46(0.60-3.56)	0.40
Sex	Male	43/120 (36 %)	Ref	-	11/58 (19 %)	Ref	-
	Female	75/140 (54 %)	2.31(1.33-4.01)	0.003	23/54 (43 %)	3.67(1.38-9.70)	0.01
Marital status	Single	49/114 (43 %)	Ref	-	16/54 (30 %)	Ref	-
	Married	69/146 (46 %)	1.34(0.71-2.55)	0.36	18/58 (31 %)	1.63(0.64-1.43)	0.30
Monthly income, PKR	<10,000	84/177 (47 %)	1.27(0.73-2.20)	0.38	18/62 (29 %)	1.0(0.42-2.40)	0.98
	≥10,000	34/83 (41 %)	Ref	-	16/50 (32 %)	Ref	-
Month of recruitment	April-September	53/137 (39 %)	Ref	-	10/53 (19 %)	Ref	-
	October-March	65/123 (53 %)	1.89(1.14-3.16)	0.01	24/59 (41 %)	2.55(1.03-6.31)	0.04

[a]Odds ratio adjusted for age, sex, marital status, monthly income and month of recruitment. *PKR* Pakistani rupees, 25(OH)D, 25-hydroxyvitamin D

Table 2 Association between participants phenotypic characteristics and susceptibility to active tuberculosis

		TB cases ($N = 260$)	Control ($N = 112$)	OR (95 % CI)	P	aOR(95 % CI)[a]	P
Age	>30 years	124 (48 %)	50 (45 %)	Ref	-	Ref	-
	≤30 years	136 (52 %)	62 (55 %)	1.01(0.58-1.42)	0.68	1.01(0.61-1.68)	0.94
Sex	Male	120 (46 %)	58 (52 %)	Ref	-	Ref	-
	Female	140 (54 %)	54 (48 %)	1.25(0.80-1.95)	0.31	1.06(0.65-1.75)	0.79
Marital status	Single	114 (44 %)	54 (48 %)	Ref	-	Ref	-
	Married	146 (56 %)	58 (52 %)	1.19(0.76-1.86)	0.43	1.13(0.67-1.90)	0.63
Monthly income, PKR	<10,000	177 (68 %)	62 (55 %)	1.72(1.10-2.71)	0.02	1.68(1.06-2.66)	0.02
	≥10,000	83 (32 %)	50 (45 %)	Ref	-	Ref	-
Season of recruitment	April-September	137 (53 %)	53 (47 %)	1.24(0.79-1.23)	0.34	1.24(0.78-1.96)	0.34
	October-March	123 (47 %)	59 (53 %)	Ref	-	Ref	-
Serum 25(OH)D, nmol/L	≤20 nmol/L	118 (45 %)	34 (30 %)	1.90(1.19-3.05)	0.02	1.87(1.15-3.04)	0.01
	>20 nmol/L	142(55 %)	78(70 %)	Ref	-	Ref	-

[a]Odds ratio adjusted for age, sex, marital status, monthly income, season of recruitment and serum 25(OH)D concentration. PKR, Pakistani rupees; 25(OH)D, 25-hydroxyvitamin D

independently with susceptibility to active TB. Risk of deficiency was independently associated with sampling in January - March and with female gender in cases and controls alike. However, we found no evidence to suggest that polymorphisms in *CYP2R1*, *VDR* or *DBP* influenced susceptibility to TB in this population, either as main effects, or in interaction with vitamin D deficiency.

Our finding of an independent association between vitamin D deficiency and susceptibility to active TB is in keeping with previous reports from Pakistan [9] and elsewhere [10]. A prospective study in Pakistan has previously reported that vitamin D deficiency precedes onset of active disease [11], and laboratory studies have reported that vitamin D metabolites induce antimycobacterial activity in vitro [12]: taken together, such reports suggest that vitamin D deficiency plays a causal role in increasing susceptibility to active TB. However, cross-sectional studies such as our own cannot distinguish causality from reverse causality, and the possibility remains that active TB may be a cause, as well as a consequence, of vitamin D deficiency.

Table 3 Association between vitamin D pathway genotype and susceptibility to active tuberculosis

SNP, gene	Genotype	TB cases, n/N (%)	TB contacts, n/N (%)	aOR (95 % CI)[a]	P
rs7312236, *VDR*	AA	84/230 (37 %)	42/100 (42 %)	Ref	-
	AG/GG	146/230 (63 %)	58/100 (58 %)	1.22(0.75-1.98)	0.42
rs154410, *VDR*	CC	53/235 (23 %)	29/106 (27 %)	Ref	-
	CT/TT	182/235 (77 %)	77/106 (73 %)	1.23(0.71-2.09)	0.45
rs228570, *VDR*	GG	137/235 (59 %)	68/107 (64 %)	Ref	-
	GA/AA	98/235 (41 %)	39/107 (36 %)	1.89(0.80-2.10)	0.28
rs7041, *DBP*	AA	55/232 (24 %)	21/102 (21 %)	Ref	-
	AC/CC	177/232 (76 %)	81/102 (79 %)	0.77(0.43-1.39)	0.39
rs4588, *DBP*	GG	122/234 (52 %)	50/107 (47 %)	Ref	-
	GT/TT	112/234 (48 %)	57/107 (53 %)	0.93(0.58-1.49)	0.77
rs10500804, *CYP2R1*	GG	59/231 (26 %)	22/103 (22 %)	Ref	-
	GT/TT	172/231 (74 %)	81/103 (78 %)	0.83(0.47-1.47)	0.53
rs2060793, *CYP2R1*	GG	112/228 (49 %)	51/101 (50 %)	Ref	-
	AG/AA	116/228 (51 %)	50/101 (50 %)	0.91(0.56-1.48)	0.72
rs10766197, *CYP2R1*	AA	52/232 (23 %)	19/104 (18 %)	Ref	-
	AG/GG	124/232 (77 %)	55/104 (82 %)	0.68(0.37-1.26)	0.23

[a]Odds ratio adjusted for monthly income and vitamin D status, *SNP* single nucleotide polymorphism, *Ref* Referent category, *VDR* Vitamin D receptor, *CYP2R1* Vitamin D 25-hydroxylase, *DBP* Vitamin D binding protein. The total number of samples is less than 260 and 112 in cases and controls respectively due to failed genotyping for some samples

Table 4 Association between vitamin D deficiency and host genotype, stratified by vitamin D status

SNP, gene	Genotype	Serum 25(OH) D ≤20 nmol/l				Serum 25(OH) D >20 nmol/l				Adjusted ratio of odds ratios[a]	P $_{interaction}$
		TB cases	Controls	OR(95 % CI)	P	TB cases	Control	OR(95 % CI)	P		
rs7312236, *VDR*	AA	30/102(29 %)	12/24(50 %)	Ref	-	54/128(42 %)	30/76(40 %)	Ref	-	Ref	-
	AG/GG	72/102(71 %)	12/24(50 %)	2.40(0.96-5.94)	0.054	74/128(58 %)	46/76(60 %)	0.89(0.50-1.59)	0.70	1.65(0.59-4.58)	0.33
rs154410, *VDR*	CC	16/105(15 %)	8/25(32 %)	Ref	-	37/130(29 %)	21/81(26 %)	Ref		Ref	-
	CT/TT	89/105(85 %)	17/25(68 %)	2.61(0.96-7.07)	0.052	93/130(71 %)	60/81(74 %)	0.88(0.47-1.64)	0.68	2.16(0.69-6.75)	0.18
rs228570, *VDR*	GG	60/105(57 %)	13/25(52 %)	Ref	-	77/130(59 %)	55/82(67 %)	Ref		Ref	-
	GA/AA	45/105(43 %)	12/25(48 %)	0.81(0.33-1.94)	0.64	53/130(41 %)	27/82(33 %)	1.40(0.78-2.5)	0.25	0.48(0.17-1.29)	0.14
rs10500804, *CYP2R1*	GG	27/102(26 %)	6/23(26 %)	Ref	-	32/129(25 %)	16/80(20 %)	Ref		Ref	-
	GT/TT	75/102(74 %)	17/23(74 %)	0.98(0.35-2.74)	0.97	97/129(75 %)	64/80(80 %)	0.75(0.38-1.49)	0.42	1.51(0.47-4.8)	0.48
rs2060793, *CYP2R1*	GG	48/104(46 %)	11/22(50 %)	Ref	-	64/124(52 %)	40/79(51 %)	Ref		Ref	-
	AG/AA	56/104(54 %)	11/22(50 %)	1.16(0.46-2.92)	0.74	60/124(48 %)	39/79(49 %)	0.96(0.54-1.69)	0.89	1.02(0.37-2.78)	0.96
rs10766197, *CYP2R1*	AA	23/104(22 %)	4/23(17 %)	Ref	-	29/128(23 %)	15/81(19 %)	Ref		Ref	-
	AG/GG	81/104(78 %)	19/23(83 %)	0.74(0.22-2.39)	0.60	99/128(77 %)	66/81(81 %)	0.77(0.38-1.55)	0.47	1.25(0.35-4.45)	0.72
rs7041, *DBP*	AA	27/104(52 %)	4/23(43.5 %)	Ref	-	26/133(20 %)	19/74(47 %)	Ref		Ref	-
	AC/CC	77/10(35 %)	19/23(43.5 %)	0.60(0.18-1.9)	0.39	107/133(80 %)	55/74(45 %)	1.42(0.72-2.79)	0.30	1.15(0.34-3.88)	0.81
rs4588, *DBP*	GG	55/105(52 %)	10/24(42 %)	Ref	-	68/135(50 %)	38/76(50 %)	Ref	-	Ref	-
	GT/TT	50/105(48 %)	14/24(58 %)	0.64(0.26-1.59)	0.34	67/135(50 %)	38/76(50 %)	0.98(0.56-1.72)	0.95	0.93(0.35-2.48)	0.89

[a]Adjusted for monthly income and vitamin D status, *SNP* single nucleotide polymorphism, *Ref* Referent category; *VDR*, Vitamin D receptor; *CYP2R1*, Vitamin D 25-hydroxylase; *DBP*, Vitamin D binding protein. The total number of samples is less than 260 and 112 in cases and controls respectively due to failed genotyping for some samples

By contrast, our study did not replicate previous reports of associations between polymorphisms in *VDR* and *DBP* and susceptibility to active TB [4, 13], either as main effects or in interaction with serum 25(OH)D concentration. Neither did we find any such associations for variants in *CYP2R1*. "A recent study in pulmonary TB in a cohort of HIV-infected and HIV exposed uninfected children in South Africa also showed no association between polymorphisms in VDR, DBP and CYP2R1 and a diagnosis of TB [5]. It should be noted, however, that our study was formally powered to detect associations between vitamin D deficiency and susceptibility to active tuberculosis, rather than genetic associations: the strength of previously reported associations is modest, and we may have lacked power to detect weaker associations. Another limitation of this study is that we collected information on a limited set of confounders. Despite adjustment for these, we cannot exclude the possibility that residual confounding may have contributed to the association seen.

Women participants in this study had lower vitamin D status that was in keeping with our previous reports that female gender is a risk factor for vitamin D deficiency; women may experiencing less sun exposure than men, and may also have lower dietary vitamin D intake [14, 15].

Conclusion

In conclusion, our study reports an independent association between vitamin D deficiency and susceptibility to active tuberculosis in Pakistani adults. However, polymorphisms in *VDR*, *DBP* and *CYP2R1* were not found to associate with susceptibility to disease in this setting.

Competing interests

The authors declare that they have no competing interests.

Authors'contributions

KJ designed the study, carried out experimental work and drafted this manuscript; AR helped in study design and drafting this manuscript; DAJ helped in drafting of this manuscript and experimental work, KW carried out genotyping, ARM contributed to study design, statistical analysis and critical review of drafts of the manuscript. All authors read and approved the final manuscript.

Acknowledgements

This study was supported by Higher Education Commission of Pakistan grant number BM7-139.

Author details

[1]Department of Microbiology and Molecular Genetics, University of the Punjab, Quaid-e-Azam Campus, Lahore 5400, Pakistan. [2]Centre for Primary Care and Public Health, Barts and The London School of Medicine and Dentistry, Queen Mary University of London, London E1 2AB, UK. [3]Gulab Devi Chest Hospital, Lahore, Pakistan. [4]Genome Centre, Barts and the London School of Medicine and Dentistry, Queen Mary University of London, London EC1M 6BQ, UK.

References

1. WHO: Global tuberculosis report In. Geneva, Switzerland: World Health Organization; 2015.
2. Martineau AR. Old wine in new bottles: vitamin D in the treatment and prevention of tuberculosis. Proc Nutr Soc. 2012;71(01):84–9.
3. Wilkinson RJ, Llewelyn M, Toossi Z, Patel P, Pasvol G, Lalvani A, Wright D, Latif M, Davidson RN. Influence of vitamin D deficiency and vitamin D receptor polymorphisms on tuberculosis among Gujarati Asians in west London: a case-control study. Lancet. 2000;355(9204):618–21.
4. Martineau AR, Leandro ACC, Anderson ST, Newton SM, Wilkinson KA, Nicol MP, Pienaar SM, Skolimowska KH, Rocha MA, Rolla VC. Association between Gc genotype and susceptibility to TB is dependent on vitamin D status. Eur Respir J. 2010;35(5):1106–12.
5. Gupta A, Montepiedra G, Gupte A, Zeldow B, Jubulis J, Detrick B, Violari A, Madhi S, Bobat R, Cotton M. Low Vitamin-D Levels Combined with PKP3-SIGIRR-TMEM16J Host Variants Is Associated with Tuberculosis and Death in HIV-Infected and-Exposed Infants. PLoS One. 2016;11(2), e0148649.
6. Wang TJ, Zhang F, Richards JB, Kestenbaum B, Van Meurs JB, Berry D, Kiel DP, Streeten EA, Ohlsson C, Koller DL. Common genetic determinants of vitamin D insufficiency: a genome-wide association study. Lancet. 2010;376(9736):180–8.
7. Martineau AR, Maclaughlin BD, Hooper RL, Barnes NC, Jolliffe DA, Greiller CL, Kilpin K, McLaughlin D, Fletcher G, Mein CA. Double-blind randomised placebo-controlled trial of bolus-dose vitamin D3 supplementation in adults with asthma (ViDiAs). Thorax. 2015;70(5):451–7.
8. Sullivan KM, Dean A, Soe MM. OpenEpi: a web-based epidemiologic and statistical calculator for public health. Public Health Rep. 2009;124(3):471.
9. Iftikhar R, Kamran SM, Qadir A, Haider E, Bin UH. Vitamin D deficiency in patients with tuberculosis. J Coll Physicians Surg Pak. 2013;23(10):780–3.
10. Nnoaham KE, Clarke A. Low serum vitamin D levels and tuberculosis: a systematic review and meta-analysis. Int J Epidemiol. 2008;37(1):113–9.
11. Talat N, Perry S, Parsonnet J, Dawood G, Hussain R. Vitamin D deficiency and tuberculosis progression. Emerg Infect Dis. 2010;16(5):853.
12. Martineau AR, Wilkinson KA, Newton SM, Floto RA, Norman AW, Skolimowska K, Davidson RN, Sørensen OE, Kampmann B, Griffiths CJ. IFN-γ-and TNF-independent vitamin D-inducible human suppression of mycobacteria: the role of cathelicidin LL-37. J Immunol. 2007;178(11):7190–8.
13. Huang L, Liu C, Liao G, Yang X, Tang X, Chen J. Vitamin D receptor gene foki polymorphism contributes to increasing the risk of tuberculosis: an update meta-analysis. Medicine. 2015;94(51):e2256.
14. Junaid K, Rehman A, Saeed T, Jolliffe DA, Wood K, Martineau AR. Genotype-independent association between profound vitamin D deficiency and delayed sputum smear conversion in pulmonary tuberculosis. BMC Infect Dis. 2015;15(1):1.
15. Junaid K, Rehman A, Jolliffe DA, Wood K, Martineau AR. High prevalence of vitamin D deficiency among women of child-bearing age in Lahore Pakistan, associating with lack of sun exposure and illiteracy. BMC Womens Health. 2015;15(1):1.

12

Rapid urine lipoarabinomannan assay as a clinic-based screening test for active tuberculosis at HIV diagnosis

Paul K. Drain[1,2,3,7*], Elena Losina[4,6,8], Sharon M. Coleman[9], Janet Giddy[10], Douglas Ross[11], Jeffrey N. Katz[8] and Ingrid V. Bassett[4,5,6]

Abstract

Background: World Health Organization (WHO) recommends tuberculosis (TB) screening at HIV diagnosis. We evaluated the inclusion of rapid urine lipoarabinomannan (LAM) testing in TB screening algorithms.

Methods: We enrolled ART-naïve adults who screened HIV-infected in KwaZulu-Natal, assessed TB-related symptoms (cough, fever, night sweats, weight loss), and obtained sputum specimens for mycobacterial culture. Trained nurses performed clinic-based urine LAM testing using a rapid assay. We used diagnostic accuracy, negative predictive value (NPV), and negative likelihood ratio, stratified by CD4 count, to evaluate screening for culture-positive TB.

Results: Among 675 HIV-infected adults with median CD4 of 213/mm^3 (interquartile range 85-360/mm^3), 123 (18%) had culture-confirmed pulmonary TB. The WHO-recommended algorithm of any TB-related symptom had a sensitivity of 77% [95% confidence interval (CI) 69-84%] and NPV of 89% (95% CI 84-92%) for identifying active pulmonary TB. Including the LAM assay improved sensitivity (83%; 95% CI 75-89%) and NPV (91%; 95% CI 86-94%), while decreasing the negative likelihood ratio (0.45 versus 0.57). Among participants with CD4 < 100/mm^3, including urine LAM testing improved the negative predictive value of symptom based screening from 83% to 87%. All screening algorithms with urine LAM performed better among participants with CD4 < 100/mm^3, compared to those with CD4 ≥ 100/mm^3.

Conclusion: Clinic-based urine LAM screening increased the sensitivity of symptom-based screening by 6% among ART-naïve HIV-infected adults in a TB-endemic setting, thereby providing marginal benefit.

Keywords: Tuberculosis, HIV/AIDS, Lipoarabinomannan (LAM), Urine, Diagnostic screening, South Africa

Background

Over 9 million people develop active *Mycobacterium tuberculosis* (TB) infection each year, and TB remains a leading cause of HIV-related mortality [1, 2]. In 2006, the World Health Organization (WHO) suggested systematic screening for active TB in HIV-infected adults by assessing the presence of a cough for at least two weeks [3]. In 2011, following a meta-analysis of 12 observational studies, WHO recommended systematic screening by assessing the presence of any TB-related symptom—current cough, fever, night sweats, and weight loss [4–7]. Symptom-based screening misses approximately one-quarter of active TB cases among HIV-infected adults [7], and a more recent study suggested this might be as high as 76% of active TB cases in western South Africa [8]. The Xpert® MTB/RIF assay has been endorsed by the WHO as the primary diagnostic test for HIV-associated pulmonary TB among those with symptoms, but is not recommended for use as a screening test. [9] A better screening strategy for HIV-associated TB is needed to accurately initiate anti-TB treatment for active disease or isoniazid preventive therapy for latent infections [10].

* Correspondence: pkdrain@uw.edu
[1]Department of Global Health, University of Washington, 325 Ninth Ave, UW Box 359927, Seattle, WA 98104-2420, USA
[2]Department of Medicine, University of Washington, Seattle, WA, USA
Full list of author information is available at the end of the article

A rapid urine lateral flow assay to detect lipoarabinomannan (LAM), a glycolipid released from the cell wall of TB, has been shown to reduce mortality among HIV-infected hospitalized patients with TB-related symptoms when used to guide anti-TB treatment [11, 12]. In two clinic-based studies, we demonstrated that the rapid urine LAM assay had poor overall diagnostic sensitivity (28-41%) to be used as a stand-alone TB screening test at HIV diagnosis [13, 14]. With similar results from another outpatient screening study [15, 16], the WHO recently recommended against using the urine LAM assay as a TB screening test. [17] However, since the rapid LAM assay can be easily performed by nurses in a clinic [13, 14], we sought to determine if urine LAM testing might augment symptom-based TB screening at HIV diagnosis in a high TB-endemic region of South Africa.

Methods

Study design and participant selection

We conducted a prospective, clinic-based study enrolling consecutive ART-naïve HIV-infected adults in the ambulatory clinical areas of two hospitals and two municipal health centers in KwaZulu-Natal, South Africa from October 2011 to January 2014. The parent study has been described in detail [18]. Eligible participants were adults (≥18 years), not known to be pregnant, and not having received anti-TB therapy within three months. Ethics committees of the two local hospitals (McCord Hospital and St. Mary's Hospital) and Partners Health-Care in Boston [Protocol #: 2006-P-001379/40] approved the study, and all participants provided written informed consent.

Study procedures

Prior to study commencement, a representative from Alere Inc., the manufacturer of the rapid LAM assay, conducted a training session for study nurses. The session reviewed the procedures and interpretation of the Determine™ TB LAM assay (Alere Inc., Waltham, USA), and study nurses practiced performing and interpreting the urine LAM assay until comfortable. Throughout the study, LAM tests and reagents were maintained in a sealed pouch and stored out of direct sunlight, in accordance with the manufacturer's specifications. Regular oversight of the nurses' LAM testing procedures ensured continued testing competence and proficiency.

At participant enrollment, trained study nurses collected demographic and clinical information, including TB-related symptoms—current cough, fever, night sweats, and weight loss. Study nurses tested urine samples for LAM using the Determine™ TB LAM assay and interpreted results after 25 minutes. Participants provided one respiratory sputum sample, and those unable to provide an expectorated sputum sample received sputum induction with 3% hypertonic saline using a nebulizer (WH-802, Yuehua Medical Instrument Factory Co.; Guangdong, China). Sputum samples were decontaminated with N-acetyl L Cysteine and NaOH to a final concentration of 1.25% before being centrifuged at 3,000 revs for 20 minutes and resuspended in 1 ml of 7H9 broth. 0.5 ml of the suspension was inoculated into Bactec™ 960 mycobacterial growth indicator tubes (MGIT™) (BD; Franklin Lakes, USA), and solid culture Middlebrook 7H11 agar medium. *M. tuberculosis* was confirmed using niacin and nitrate testing. Participants received chest radiography, as indicated, which was interpreted by a certified radiologist. All participants were offered treatment in accordance with local and South African Department of Health guidelines [19].

Statistical analyses

Participants were considered culture-positive if *M. tuberculosis* was identified from either liquid or solid culture media, and we used culture of sputum as the accepted gold-standard diagnostic test. [20] We categorized LAM test results as positive vs. negative, using the manufacturer's 5-grade reference card. We defined a positive LAM test as grade 1 or higher, since this study was conducted before the reference card was changed to grade 2 or higher and in order to maximize diagnostic sensitivity for screening algorithms. We calculated diagnostic sensitivity, specificity, and negative predictive values of various screening algorithms, both with and without the urine LAM assay. Combined algorithms allowed for either screening test modality to be positive, since requiring multiple modalities to be positive lowered diagnostic sensitivity to an unacceptable level (29%) for a screening algorithm. We stratified algorithms above and below CD4 100/mm^3. We used Fisher's exact test to compare diagnostic sensitivity, specificity, and negative predictive value between groups. We also calculated negative likelihood ratios [the probability of a person who has the disease testing negative divided by the probability of a person who does not have the disease testing negative; (1-sensitivity/specificity)] to determine whether a test result changed the probability of excluding disease. The formula for calculating negative likelihood ratio includes both sensitivity and specificity, so a reduced value (< 1) indicates a favorable balance between sensitivity and specificity for a diagnostic screening "rule out" test. The WHO considers the negative predictive value (NPV; the proportion of algorithm-negative subjects who proved NOT to have TB) to be the most important parameters for a screening algorithm to exclude active TB disease [6]. We used the likelihood ratio to generate post-test probabilities based on estimated population TB prevalences of 5%, 10% and 20%. We calculated exact 95% confidence intervals (CI), reported two-tailed p-values ($\alpha = 0.05$), and used SAS 9.4 (Cary, USA).

Results

We enrolled 757 ART-naïve HIV-infected adults. After excluding 31 people without a urine specimen, and 51 people who had no mycobacterial culture results, our analyses included 675 adults. Mean age was 34 years (standard deviation ±10 years), 359 (53%) participants were male, 58 (9%) participants reported a prior TB infection, 165 (24%) participants were current smokers, and 3 (< 1%) participants were taking a diuretic medication (Table 1). The median CD4 count was 213/mm^3 (interquartile range 85-360/mm^3).

Overall, 425 (63%) participants reported ≥ 1 TB-related symptom, and each TB-related symptom was reported by 31-39% of participants. Fifty-two (8%) participants had an abnormal chest x-ray, 36 (5%) people were sputum smear AFB positive, and 89 (13%) participants were positive by a single urine LAM assay. 123 people had culture confirmed pulmonary TB, and the estimated prevalence of culture-confirmed pulmonary TB was 18.2% (95% CI 15-21%). Prevalence of TB was 30% (71/238) and 12% (52/437) among those with CD4 < 100/mm^3 and CD4 ≥ 100/mm^3, respectively.

Table 1 Cohort characteristics of HIV-infected adults ($N = 675$).

	Mean ± SD or N (%)
Demographics	
Age (years)	34 ± 10
Male gender	359 (53)
Clinical	
Prior TB infection	58 (9)
Currently Smoke	165 (24)
Taking a Diuretic Medication	3 (1)
TB-related Symptoms	
Any TB-related Symptom	425 (63)
Current cough	242 (36)
Fever	220 (33)
Night sweats	211 (31)
Weight loss	264 (39)
CD4 Cell Count (median/IQR)/mm^3 ($N = 611$)	213 (85, 360)
≥ 100 cells/mm^3	437 (74)
< 100 cells/mm^3	174 (29)
Radiography	
Abnormal chest x-ray	52 (8)
Rapid Urine LAM testing	
Positive by Rapid Urine LAM Test	89 (13)
Tuberculosis test results	
Sputum smear acid-fast bacilli positive	36 (5)
Culture-confirmed pulmonary TB positive	123 (18)

IQR interquartile range, *LAM* lipoarabinomannan, *SD* standard deviation, *TB* tuberculosis

The diagnostic sensitivity of presence of a cough alone was 54% (95% CI 44-63%) (Table 2). The WHO-recommended symptom-based screening algorithm (i.e. presence of any TB-related symptom) had a diagnostic sensitivity of 77% (95% CI 69-84%) and specificity of 40% (95% CI 36-44%). The combination of any TB-related symptom or abnormal chest radiography had 83% (95% CI 75-89%) sensitivity. The negative predictive value was 89% (95% CI 84-92%) for symptom-based screening, and 91% (95% CI 87-95%) when including chest radiography.

The urine LAM assay identified 25% (7/28) of TB-infected adults who did not have any TB-related symptom. The diagnostic sensitivity when incorporating the urine LAM assay with symptom-based screening was 83% (95% CI 75-89%), and with symptom-based screening plus chest radiography was 87% (95% CI 80-92%). Diagnostic specificity decreased by 2-3% in both algorithms, and was 95% among participants without TB-related symptoms. The addition of the urine LAM assay increased the negative predictive value by 2% in both screening algorithms. The highest negative predictive values were any TB-related symptom or urine LAM positive (91%; 95% CI 86-94%), and a combination of symptom screening, urine LAM, and chest radiography (93%; 95% CI 89-96%).

All screening algorithms, except those with current cough as the only TB-symptom, had higher diagnostic sensitivity among participants with CD4 < 100/mm^3, as compared to those with CD4 ≥ 100/mm^3 (Table 3). These differences were significant for symptom-based screening ($p = 0.05$) and symptoms plus chest radiography ($p = 0.03$). All algorithms had significantly lower diagnostic specificities among participants with CD4 < 100/mm^3 (p-values <0.001). A combination of symptom screening, urine LAM, and chest radiography had a negative predictive value of 94% (95% CI 89-97%) among participants with CD4 ≥ 100/mm^3, and 91% (95% CI 80-97%) among participants with CD4 < 100/mm^3.

We calculated negative likelihood ratios, which include sensitivity and specificity in a single formula, to identify the algorithm with lowest and therefore most favorable screening profile (Table 4). Overall, presence of any TB-related symptom had a negative likelihood ratio of 0.57 (95% CI 0.40-0.80), which reduces the post-test probability of a patient having active TB from 18% to 11%. The combination of symptom-based screening and chest radiography had a negative likelihood ratio of 0.43 (95% CI 0.29-0.64), which was not significantly better than

Table 2 Diagnostic accuracy of symptoms and rapid testing for diagnosing culture-confirmed pulmonary tuberculosis.

	Sensitivity		Specificity		Positive PV	Negative PV
	Positive/Total	% (95% CI)	Negative/Total	% (95% CI)	% (95% CI)	% (95% CI)
Existing screening algorithms						
Cough	66/123	54 (44–63)	376/552	68 (64–72)	27 (22–33)	87 (83–90)
Any TB-related Symptom[a]	95/123	77 (69–84)	222/552	40 (36–44)	22 (18–27)	89 (84–92)
Any TB-related Symptom[a] or Abnormal chest x-ray	102/123	83 (75–89)	219/552	40 (36–44)	23 (20–28)	91 (87–95)
Urine LAM alone						
Urine LAM Test Positive	38/123	31 (23–39)	508/552	92 (89–94)	46 (35–58)	86 (83–88)
Adding urine LAM to existing screening algorithms						
Cough or Urine LAM Positive	84/123	68 (59–76)	353/552	63 (60–68)	30 (24–35)	90 (87–93)
Any TB-related Symptom[a] or Urine LAM Positive	102/123	83 (75–89)	205/552	37 (33–41)	23 (19–27)	91 (86–94)
Any TB-related Symptom[a] or Abnormal chest x-ray or Urine LAM Positive	107/123	87 (80–92)	208/552	38 (34–42)	24 (20–28)	93 (89–96)

CI confidence interval, *LAM* lipoarabinomannan, *PV* predictive value, *TB* tuberculosis
[a] TB-related symptoms were current cough, fever, night sweats, and weight loss

symptom-based screening alone. Incorporating the urine LAM assay into these screening algorithms lowered the negative likelihood ratios to 0.45 (95% CI 0.30-0.68) and 0.34 (95% CI 0.22-0.55), respectively. Including urine LAM in the symptom-based screening algorithm lowered the probability of active TB from 11% (using symptom-based screening alone) to 9%. All negative likelihood ratios were more favorable for participants with CD4 < 100/mm^3, compared to those with CD4 ≥ 100/mm^3.

All clinical screening algorithms improved the ability to exclude pulmonary TB, but those benefits varied by

Table 3 Diagnostic accuracy of TB-related symptoms with and without urine LAM testing for diagnosing culture-confirmed pulmonary tuberculosis by CD4 count ≥ and <100 cell/mm^3

	Sensitivity			Specificity			Negative PV	
	Positive/Total	% (95% CI)	*p*-value	Negative/Total	% (95% CI)	*p*-value	% (95% CI)	*p*-value
Cough			0.35			0.005		<0.0001
CD4 ≥ 100 cells/mm^3	25/52	48 (34–62)		270/385	70 (65–75)	—	91 (87–94)	—
CD4 < 100 cells/mm^3	41/71	58 (45–69)		106/167	63 (56–71)	—	78 (70–85)	—
Cough or Urine LAM Positive			0.24			0.007		0.0002
CD4 ≥ 100 cells/mm^3	32/52	62 (47–75)	—	255/385	66 (61–71)	—	93 (90–96)	—
CD4 < 100 cells/mm^3	52/71	73 (61–83)	—	98/167	59 (51–66)	—	84 (76–90)	—
Any TB-related Symptom[a]			0.05			<0.0001		0.0007
CD4 ≥ 100 cells/mm^3	35/52	67 (53–80)	—	168/385	44 (39–49)	—	91 (86–95)	—
CD4 < 100 cells/mm^3	60/71	85 (74–92)	—	54/167	32 (25–40)	—	83 (72–91)	—
Any TB-related Symptom[a] or Urine LAM Positive			0.09			<0.0001		0.004
CD4 ≥ 100 cells/mm^3	39/52	75 (61–86)	—	159/385	41 (36–46)	—	92 (87–96)	—
CD4 < 100 cells/mm^3	63/71	89 (79–95)	—	52/167	31 (24–39)	—	87 (75–94)	—
Any TB-related Symptom[a] or Abnormal chest x-ray			0.03			<0.0001		0.007
CD4 ≥ 100 cells/mm^3	38/52	73 (59–84)	—	168/385	44 (39–49)	—	92 (88–96)	—
CD4 < 100 cells/mm^3	64/71	90 (81–96)	—	51/167	31 (24–38)	—	88 (77–95)	—
Any TB-related Symptom[a] or Abnormal chest x-ray or Urine LAM Positive			0.06			<0.0001		0.03
CD4 ≥ 100 cells/mm^3	41/52	79 (65–89)	—	159/385	41 (36–46)	—	94 (89–97)	—
CD4 < 100 cells/mm^3	66/71	93 (84–98)	—	49/167	29 (23–37)	—	91 (80–97)	—

CI confidence interval, *LAM* lipoarabinomannan, *TB* tuberculosis
[a]TB-related symptoms were current cough, fever, night sweats, and weight loss

Table 4 Screening strategies for diagnosing culture-confirmed pulmonary tuberculosis

	Screening without Urine LAM LR- (95% CI)	Screening with Urine LAM LR- (95% CI)	Difference
Entire Cohort			
Cough	0.68 (0.56–0.83)	0.50 (0.38–0.65)	−0.18
Any TB-related Symptom[a]	0.57 (0.40–0.80)	0.45 (0.30–0.68)	−0.12
Any TB-related Symptom[a] or Abnormal chest x-ray	0.43 (0.29–0.64)	0.34 (0.22–0.55)	−0.09
Cohort with CD4 ≥ 100 cells/mm^3			
Cough	0.74 (0.57–0.97)	0.58 (0.41–0.83)	−0.16
Any TB-related Symptom[a]	0.75 (0.50–1.12)	0.61 (0.37–0.98)	−0.14
Any TB-related Symptom[a] or Abnormal chest x-ray	0.62 (0.39–0.98)	0.51 (0.30–0.88)	−0.11
Cohort with CD4 < 100 cells/mm^3			
Cough	0.66 (0.50–0.89)	0.46 (0.30–0.68)	−0.20
Any TB-related Symptom[a]	0.48 (0.27–0.86)	0.36 (0.18–0.72)	−0.12
Any TB-related Symptom[a] or Abnormal chest x-ray	0.32 (0.15–0.68)	0.24 (0.10–0.58)	−0.08

CI confidence interval, *LAM* lipoarabinomannan, *LR* likelihood ratio, *TB* tuberculosis
[a]TB-related symptoms were current cough, fever, night sweats, and weight loss

the estimated population TB prevalence (Fig. 1). Assuming a population TB prevalence of 20%, screening negative for any TB-related symptom decreased the post-test probability of active TB disease by 37.6%. In comparison, including urine LAM in the symptom screening algorithm decreased the post-test probability by 49.4%, and including both urine LAM and chest radiography decreased the post-test probability by 60.8%. These differences were more apparent among populations with a high TB prevalence (20%) as compared to populations with a low (≤ 5%) or moderate TB prevalence (10%).

Discussion

In this high TB-burden region of South Africa, the current symptom-based TB screening algorithm performed at initial HIV diagnosis missed nearly one-quarter of active TB cases, and had many false positive results. In particular, the WHO's recommended symptom-based screening algorithm had a sub-optimal negative predictive value for detecting active HIV-associated TB among patients with CD4 < 100 cells/mm^3 in this setting. Additional screening with the urine LAM assay at HIV diagnosis had marginal benefits to the existing symptom-based screening algorithm. Urine LAM testing identified one-quarter (7/28) of TB-infected adults who did not endorse any TB-related symptom, which increased the overall diagnostic sensitivity by 6%. This combined screening algorithm still missed 17% of active TB cases (83% sensitivity) among all patients, which does not meet the minimum requirements established by the WHO [21, 22]. In addition, this combination had a high rate of false positive screening results, due mostly to symptom-based screening. The overall utility of urine LAM screening improved the negative likelihood ratios, but the changes were modest. Any benefit of urine LAM appeared to be greatest in populations with a high estimated TB prevalence and CD4 < 100/mm^3.

Our findings are consistent with a meta-analysis of 12 clinical studies that reported a similar diagnostic sensitivity (79%), but higher diagnostic specificity (50%), of symptom-based screening for culture-confirmed active TB among HIV-infected adults [7]. The meta-analysis included observational studies that collected sputum regardless of symptoms, assessed TB-related symptoms and HIV status, and used mycobacterial culture as the gold standard diagnostic test. The addition of chest radiography in the meta-analysis (defined as positive symptoms OR chest radiography) increased sensitivity to 90%, which was higher than our cohort (83%), but decreased specificity to 39%. Taken together, their calculated negative likelihood ratio was 0.43 by symptom screening alone and 0.26 when including chest radiography, which was lower (better) than our findings. However, only 3 studies included in the meta-analysis were conducted in a setting with a TB prevalence >10%—two were in Southeast Asia [23, 24], and one South African study had a small sample size with 58 culture-positive TB participants [25]. Our results further highlight the urgent need for a better TB screening algorithm among HIV-infected adults.

The negative predictive value, which changes a pre-test probability of disease into a post-test probability of disease, is a critical clinical measure for excluding TB disease by a screening algorithm [6]. When screening a population with a high estimated TB prevalence (20%), the meta-analysis reported a negative predictive value of the WHO algorithm at 90%, similar to our cohort

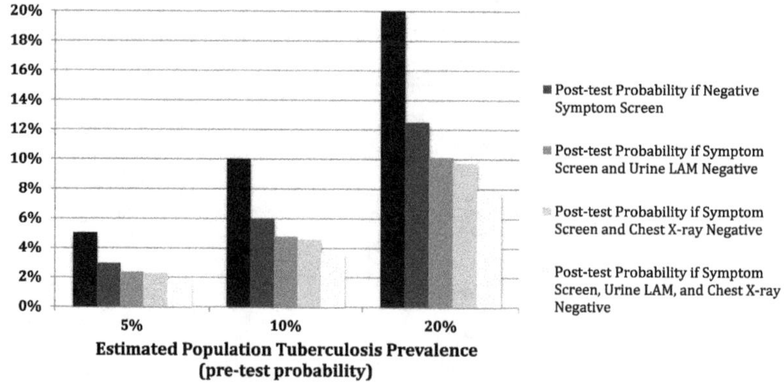

Fig. 1 Pre- and post-test probabilities for various screening algorithms for HIV-infected populations with TB prevalence of 5%, 10%, and 20%

(89%). While our cohort had a more modest increase with the addition of chest radiography (89% to 91%), the most significant impact was achieved when adding both urine LAM and chest radiography (93%). In this algorithm, 7% of those who screening negative will still have active TB disease, which highlights the continued need for an improved screening algorithm.

The consequences of inaccurate TB screening among HIV-infected adults are severe, and include missed diagnosis and inappropriate treatment of active TB, unnecessary delays for antiretroviral therapy and isoniazid preventive therapy (IPT) initiation while awaiting sputum-based diagnostic testing, inadequate provision of IPT, overprescribing of empiric TB therapy, and high loss to follow-up rates with increased program costs [8, 26]. For these reasons, the WHO has prioritized a rapid screening test that can be used by first-contact health care providers to screen for active TB, which will "triage" patients to either receive immediate IPT or diagnostic sputum-based testing with the Xpert MTB/RIF assay [21, 22]. Since the urine LAM test meets several of the WHO requirements (specificity > 70%, point-of-care test with minimal steps, time to result < 30 minutes) [21, 22], but falls short of having > 90% diagnostic sensitivity [13–15], groups are working to develop a more sensitive urinary LAM assay. In an Ethiopian cohort, increasing the LAM assay detection 50-fold by using high-avidity monoclonal antibodies improved the diagnostic sensitivity of urine LAM testing to 93% [27].

Our study had several additional strengths and limitations. Primary strengths were evaluating the urine LAM assay when used by trained nurses in ambulatory settings, which is similar to a real-world application, assessing both liquid and solid mycobacterial culture as the gold standard, enrolling people prior to HIV diagnosis and ART initiation, and assessing urine LAM among people with a range of CD4 counts. Limitations included obtaining a single sputum sample for mycobacterial culture and not performing a comprehensive evaluation for extrapulmonary TB, both of which could have misclassified people as not having TB due to an imperfect reference standard. We excluded the patients who did not provide a urine or sputum sample. Although this study was among the largest TB screening studies in HIV-infected adults [7], a limited sample size prevented the detection of statistically significant differences in improved diagnostic sensitivity and negative predictive values, or reduced negative likelihood ratios, for new screening algorithms. The WHO guidelines recommend that HIV-infected adults be screened for TB at every visit to a health facility or contact with a health worker, which we did not evaluate in our study.

Conclusions

In conclusion, our results demonstrate a marginal benefit from the inclusion of rapid urine LAM screening to clinical symptom screening among ART-naïve HIV-infected adults in resource-constrained TB-endemic regions. Future studies should examine the role of point-of-care testing to expedite initiation of anti-TB therapy and include a cost-effectiveness analysis for clinic-based LAM screening. The current urine LAM assay is imperfect and does not solve the public health challenge of screening or diagnosing TB. However, since the principles behind the urine LAM assay are sound, an improved, next-generation urinary LAM assay could meet the criteria for a rapid, clinic-based TB screening test among HIV-infected adults in TB-endemic settings.

Abbreviations

ART: Antiretroviral therapy; CI: Confidence interval; IPT: Isoniazid preventive therapy; IQR: Interquartile range; LAM: Lipoarabinomannan; LR: Likelihood ratio; NPV: Negative predictive value; SD: Standard deviation; TB: Tuberculosis; WHO: World Health Organization

Acknowledgements

We thank the women and men who participated in this study, each of the clinical sites for sharing their space, and our research staff and nurses who carried out the study.

Funding
This work was supported by the Harvard Global Health Institute (PKD); the Fogarty International Clinical Research Scholars and Fellows Program at Vanderbilt University [R24 TW007988] (PKD); the Infectious Disease Society of America Education & Research Foundation and National Foundation for Infectious Diseases (PKD); Massachusetts General Hospital Executive Committee on Research (PKD); the Program in AIDS Clinical Research Training Grant [T32 AI007433] (PKD); the National Institute of Mental Health [R01 MH090326] (IVB); the National Institute of Allergy and Infectious Diseases [K23 AI108293] (PKD); the Harvard University Center for AIDS Research [P30 AI060354] (PKD); the National Institute of Arthritis and Musculoskeletal and Skin Diseases [K24 AR057827] (EL); and the National Center for Research Resources [Harvard Catalyst UL1 RR 025758]. The content is solely the responsibility of the authors and does not represent the official views of the National Institutes of Health or other funding agencies.

Authors' contributions
PKD designed the study with input from IVB and EL; PKD, EL and SMC conducted and reviewed the statistical analyses; PKD, JG, DG, JNK and IVB participated in overseeing the conduct of the clinical trial; PKD prepared the first draft of the manuscript. All authors reviewed and approved the final draft of the manuscript.

Competing interests
The authors declare that they have no competing interest.

Consent for publication
Not Applicable.

Author details
[1]Department of Global Health, University of Washington, 325 Ninth Ave, UW Box 359927, Seattle, WA 98104-2420, USA. [2]Department of Medicine, University of Washington, Seattle, WA, USA. [3]Department of Epidemiology, University of Washington, Seattle, WA, USA. [4]Medical Practice Evaluation Center, Harvard Medical School, Boston, USA. [5]Division of Infectious Diseases, Harvard Medical School, Boston, USA. [6]Division of General Internal Medicine, Harvard Medical School, Boston, USA. [7]Department of Surgery, Massachusetts General Hospital, Harvard Medical School, Boston, USA. [8]Department of Orthopedic Surgery, Brigham and Women's Hospital, Harvard Medical School, Boston, USA. [9]Boston University School of Public Health, Boston, USA. [10]Department of Medicine, McCord Hospital, Durban, South Africa. [11]Department of Medicine, St. Mary's Hospital, Durban, South Africa.

References
1. World Health Organization. Global tuberculosis report 2015. Geneva: World Health Organization; 2015.
2. World Health Organization. WHO policy on collaborative TB/HIV activities. Geneva: World Health Organization; 2012.
3. World Health Organization. Improving the diagnosis and treatment of smear-negative pulmonary and extrapulmonary tuberculosis among adults and adolescents. Geneva: World Health Organization; 2006.
4. Stop TB Partnership, World Health Organization Global TB Programme. Reach the 3 million: Find. Treat. Cure TB. Geneva: World Health Organization; 2014.
5. World Health Organization. Systematic screening for active tuberculosis: principles and recommendations. Geneva: World Health Organization; 2013.
6. World Health Organization. Guidelines for intensified tuberculosis case-finding and isoniazid preventive therapy for people living with HIV in resource-constrained settings. Geneva: World Health Organization; 2011.
7. Getahun H, Kittikraisak W, Heilig CM, et al. Development of a standardized screening rule for tuberculosis in people living with HIV in resource-constrained settings: individual participant data meta-analysis of observational studies. PLoS Med. 2011;8:e1000391.
8. Rangaka M, Wilkinson RJ, Glynn JR, et al. Effect of antiretroviral therapy on the diagnostic accuracy of symptom screening for intensified case finding in a South African HIV clinic. Clin Infect Dis. 2012;55:1698–706.
9. World Health Organization. Rapid Implementation of the Xpert MTB/RIF diagnostic test: Technical and Operational 'How-to'; Practical considerations. Geneva: World Health Organization; 2011.
10. Lester R, Hamilton R, Charalambous S, et al. Barriers to implementation of isoniazid preventive therapy in HIV clinics: a qualitative study. AIDS. 2010;24 Suppl 5:S45–8.
11. Lawn SD. Point-of-care detection of lipoarabinomannan (LAM) in urine for diagnosis of HIV-associated tuberculosis: a state of the art review. BMC Infect Dis. 2012;12:103.
12. Peter JG, Zijenah LS, Chanda D, et al. Effect on mortality of point-of-care, urine-based lipoarabinomannan testing to guide tuberculosis treatment initiation in HIV-positive hospital inpatients: a pragmatic, parallel-group, multicountry, open-label, randomized controlled trial. Lancet. 2016; Published online 9 March 2016.
13. Drain PK, Losina E, Coleman SM, et al. Diagnostic accuracy of a point-of-care urine test for tuberculosis screening among newly-diagnosed HIV-infected adults: a prospective, clinic-based study. BMC Infect Dis. 2014;14:110.
14. Drain PK, Losina E, Coleman SM, et al. Value of Urine Lipoarabinomannan Grade and Second Test for Optimizing Clinic-Based Screening for HIV-Associated Pulmonary Tuberculosis. J Acquir Immune Defic Syndr. 2015;68:274–80.
15. Lawn SD, Kerkhoff AD, Vogt M, Wood R. Diagnostic accuracy of a low-cost, urine antigen, point-of-care screening assay for HIV-associated pulmonary tuberculosis before antiretroviral therapy: a descriptive study. Lancet Infect Dis. 2012;12:201–9.
16. Shah M, Hanrahan C, Wang Z, Dendukuri N, Lawn SD, Denkinger CM, Steingart KR. Lateral flow urine lipoarabinomannan assay for detecting active tuberculosis in HIV-positive adults. Cochrane Database of Systematic Reviews. 2016; (Issue 5). Art. No.: CD011420. DOI: 10.1002/14651858. CD011420.pub2
17. World Health Organization. The use of lateral flow urine lipoarabinomannan assay (LF-LAM) for the diagnosis and screening of active tuberculosis in people living with HIV; Policy guidance. Geneva: World Health Organization; 2015.
18. Bassett IV, Giddy J, Chaisson CE, et al. A randomized trial to optimize HIV/TB care in South Africa: design of the Sizanani trial. BMC Infect Dis. 2013;13:390.
19. Department of Health, Republic of South Africa. The South African Antiretroviral Treatment Guidelines 2013. Pretoria: Department of Health; 2013.
20. Liu TT, Wilson D, Dawood H, Cameron DW, Alvarez GG. Inaccuracy of death certificate diagnosis of tuberculosis and potential underdiagnosis of TB in a region of high HIV prevalence. Clin Dev Immunol. 2012;2012:937013.
21. Denkinger CM. High-priority target product profiles for new tuberculosis diagnostics: report of a consensus meeting. Geneva: World Health Organization; 2014.
22. Denkinger CM, Kik SV, Cirillo DM, et al. Defining the needs for next generation assays to Tuberculosis. J Infect Dis. 2015;211(Suppl 2):S29–38. doi:10.1093/infdis/jiu821.
23. Cain KP, McCarthy KD, Heilig CM, et al. An algorithm for tuberculosis screening and diagnosis in people with HIV. N Engl J Med. 2010;362:707–16.
24. Chheng P, Tamhane A, Natpratan C, et al. Pulmonary tuberculosis among patients visiting a voluntary confidential counseling and testing center, Cambodia. Int J Tuberc Lung Dis. 2008;12:54–62.
25. Lawn SD, Edwards DJ, Kranzer K, Vogt M, Bekker LG, Wood R. Urine lipoarabinomannan assay for tuberculosis screening before antiretroviral therapy diagnostic yield and association with immune reconstitution disease. AIDS. 2009;23:1875–80.
26. Van't Hoog A, Cobelens FG, Vassall A, et al. Optimal triage test characteristics to improve the cost-effectiveness of the Xpert MTB/RIF assay for TB diagnosis: a decision analysis. PLoS One. 2013;8:e82786.
27. Hamasur B, Bruchfeld J, van Helden P, Kallenius G, Svenson S. A sensitive urinary lipoarabinomannan test for tuberculosis. PLoS One. 2015;10:e0123457.

13

Knowledge, attitudes and practices regarding tuberculosis care among health workers in Southern Mozambique

Andrés Noé[1], Rafaela M. Ribeiro[2], Rui Anselmo[2], Maria Maixenchs[2], Layce Sitole[3], Khatia Munguambe[2,4], Silvia Blanco[2,5], Peter le Souef[1] and Alberto L. García-Basteiro[2,5,6*]

Abstract

Background: Tuberculosis (TB) control is more likely to be achieved if the level of knowledge regarding TB is increased among health workers managing high-risk groups. No formal assessments regarding knowledge, attitudes and practises of health workers about TB have been published for Mozambique, a country facing challenges in the fight against TB, with a fragile health system and considerable work overload of health personnel. The main objective of the study was to determine the level of knowledge, identify attitudes and assess practices regarding TB care and control among health care workers of the district of Manhiça.

Methods: A descriptive cross-sectional study was performed through the use of a specifically designed Knowledge, Attitudes and Practices (KAP) questionnaire in the district of Manhiça, a high tuberculosis and HIV burden rural area in Southern Mozambique. In this district, 14 health care facilities service a population of approximately 160,000 people. The questionnaire took 30–45 min to administer with external assistance not permitted. The survey contained 79 questions pertaining to four different areas: demographics, TB knowledge, attitudes and practices.

Results: The study sample included 170 health care workers. The average knowledge score was 14.89 points (SD = 3.61) out of a total possible 26 points. Less than 30% of respondents had heard of Xpert MTB/RIF®. Seventy per cent agreed there was stigma associated with TB and 48.2% believed this stigma was greater than that associated with HIV. The average practice score was 3.2 out of 9 points (35.6%, SD = 2.4).

Conclusion: Health care worker's knowledge gaps identified in this study may result in substandard patient care. Specific deficiencies in understanding existed in terms of paediatric TB and Xpert MTB/RIF® testing. The present study provides impetus for tailored TB education among health care workers from a high TB burden rural area in Southern Mozambique.

Keywords: Tuberculosis, Control, Health care workers, Mozambique, Knowledge, Attitudes, Practises

Background

The World Health Organisation (WHO) has deemed tuberculosis (TB) a global public health emergency since 1993 [1]. TB ranks as the leading cause of death from infectious disease [2]. In 2014, there were 9.6 million new cases and 1.5 million deaths due to TB [2]. Mozambique has been among the 22 high TB-burden countries for many years, ranking sixth in TB incidence [2]. The estimated incidence for the country is 551 per 100,000 [2].

TB control is more likely to be achieved if the level of knowledge regarding TB is increased among health care workers (HCWs) managing high-risk groups [3]. HCWs need to be adequately educated and trained in order to effectively treat TB [4]. In particular, front-line staff members are intrinsically linked to the success of TB control programs through their involvement in treatment services and supervision, and patient support (element three of WHO's Directly Observed Treatment Short-course approach) [5]. As such, assessing the

* Correspondence: alberto.garcia-basteiro@manhica.net
[2]Centro de Investigação em Saúde de Manhiça (CISM), CP 1929 Maputo, Mozambique
[5]ISGlobal, Barcelona Ctr. Int. Health Res. (CRESIB), Hospital Clínic - Universitat de Barcelona, Barcelona, Spain
Full list of author information is available at the end of the article

knowledge, attitudes and practices (KAP) about TB in front-line TB HCWs is essential in order to optimise difficulties, limitations and capacities for enhancement.

KAP-style surveys can be used to establish a baseline or measure intervention-related changes in a person's understanding, related thoughts and skills. Some studies have found that TB knowledge among HCWs was in general poor, especially in terms of diagnosis and treatment [6–8]. Good understanding of TB disease management is often inadequate even in the context of recent TB training [4]. By contrast, other studies suggest that TB knowledge pre-training is satisfactory and may even improve following brief education [9–11]. While the results of a once-off training program can be inconsistent, there are examples of how periodic training and supervision can improve HCWs' TB knowledge and skills [12, 13].

No KAP-style TB assessments among HCWs have been published in Mozambique, a country facing challenges in the fight against TB, with a fragile health system and considerable work overload of health personnel [14, 15]. Therefore we aimed to determine the level of knowledge, attitudes and practices regarding TB care among HCWs in a rural area in Southern Mozambique.

Methods

Study setting

We conducted a descriptive cross-sectional study over January-March 2015.

The study was conducted in the district of Manhiça, a high TB- and HIV-burden, low-resource, rural area in Southern Mozambique. [16–18] Manhiça district has very high TB incidence and TB associated mortality rates with a low case detection rate [19, 20]. In the district there is one district hospital (Hospital Distrital da Manhiça), one rural hospital (Hospital Rural de Xinavane) and 12 peripheral primary Health Care Centres (HCC). Altogether, these centres service, at the time of the survey, a population of approximately 160,000 people [21–23].

Survey and data collection

The survey was designed selecting relevant questions from previous published studies [4, 6, 9–11], and based on current Mozambican National Tuberculosis Program (NTP) guidelines, after consensus from a team including clinicians, a social scientist and an epidemiologist with experience in TB and KAP studies. The survey was conducted in an interview format as a standard, but self-administered if the HCW repeatedly (more than two times) reported they had insufficient time for an interview. The questionnaire took 30–45 min to administer with external assistance not permitted. The survey contained 79 questions pertaining to four different areas: demographics, TB knowledge, attitudes and practices. The questionnaire was written first in English and then translated to Portuguese. The demographics collected included age, gender, profession and TB-specific training.

The knowledge section contained 31 questions and was sub-divided into three sections: transmission (8 questions), diagnosis (9 questions) and treatment of TB (14 questions). Responses were established as correct or incorrect. If participants indicated more than one choice for a question or if a question was left unanswered, the question was marked as incorrect. The attitudes section posed 29 questions encompassing the subjects of quality of education of NTP HCWs, community awareness, access and barriers to the NTP, resources devoted to the NTP, treatment adherence and local TB control program priorities. The responses to these questions were obtained using a 5-point Likert scale and were collapsed into agreement, neutral or disagreement for analysis. Practices were not directly observed, rather three common practice scenarios were presented and one open question and two multiple-choice questions were posed regarding the management of these scenarios. Additional file 1 includes the questionnaire (with possible answers) in its entirety.

Data analysis

Completed questionnaires were double entered into an electronic database using the REDCap software (version 5.7.3 Copyright © RedCap Creative Group, Amarillo, TX, USA). Data was exported from completed questionnaires and prepared for analysis. Answers were scored and means were treated as continuous variables. Means and/or proportions with corresponding 95% confidence intervals were calculated for each question. These were then stratified by category of health care worker. The knowledge and practice scores were analysed using a one way analysis of variance test to study mean score differences among different groups. Tukey HSD test was used for pairwise comparisons where the analysis of variance (ANOVA) demonstrated a significant difference between the groups.

Results

In total, 170 HCWs participated in the study. This represented over 90% of the HCWs in the Manhiça district. There were eight HCWs who refused to take part in the survey. The most common reason for refusal was a lack of time to participate in the study. Fifty-one per cent of respondents were female with medical technicians (medical professionals who attended technical college) and nurses being the most common profession taking part (34.1% and 30.5%, respectively). Over half of the sample worked in Manhiça District Hospital. Seventy-five per cent of respondents reported never having had

TB-specific training. Table 1 illustrates the demographic characteristics of the study participants.

Knowledge

The average knowledge score was 14.89 points (57.3%, standard deviation (SD) = 3.61) out of a total possible score of 26 points. Greater educational attainment levels were associated with higher knowledge scores (Fig. 1a). Respondents that had attended secondary school and technical college had lower mean knowledge scores than university-educated respondents (by 3.1 points, $p = 0.01$ and 2.3 points, $p = 0.02$, respectively).

Profession affected knowledge scores (Fig. 1b). Medical doctors had the greatest knowledge score (17.5 points, SD = 3.34) while midwives had the lowest knowledge scores (13.05 points, SD = 3.61), with this difference being statistically significant ($p = 0.02$).

Working with TB patients for one year and between one and five years were both associated with a 2.3 point increase in knowledge score (Fig. 1c), compared to having never worked with TB patients ($p = 0.04$ and $p = 0.01$, respectively). Having cared for more than 40 TB patients over the HCWs' career was associated with a 1.57 point score increase over those who had cared for less than 10 patients ($p = 0.049$). Gender, place of work and age did not significantly affect knowledge scores.

Less than 30% of respondents had heard of Xpert MTB/RIF®. Of the 50 that were aware of this diagnostic test, 35 identified that it was a test used to diagnose TB and 7 HCWs acknowledged that it could also detect rifampicin resistance. Less than half of respondents accurately stated that paediatric TB was more difficult to diagnose than adult TB. When asked specifically, less than 25% of respondents correctly identified the difference in treatment time required between children and adults.

Attitudes

Ninety-five per cent of respondents agreed with the statement that community engagement was essential for the control of TB. More than 90% concurred with the idea that one should know one's own HIV serostatus. Infection control was seen as an important means to prevent the contraction of TB by 89.4% of the participants.

Seventy per cent of respondents agreed that there was a stigma associated with TB and 48.2% of them believed that this stigma was greater than that which is associated with HIV. Thirty-five per cent of the sample disagreed with the assertion, "The way I interact with TB patients contributes to TB-related stigma." Forty-four per cent of HCWs agreed with the statement, "In Mozambique, there are many barriers to TB treatment", with 35.9% disagreeing.

The statement "traditional or alternative medicine assists in the wellbeing of TB patients" led to a 71.8% disagreement rate.

Practices

Overall practice competency was low with the average practice score being 3.2 points out of 9 (35.6%, SD = 2.44).

The highest level of educational attainment and profession were associated with higher mean practice scores. University educated respondents had greater practice scores (average 4.71 points, SD = 2.49) when compared to technical college educated respondents (average 2.97 points, SD = 2.37, $p = 0.009$). Doctors on average scored 2.77 and 3.50 points greater than midwives and other HCWs, respectively ($p = 0.033$ and $p = 0.015$). Those that had never worked with TB patients had lower practice scores than those that had been working with the patients for less than one year and between one and five years (2.31 points, $p < 0.001$ and 1.66 points, $p = 0.004$, respectively; Fig. 1d).

Only 26.4% correctly identified TB as one of the most likely diagnoses in a patient vignette with a persistent cough, night sweats and fatigue in the context of a close relative with similar symptoms. While 30% of professionals noted that fixed dose combinations was used in the intensive phase of TB treatment, only 50% of these could correctly name all four drugs used, as well as the amount of time that this phase lasts. Over 58% of the participants could not identify the drugs or the time frame for the maintenance phase of treatment. Only 20 respondents correctly identified the course of action to take when a patient presents with jaundice after recently commencing TB intensive phase treatment. While the majority of respondents (79 HCWs) noted that they would monitor the liver enzymes, they failed to relate the occurrence of jaundice to TB treatment.

Discussion

This study, identifies key areas for training on TB and stresses the need for continuous re-training of all TB front-line health personnel. The present study's main findings were: a) knowledge regarding TB patient characteristics, diagnosis and treatment was poor among HCWs; b) specific deficiencies in understanding existed in terms of paediatric TB and Xpert MTB/RIF® testing; c) there was disagreement in attitudes regarding stigma and traditional/alternative medicine, and d) practice competencies were poor.

Across all professions, knowledge in the study sample relating to TB was low. While this finding contrasts some studies from larger African centres [24–26], it is consistent with similar rural low-resource high-TB burden samples in Uganda, Tanzania, South Africa and Kenya [7, 8, 27, 28]. Although context dependent, the

Table 1 Characteristics of health care workers included in the study

	Category	Number	Per cent
Gender	Male	38	48.7
	Female	40	51.3
	No response	92	
Time spent working	Less than one year	24	14.2
	One to five years	64	37.9
	Five to ten years	35	20.7
	More than ten years	46	27.2
	No response	1	
Profession	Medical Agent	23	14.0
	Counsellor	1	0.6
	Nurse	50	30.5
	Midwife	21	12.8
	Dentist	1	0.6
	Doctor	10	6.1
	Microscopist	2	1.2
	Medical Technician	56	34.1
	No response	6	
Level of education	Primary school	4	2.4
	Secondary school	28	17.1
	Technical college	108	65.9
	University	24	14.6
	No response	6	
Age	20 - 25	30	19.2
	26 - 30	47	30.1
	31 - 35	34	21.8
	36 - 40	12	7.7
	41 - 45	12	7.7
	46 - 50	6	3.8
	51 - 55	14	9.0
	56 - 60	1	0.6
	No response	14	
Place of work	Manhiça	90	54.2
	Xinavane	37	22.3
	Peripheral HCC	39	23.5
	No response	4	
Participated in TB training in the past?	Yes	43	25.9
	No	123	74.1
	No response	4	
TB training in past 6 months?	Yes	3	1.76
	No	166	97.6
	No response	1	

Table 1 Characteristics of health care workers included in the study *(Continued)*

Diagnosed with active TB in the past?	Yes	14	8.4
	No	153	91.6
	No response	3	
Directly involved in TB control?	Yes	52	32.1
	No	110	67.9
	No response	8	

low knowledge might reflect the difficulty of training HCWs and keeping them updated with current NTP guidelines in low resource settings [29]. As would be expected, doctors had the highest knowledge scores, and nurses and midwives were the two poorest performing professions in the knowledge section. Naidoo et al. also noted the knowledge gap between professions [30]. This has important clinical implications; in Manhiça doctors develop care plans that nurses then implement, as a result patient care may be adversely affected if a nurse fails to comprehend the fundamentals behind clinical decisions. Likewise, the clinical implications of midwives' knowledge scores are likely to be minimal if they are not regularly involved in TB patient care.

The present study was the first to look at knowledge regarding Xpert MTB/RIF®, a relatively new nucleic acid amplification test used for diagnosis of TB and resistance testing, in a low-resource high-TB burden setting. Despite the WHO issuing recommendations endorsing Xpert MTB/RIF® technology in December 2010 and the widespread uptake of its use worldwide since [1], knowledge of its existence and purpose remains low in the present study. The use of Xpert in Mozambique at the time of the survey was limited, although it was available in the district of Manhiça (among others) for specific high risks groups where it has been broadly used as part of surveillance based studies. This perhaps suggests that the roll out of Xpert MTB/RIF® might not have been accompanied with sufficient education for HCWs. While this technology is lauded as "a major advance for TB diagnostics", without a widespread understanding of its potential among HCWs and the critical operational requirement of trained laboratory and clinical staff, Xpert MTB/RIF® may not be fully adopted [31]. There is a paucity of evidence investigating HCWs' knowledge regarding paediatric TB. Regardless of demographic characteristics, respondents were not aware of the treatment duration or the diagnostic differences between children and adults. These findings provide impetus for further research into paediatric TB HCWs' knowledge and education.

The HCWs identified that there was clearly a stigma associated with TB. About a third of HCWs in the

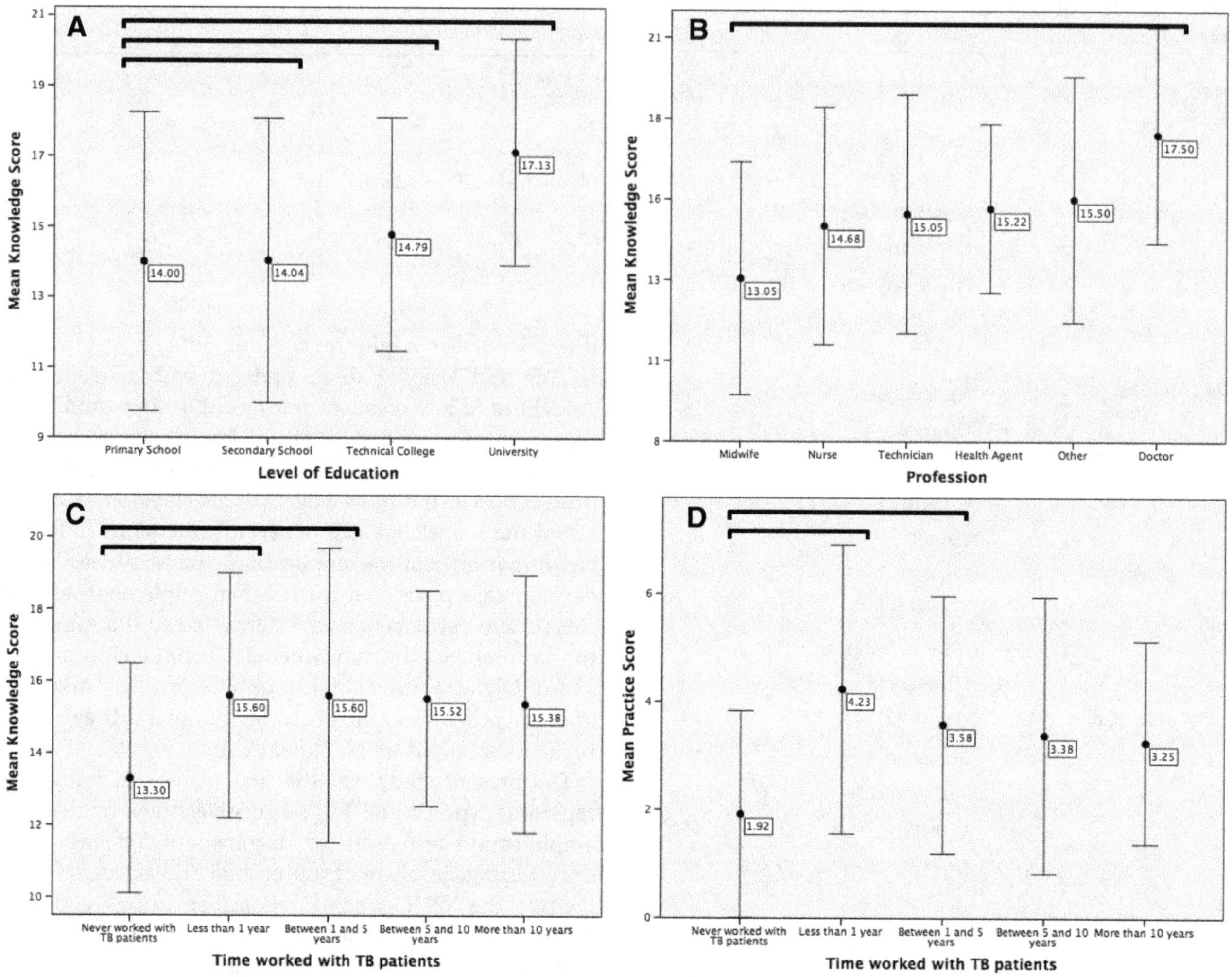

Fig. 1 Panels **a**) Mean of knowledge score against highest level of educational attainment. **b**) Mean of knowledge score against profession. **c**) Mean of knowledge score against time worked with TB patients. **d**) Mean of practice score against time worked with TB patients. Error bars: ± 1 x SD. The square brackets denote a statistically significant difference between the two groups bounded by the bracket

present study believed that their clinical conduct did not contribute to this stigma, while, conversely, many believed that their actions did stigmatise TB patients citing their use of personal protective equipment as sufficient to perpetuate the stigma. Two studies from Ghana found that fear of infection is a major cause of TB stigma and this fear results in TB patients being shunned, avoided and segregated [32, 33]. The exact cause of the stigma in the present study warrants further investigation as a review of 83 studies by Chang et al. revealed that there are significant cultural variations with respect to TB and the development of stigma [34]. Attitudes towards traditional and/or alternative medicine were largely negative or neutral. Over 70% of the HCWs disagreed with the statement that "Access to traditional and alternative medicine improves patient wellbeing" and many HCW believed that they were in fact a hindrance to TB management. These sentiments are in line with the conclusions by Islam et al. who showed that allopathic providers lack knowledge and irrationally use antibiotics, adding to the challenge of TB control and prevention [35]. It is unclear whether combining traditional and medical management leads to poorer treatment outcomes [36, 37], as this probably depends on the relationship between formal and informal healthcare providers.

Practice competency as measured by the survey was low. The questions asked were deemed essential knowledge that most HCWs should be familiar with. The low scores may relate to the fact that the survey was administered among all HCWs from the Manhiça district, regardless of profession or department; as such professionals may have a lack of experience in dealing with common TB scenarios. Chakaya et al. assessed practice competency in HCWs with comparable methods, finding similar deficiencies in the initial investigation of TB suspects as well as an unfamiliarity with anti-TB drugs and regimens [27].

This study has several limitations. Firstly, the external validity might be affected by its cross-sectional analysis and relatively small sample size. Seventy per cent of the population in Southern Mozambique lives in rural areas, as such, we believe the Manhiça District might be a reliable reflection of the rest of the region. Secondly, the semi-qualitative analysis approach may have resulted in sections of data being misinterpreted due to thematic aggregation. Thirdly, practice competency was approximated by self-reporting, rather than direct observation, which may overstate adherence to guidelines. Reinforcing the fact that the survey was not an assessment of individual's knowledge and performance reduced the potential for them to seek external help and affect results. Nonetheless, this study offers novel findings that may be applied to similar settings.

Conclusion

The assessment of TB HCWs' knowledge, attitudes and practises provides valuable baseline information concerning insufficiencies and obstacles to sound TB care and control. The present study provides impetus for tailored education among HCWs regarding TB in general, in children and diagnostic testing, such as Xpert MTB/RIF®, as well as reassessment of TB HCW KAP following education. Further qualitative assessment is also indicated to establish the grounding for TB-associated stigma.

Abbreviations

ANOVA: Analysis of variance; CISM: Manhiça health research center; CNBS: National bioethics committee; HCC: Health care centers; HCW: Health care workers; HIV: Human immunodeficiency virus; KAP: Knowledge, attitudes, practices; NTP: National tuberculosis program; SD: Standard deviation; TB: Tuberculosis; WHO: World health organization

Acknowledgements

The authors would like to thank all the study participants and the National Tuberculosis Program, for their cooperation, as well as Alberto Junior (CISM), Sebastian Mabunda (CISM), and Ruben Langa (NTP) for their assistance in the conduct of the study. Special thanks to all CISM's staff and Dr Eusebio Macete for making this study possible. We are also thankful to Prof Frank Cobelens (AIGHD) for his comments to the manuscript.

Funding

All funding needed for the conduct of this study came from internal resources at CISM

Authors' contributions

ALGB, PIS, AN conceived the study. AN, RMR, LS, RA, MM participated in data collection. AN, ALGB conducted the analysis. SB, KM, AN, RMR, ALGB contributed to data interpretation. ALGB provided direction throughout the research process. All authors have been involved in drafting the manuscript. All authors approved the last version as sent to the journal.

Competing interests

The authors declare that they have no competing interests.

Consent for publication

The manuscript does not contain individual person's data.

Author details

[1]School of Paediatrics and Child Health, University of Western Australia, Crawley, Australia. [2]Centro de Investigação em Saúde de Manhiça (CISM), CP 1929 Maputo, Mozambique. [3]Maternal and Infant Health Service, Manhiça District, Maputo, Mozambique. [4]Faculdade de Medicina, Eduardo Mondlane University (UEM), Maputo, Mozambique. [5]ISGlobal, Barcelona Ctr. Int. Health Res. (CRESIB), Hospital Clínic - Universitat de Barcelona, Barcelona, Spain. [6]Amsterdam Institute for Global Health and Development (AIGHD), Amsterdam, The Netherlands.

References

1. WHO. Global tuberculosis report. Geneva: World Health Organisation; 2014.
2. WHO. Global tuberculosis report. Geneva: World Health Organisation; 2015.
3. Brassard P, Anderson KK, Menzies D, Schwartzman K, Macdonald ME. Knowledge and perceptions of tuberculosis among a sample of urban aboriginal people. J Community Health. 2008;33(4):192–8.
4. Hoa NP, Diwan VK, Thorson AE. Diagnosis and treatment of pulmonary tuberculosis at basic health care facilities in rural Vietnam: a survey of knowledge and reported practices among health staff. Health Policy. 2005;72(1):1–8.
5. Stop TB Policy Paper: Contributing to Health System Strengthening: Guiding Principles for National Tuberculosis Programmes. Geneva: World Health Organization; 2008 Jan. THE STOP TB STRATEGY. Available from: http://www.who.int/tb/dots/whatisdots/en/index2.html
6. Minnery M, Contreras C, Perez R, et al. A cross sectional study of knowledge and attitudes towards tuberculosis amongst front-line tuberculosis personnel in high burden areas of Lima, Peru. PLoS ONE. 2013;8(9):e75698.
7. Buregyeya E, Kulane A, Colebunders R, et al. Tuberculosis knowledge, attitudes and health-seeking behaviour in rural Uganda. Int J Tuberc Lung Dis. 2011;15(7):938–42.
8. Haasnoot PJ, Boeting TE, Kuney MO, van Roosmalen J. Knowledge, attitudes, and practice of tuberculosis among maasai in simanjiro district, Tanzania. Am J Trop Med Hyg. 2010;83(4):902–5.
9. Kanjee Z, Catterick K, Moll AP, Amico KR, Friedland GH, 4. Tuberculosis infection control in rural south Africa: survey of knowledge, attitude and practice in hospital staff. J Hosp Infect. 2011;79:333–8.
10. Naidoo S, Taylor M, Esterhuizen TM, et al. Changes in healthcare workers' knowledge about tuberculosis following a tuberculosis training programme. Educ Health (Abingdon). 2011;24(2):514.
11. Roy A, Abubakar I, Chapman A, et al. A controlled trial of the knowledge impact of tuberculosis information leaflets among staff supporting substance misusers: pilot study. PLoS ONE. 2011;6(6):e20875.
12. Awofeso N, Schelokova I, Dalhatu A. Training of front-line health workers for tuberculosis control: lessons from Nigeria and Kyrgyzstan. Hum Resour Health. 2008;6:20.

13. Vanden Driessche K, Sabue M, Dufour W, Behets F, Van Rie A. Training health care workers to promote HIV services for patients with tuberculosis in the democratic republic of Congo. Hum Resour Health. 2009;7:23.
14. Pfeiffer J, Chapman R. An anthropology of aid in Africa. Lancet. 2015;385(9983):2144–5.
15. Garcia-Basteiro AL, Lopez-Varela E, Manhica I, Macete E, Alonso PL, 9913. Mozambique faces challenges in the fight against tuberculosis. Lancet. 2014;18:215–6.
16. Garcia-Basteiro AL, Lopez-Varela E, Augusto OJ, et al. Radiological findings in young children investigated for tuberculosis in mozambique. PLoS ONE. 2015;10(5):e0127323.
17. Garcia-Basteiro AL, Lopez-Varela E, Respeito D, et al. High tuberculosis burden among people living with HIV in southern Mozambique. Eur Respir J. 2015;45(2):547–9.
18. Lopez-Varela E, Augusto OJ, Gondo K, et al. Incidence of tuberculosis among young children in rural Mozambique. Pediatr Infect Dis J. 2015;34(7):686–92.
19. García-Basteiro AL, Respeito D, Augusto OJ, et al. Poor tuberculosis treatment outcomes in southern Mozambique (2011–2012). BMC Infect Dis. 2016;16(1):214.
20. García-Basteiro AL, Ribeiro RM, Brew J, et al. Tuberculosis on the rise in southern Mozambique (1997–2012). Eur Respir J. 2016; In Publication.
21. Sacoor C, Nhacolo A, Nhalungo D, et al. Profile: Manhica Health Research Centre (Manhica HDSS). Int J Epidemiol. 2013;42(5):1309–18.
22. Instituto Nacional de Estatística. Estatísticas Distritais (Estatísticas do Distrito de Manhiça). Maputo: Instituto Nacional de Estatística; 2013.
23. Instituto Nacional de Estatística. Projecções anuais da população total, Urbana e rural, dos distritos da província de Maputo 2007 – 2010. Instituto Nacional de Estatística: Maputo; 2010.
24. Kanjee Z, Catterick K, Moll AP, Amico KR, Friedland GH. Tuberculosis infection control in rural south Africa: survey of knowledge, attitude and practice in hospital staff. J Hosp Infect. 2011;79(4):333–8. Available from: MEDLINE.
25. Heunis C, Wouters E, Kigozi G, Van Rensburg-Bonthuyzen EJ, Jacobs N, 2. TB/HIV-related training, knowledge and attitudes of community health workers in the free state province, south Africa. Afr J AIDS Res. 2013;12:113–9. Available from: Scopus.
26. Temesgen C, Demissie M. Knowledge and practice of tuberculosis infection control among health professionals in northwest Ethiopia; 2011. BMC Health Serv Res. 2014;14:593.
27. Chakaya JM, Meme H, Kwamanga D, et al. Planning for PPM-DOTS implementation in urban slums in Kenya: knowledge, attitude and practices of private health care providers in Kibera slum, Nairobi. Int J Tuberc Lung Dis. 2005;9(4):403–8. Available from: MEDLINE.
28. Peltzer K, Mngqundaniso N, Petros G, 6. HIV/AIDS/STI/TB knowledge, beliefs and practices of traditional healers in KwaZulu-Natal, south Africa. AIDS Care. 2006;18:608–13. Available from: Scopus.
29. Bell CA, Duncan G, Saini B. Knowledge, attitudes and practices of private sector providers of tuberculosis care: a scoping review. Int J Tuberc Lung Dis. 2011;15(8):1005–17.
30. Naidoo S, Taylor M, Esterhuizen TM, 2, et al. Changes in healthcare workers' knowledge about tuberculosis following a tuberculosis training programme. Educ Health. 2011;24:514. Available from: MEDLINE.
31. Piatek AS, Van Cleeff M, Alexander H, et al. GeneXpert for TB diagnosis: planned and purposeful implementation. Glob Health Sci Pract. 2013;1(1):18–23.
32. Dodor EA, Kelly SJ. Manifestations of tuberculosis stigma within the healthcare system: the case of Sekondi-Takoradi metropolitan district in Ghana. Health Policy. 2010;98(2–3):195–202. Available from: MEDLINE.
33. Dodor EA, Neal K, Kelly S. An exploration of the causes of tuberculosis stigma in an urban district in Ghana. Int J Tuberc Lung Dis. 2008;12(9):1048–54. Available from: MEDLINE.
34. Chang SH, Cataldo JK. A systematic review of global cultural variations in knowledge, attitudes and health responses to tuberculosis stigma. Int J Tuberc Lung Dis. 2014;18(2):168–73. i-iv.
35. Islam QS, Ahmed SM, Islam MA, Chowdhury AS, Siddiquea BN, Husain MA. Informal allopathic provider knowledge and practice regarding control and prevention of TB in rural Bangladesh. Int Health. 2014;6(3):225–31. Available from: MEDLINE.
36. Rowe KA, Makhubele B, Hargreaves JR, Porter JD, Hausler HP, Pronyk PM. Adherence to TB preventive therapy for HIV-positive patients in rural South Africa: implications for antiretroviral delivery in resource-poor settings? Int J Tuberc Lung Dis. 2005;9(3):263–9.
37. Greene JA. An ethnography of nonadherence: culture, poverty, and tuberculosis in urban Bolivia. Cult Med Psychiatry. 2004;28(3):401–25.

14

Risk of incident active tuberculosis disease in patients treated with non-steroidal anti-inflammatory drugs

Chun-Wei Wu[1], Jiunn-Yih Wu[1], Meng-Tse Gabriel Lee[2], Chih-Cheng Lai[3], I-Lin Wu[4], Yi-Wen Tsai[5], Shy-Shin Chang[6,7*†] and Chien-Chang Lee[2*†]

Abstract

Background: *Mycobacterium tuberculosis* (TB) is one of the world's most devastating public health threats. Our goal is to evaluate whether the use of non-steroidal anti-inflammatory drugs (NSAIDs) affect the risk of new incident active TB disease.

Methods: We conducted a nested case-control analysis by using a 1 million longitudinally followed cohort, from Taiwan's national health insurance research database. Effects of NSAIDs on active TB were estimated by conditional logistic regression and adjusted using a TB-specific disease risk score (DRS). NSAIDs exposures were defined as having a prescription record of NSAIDs ≧ 7 days that ended between 31 and 90 days prior to the index date.

Results: A total of 123,419 users of traditional NSAIDs, 16,392 users of cyclooxygenase-2 selective inhibitor (Coxibs), and 4706 incident cases of active TB were identified. Compared with nonusers, use of traditional NSAIDs was associated with an increased risk of TB in the unadjusted analysis ([RR], 1.39; 95% [CI], 1.24 – 1.57 and DRS adjusted analysis ([ARR], 1.30; 95% [CI], 1.15– 1.47). However, use of Coxibs was not associated with a significant increase in the risk of TB after DRS adjustment ([ARR], 1.23; 95% [CI], 0.89 – 1.70).

Conclusions: In this large population-based study, we found that subjects using traditional NSAIDs were associated with increased risk for active TB. We did not find evidence for a causative mechanism between traditional NSAIDs and TB, and more research is required to verify whether the association between traditional NSAIDs and TB is causal, or simply reflects an increased use of anti-inflammatory drugs in the early phases of TB onset.

Keywords: Tuberculosis, NSAIDs, Coxibs

Background

Mycobacterium tuberculosis (TB), the causative bacterium pathogen, is one of the world's most devastating public health threats. In 2013, there are approximately 9 million cases of new active TB, and an associated death of 1.5 million [1, 2]. It is WHO's Global Plan to eradicate TB by the year of 2050, but it is difficult to achieve that goal by the current rate of decrease in TB infection. Our goal is to find out whether Non-steroidal anti-inflammatory drugs (NSAIDs), which is one of the most commonly used drugs in the world, might affect the risk of active TB [3–5]. Use of traditional NSAIDs is considered safe and they can be bought over the counter to relieve pain and fever. The therapeutic effects of traditional NSAIDs are primarily attained through the inhibition of the cyclooxygenase-1 (COX-1) and cyclooxygenase-2 (COX-2) enzymes, which are critical mediators of pain, inflammation, and fever [6–8]. Specific COX-2 inhibitors (Coxibs)

* Correspondence: sschang0529@gmail.com; cclee100@gmail.com
†Equal contributors
[6]Department of Family Medicine, Taipei Medical University Hospital and School of Medicine, Taipei Medical University, Taipei 110, Taiwan
[2]Department of Emergency Medicine, National Taiwan University Hospital, Number 7, Chung-Shan South Road, Taipei 100, Taiwan
Full list of author information is available at the end of the article

are the newer generation of NSAIDs that selectively inhibit the COX-2 enzyme. Use of Coxibs is associated with less gastrointestinal complication than traditional NSAIDs and their use often requires a prescription [9–11].

As far as we were aware of, there is only one small-scale observation study that investigates the direct relationship between use of NSAIDs and active TB onset, and two small-scale observation studies that we can infer the relationship between NSAIDs and active TB onset [12–14]. In 1984, the Bass group showed that in 38 latent TB patients, the chance of developing active TB is directly increased with the use of NSAIDs [13]. Unfortunately, no risk estimate was provided due to the small sample size. In the 2009 Brassard paper, the group reported that NSAID is the most frequently used nonbiologic anti- rheumatoid arthritis medication for the 50 rheumatoid arthritis patients that developed TB. In addition, use of NSAID is associated with 1.2 fold increase in the risk of active TB [14]. In a more recent study by Chang et al., the group reported that NSAID is the most frequently used traditional systemic antipsoriatic drugs for the 497 psoriasis patients that developed TB, and frequent users of traditional NSAIDs were found to have 1.85 fold increase in TB risk [12]. Just like the bass study, the Chang study has a limited sample size and only looked at patients with psoriasis. Hence, we wish to investigate the influence of NSAIDs on active TB in the general population.

Taiwan has one of the most affordable single-payer universal public health insurance and the claim history is completely recorded in a public database. Since the cost of a physician prescribed NSAID (about $4-8US) is often similar to the self acquisition cost of NSAID over the counter, we believe that there are minimal over the counter use of traditional NSAIDs [15]. As a result, the Taiwanese National Health Insurance Research Database (NHIRD) of Taiwan, a national representative longitudinal cohort, is a great data source for analyzing the risk of new incident active tuberculosis disease in patients treated with NSAIDs or Coxibs. We, therefore, carried out a population-based study using the 1 million national cohort samples.

Methods

Data source

We carried out a population-based study using the National Health Insurance Research Database (NHIRD) of Taiwan, done under the approval of the institutional review board of National Taiwan University Hospital. The NHIRD database contains de-identified secondary data, and met the requirements of the "Personal Information Protection Act" in Taiwan. Thus, the data were analyzed anonymously and the need for informed consent was waived. NHIRD records the complete claim history of 1 million randomly selected participants enrolled in Taiwan's National Health Insurance (NHI), which is a single-payer universal public health insurance [15]. These 1 million participants are believed to be representative of the entire Taiwanese population.

Several studies showed that the NHIRD database is appropriate for use in pharmacoepidemiologic research [12, 16, 17]. The NHIRD database contains participant demographics and detail claim history, which includes medications prescribed, medications quantity, route of administration, individual diagnoses, operations, and outpatient and inpatient electronic claim records.

Study cohort

We used a study cohort that consists of a longitudinally followed Taiwanese' population from January 1999 to December 2011. A new-user cohort design was adopted by excluding existing users of NSAID and prevalent cases of TB in the year 1999 (pre-enrollment period) [18]. Patients entered the cohort on the first day of the year 2000 and were followed up until the first occurrence of any of these events: diagnosis of active TB, termination of health insurance coverage, death, or end of the study period. People who were less than 18 years old on January 1, 2000, were not eligible for entering the cohort until they became 18 years old in later years. This cohort design thus allows a clean selection of case and controls, in which all patients investigated are new users of NSAIDs and have new cases of active TB.

Selection of cases and controls

Patients with new onset active TB disease were identified using the following criteria: at least one outpatient visit or one hospital admission with ICD-9-CM codes of TB (010-018, including all subcategories), plus the prescription of more than two anti-tuberculosis medications for more than 28 days. We excluded patients with a subsequent diagnosis of nontuberculosis mycobacterial infection or lung cancer. This is because the diagnosis of nontuberculosis lung cancer is clinically difficult, and lung cancer has been associated with an increase in the risk of TB. Our case definition had been used in previous studies and had been validated in a linked survey database [19, 20]. One hundred controls were selected to match cases on index date, 5-year age group, and gender using risk set sampling scheme. Index date referred to the first date of TB diagnosis. The one-year period preceding index date was used for assessment of NSAID exposure status.

Medication exposure

NSAIDs exposures were defined as having a prescription record of NSAID ≧ 7 days. By restricting to NSAID users having a drug prescription record ≧ 7 days, we found that most of the NSAID users were associated with codes for arthritis and other rheumatic conditions. Few patients were associated with codes for fever. As NSAID may be used to treat the early symptoms of active TB, we defined use of NSAID as a prescription that ended between 31 and 90 days prior to TB diagnosis to avoid the possible reverse causation between use of NSAID and active TB. Traditional NSAIDs are defined as drugs with any of the following compounds: ibuprofen, naproxen, ketoprofen, dexibuprofen, piroxicam, tolfenamic acid, diclofenac, etodolac, nabumetone, and meloxicam. However, aspirin is not included as a drug in the traditional NSAIDs. This is because aspirin has a unique mechanism of action and are usually used on cardiovascular patients. Specific COX-2 inhibitors (COXIBs) are defined as drugs with any of the following compound: celeCoxib, rofeCoxib, valdeCoxib, pareCoxib and etoriCoxib.

Covariates

In order to be as comprehensive as possible in adjusting for factors that might affect the outcome, we looked at published risk factors for TB and identified 71 covariates (Table 1) [1, 19, 20]. All covariates were assessed before NSAID exposure, except for the one-year period used for exposure assessment. Using ICD9-CM codes, the following covariates were assessed: age, sex, burden of comorbid conditions, indicators for frailty, risk factors for TB disease and use of specific medications. Risk factors for TB included alcoholism-related disease (291, 303, 305.0, 357, 425, 535.3, 571.0-571.3, 577.1), diabetes mellitus (DM) (250), chronic renal failure or hemodialysis (585, V56.0), solid organ transplantation (V42), COPD (491,492, 496), silicosis (502), presence of cancer (140-239), malnutrition-related disorders such as cachexia, anorexia, abnormal loss of weight (799.4, 263, 783.2, 783.3), and postgastric surgery (564.2). Use of specific medications included aspirin (N02BA), systemic immunosuppressive agents and biologics (L04A), systemic corticosteroids, and disease modifying anti-rheumatic drugs (M01B, M01C). Each individual's burden of comorbidity was quantified by a combined weighted comorbidity index. This index is an improved Charlson Index that combines the Elixhauser system [21]. The score contains common comorbidities such as myocardial infarction, congestive heart failure, peripheral vascular disease, cerebrovascular disease, dementia, chronic pulmonary disease, connective tissue disease, ulcer disease, liver disease, diabetes, hemiplegia, renal disease, neoplasms and AIDS.

Data analysis

We estimated the rate ratio by using a time matched case control-sampling scheme [22]. Incidence rate ratios of active TB (plus 95% confidence intervals [CIs]) were estimated by conditional logistic regression analysis adjusted for all covariates. Disease risk score (DRS) was used to adjust for confounders, and compared the different exposures in a case-control study design [23]. A study-specific DRS was constructed to balance disease risks between different drug exposure groups. On Additional file 1, we reported the c- statistic (0.81) of the DRS model, component variables, and the respective weights of the component variables. The DRS was defined as the probability of developing active TB among the participants unexposed to NSAID or Coxibs based on the individual's baseline covariates. To estimate DRS, we carried out multivariate logistic regression analysis, where active TB was treated as the dependent variable, and all empirical clinical predictors were treated as independent variables. Hence, the DRS characterize the relationship between potential risk factors and active TB. To avoid the potential unrealistic linear assumption of continuous variables in the regression model, we carried out a fractional polynomial DRS (fpDRS) adjustment.

We also carried out a dose response analyses and subgroup analyses in high-risk patients, to further assess the robustness of our results. Predefined subgroups included sex and age of 70 years. Attributable risk percentage and population attributable risk percentage were also calculated (Additional file 2). All analyses were carried out with SAS 9.3 for Windows (SAS Institute Inc, Cary, NC) and the data are reported in accordance with STROBE guidance.

Results

Participant enrollment and baseline characteristics

Table 1 shows the baseline characteristics of the cohort. The source population comprises of 1,000,000 participants. After exclusion of prevalent users of NSAIDs and prevalent cases of TB in the 1 year pre-enrollment period, 123,419 person years were exposed to traditional NSAIDs and 16,392 person years were exposed to Coxibs. Coxibs users were found to increase steadily from 2001 to 2004. However, there is a sharp decline in Coxib users after 2004, when rofecoxib revealed safety concerns and was pulled off the market. The use of Coxib was found to increase steadily again from 2007 to 2011. There were significant differences in the age, and Charlson index comorbidity score of the different participants. In general, Coxibs users were the oldest (75.5 ± 9.8 years old) and had the highest comorbidity score (2.54 ± 2.43), while the unexposed control was the youngest (55.9 ± 19.9 years old) and had the lowest comorbidity score (0.84 ± 1.54). Traditional NSAIDs users had an average age and comorbidity score in between that of Coxibs users and unexposed control. The number of comorbidities, known risk factors and medications

Table 1 Participant enrollment and baseline characteristics

	Total number of control= 470600 person-years			
	Traditional NSAIDs (*N*=123,419 person years)	Coxibs (*N*=16,392 person years)	Unexposed (*N*=340,396 person years)	*P*-value
Number of TB cases	1407	206	3206	N.A
Demographics				
Male sex (%)	84623 (68.6)	10420 (63.6)	245077 (72.0)	<.0001
Age mean (year)	63.1±17.5	75.5±9.8	55.9±19.9	<.0001
Index year (%)				
1999	8740 (7.1)	0	24660 (7.2)	<.0001
2000	10496 (8.5)	0	28004 (8.2)	
2001	10168 (8.2)	80 (0.5)	26409 (7.8)	
2002	11097 (8.9)	990 (6.0)	29178 (8.6)	
2003	11271 (9.1)	2104 (12.8)	29385 (8.6)	
2004	10658 (8.6)	2463 (15.0)	28264 (8.3)	
2005	11368 (9.2)	2122 (13.0)	30022 (8.8)	
2006	9328 (7.6)	1143 (6.9)	26013 (7.6)	
2007	8046 (6.5)	1091 (6.7)	22810 (6.7)	
2008	9164 (7.4)	1429 (8.7)	26625 (8.1)	
2009	7438 (6.0)	1452 (8.9)	22080 (6.5)	
2010	7942 (6.4)	1704 (10.4)	23837 (7.0)	
2011	7585 (6.2)	1814 (11.1)	21827 (6.4)	
Area : urban region	52030 (42.2)	6788 (41.4)	169458 (49.8)	<.0001
Area : metro area	31446 (25.5)	3897 (23.8)	85565 (25.1)	
Area : suburban area	26117 (21.2)	3531 (21.5)	59604 (17.5)	
Area : countryside area	13826 (11.2)	2176 (13.3)	25769 (7.6)	
Annual insurance premium				
Dependent	10446 (8.6)	2349 (14.6)	28046 (8.3)	<.0001
<666 USD	37517 (30.7)	6355 (39.5)	90984 (26.9)	
666-1331 USD	52657 (43.2)	5914 (36.8)	139440 (41.3)	
>= 1331 USD	21424 (17.6)	1462 (9.1)	79315 (23.5)	
Comorbidity score				
Baseline combined comorbidity score	1.41±1.94	2.54±2.43	0.84±1.54	<.0001
Individual comorbidity				
Peripheral vascular disease	9704 (7.9)	2539 (15.8)	13440 (4.0)	<.0001
Congestive heart failure	14689 (12.0)	4049 (25.2)	20203 (6.0)	<.0001
Myocardial infarction/acute coronary syndromes	3842 (3.2)	947 (5.9)	6008 (1.8)	<.0001
Cerebrovascular disease	25397 (20.8)	6550 (40.7)	40531 (12.0)	<.0001
Dementia	4412 (3.6)	1439 (8.9)	9242 (2.7)	<.0001
Chronic pulmonary disease	51073 (41.9)	10138 (63.1)	86738 (25.7)	<.0001
Rheumatologic disease	4587 (3.8)	1231 (7.7)	5615 (1.7)	<.0001
Peptic ulcer disease	51084 (41.9)	10386 (64.6)	84019 (24.9)	<.0001
Mild liver disease	39309 (32.2)	6968 (43.3)	68469 (20.3)	<.0001
Diabetes without chronic complications	26942 (22.1)	5782 (35.9)	45868 (13.6)	<.0001
Diabetes with chronic complications	8356 (6.9)	2053 (12.8)	13954 (4.1)	<.0001
Hemiplegia or paraplegia	5199 (4.3)	1263 (7.9)	9365 (2.8)	<.0001

Table 1 Participant enrollment and baseline characteristics *(Continued)*

Renal disease	11377 (9.3)	2978 (18.5)	16967 (5.0)	<.0001
Any malignancy, including leukemia and lymphoma	11991 (9.8)	2900 (18.0)	19535 (5.8)	<.0001
Moderate or severe liver disease	690 (0.6)	157 (1.0)	1252 (0.4)	<.0001
Metastatic solid tumor	1245 (1.0)	271 (1.7)	2041 (0.6)	<.0001
AIDS/HIV	84 (0.07)	15 (0.09)	154 (0.05)	0.003
Alcohol/drug use	3425 (2.8)	549 (3.4)	6826	<.0001
Psychiatric disorder	43667 (35.8)	8652 (53.8)	66012 (19.5)	<.0001
Neurologic disorder	7046 (5.8)	2069 (12.9)	12232 (3.6)	<.0001
Obesity	1194 (0.9)	223 (1.4)	1892 (0.6)	<.0001
Other Cancer except Metastatic solid tumor	36548 (29.9)	7072 (43.9)	68592 (20.3)	<.0001
COPD	37556 (30.8)	8128 (50.6)	58896 (17.4)	<.0001
Silicosis	218 (0.2)	32 (0.2)	258 (0.1)	<.0001
Gastrointestinal or esophageal hemorrhage	7319 (6.0)	1865 (11.6)	12848 (3.8)	<.0001
Risk factors				
Pregnancy	913 (0.8)	49 (0.3)	3171 (0.9)	<.0001
bed-ridden status	1561 (1.3)	361 (2.3)	2408 (0.7)	<.0001
Solid organ transplantation such as renal or heart transplantation	15 (0.01)	2 (0.01)	77 (0.02)	0.04
Malnutrition	678 (0.6)	129 (0.8)	928 (0.3)	<.0001
Postgastric surgery	34 (0.03)	7 (0.04)	30 (0.01)	<.0001
Healthcare service utilization in the previous year				
The number of outpatient department visits	32.4±25.1	42.1±27.6	14.1±15.9	<.0001
The number of emergency department visits	0.2±0.87	0.4±1.26	0.1±0.51	<.0001
The number of hospitalizations	0.3±0.87	0.5±1.12	0.2±0.9	<.0001
Medication use				
Aspirin	25603 (20.9)	5118 (31.8)	32912 (9.7)	<.0001
Systemic immunosuppressive agents and biologics	416 (0.3)	284 (1.8)	336 (0.1)	<.0001
Systemic corticosteroids	26268 (21.5)	4526 (28.2)	23802 (7.1)	<.0001
DMARDs (disease modifying anti-rheumatic drugs)	2165 (1.8)	694 (4.3)	2150 (0.6)	<.0001
Statin	9380 (7.7)	2233 (13.9)	14224 (4.2)	<.0001
ACE inhibitors	17324 (14.2)	2925 (18.2)	23278 (6.9)	<.0001
Beta blockers	21155 (17.3)	3771 (23.5)	27789 (8.2)	<.0001
Loop diuretics	8569 (7.0)	2295 (14.3)	9196 (2.7)	<.0001
Angiotensin II antagonists	12596 (10.3)	3789 (23.6)	19482 (5.8)	<.0001
Digoxin	2925 (2.4)	690 (4.3)	4265 (1.3)	<.0001
Nitrates	9178 (7.5)	2133 (13.3)	11539 (3.4)	<.0001
Antipsychotics	434 (0.4)	129 (0.8)	1190 (0.4)	0.01
Proton-pump inhibitors(PPI)	5977 (4.9)	1606 (9.9)	8098 (2.4)	<.0001
CA channel blocker	33842 (27.7)	7126 (44.3)	47053 (13.9)	<.0001
Acetaminophen	63673 (52.2)	8965 (55.8)	78967 (23.4)	<.0001

also tend to agree with the pattern observed in the comorbidity score. Coxibs users generally had a higher number of comorbidities, known risk factors and medications usage, then followed by traditional NSAIDs users and finally unexposed users.

Use of NSAIDs and risk of active TB onset

We identified 340,396 number of participants unexposed to traditional NSAIDs and Coxibs in our cohort, of which 3,206 developed active TB. The crude TB incidence rate for the unexposed control is 0.93% (3,206/343,602 person-years). (Table 1) In our cohort, 1,407 traditional NSAIDs users were found to be associated with active TB, resulting in a crude incidence rate of 1.13% (1,407/124,826 person-years). We also identified 206 Coxibs users associated with active TB, resulting in a crude incidence rate of 1.24% (206/16,598 person-years).

Table 2 shows the rate ratios associating the use of NSAIDs within 31-90 days, on the risk of new active TB onset. The first method, which is matching only on agegroup, gender, and calendar year, can be considered an unadjusted way of obtaining rate ratio (RR). The age-sex-year matched RR is 1.39 (95%CI, 1.24 – 1.57) for traditional NSAIDs and 1.40 (95%CI, 1.03 – 1.92) for Coxibs. Adjustment for individual confounders attenuated the RR to 1.31 (95%CI, 1.15 – 1.49) for use of traditional NSAIDs and 1.18 (95%CI, 0.85 – 1.63) for use of Coxibs. To balance the disease risk in multiple drug exposure groups independent of the changing indications for NSAIDs, a disease risk score (DRS) was created. The effect estimates after DRS adjustment or fractional polynomial (fp) DRS adjustment was similar to the adjustment by individual confounders. In all the different type of adjustment, use of traditional NSAIDs was associated with a significantly increased risk for TB, but the use of Coxibs was not associated with a significantly increased risk for TB.

Duration-response analysis

Table 3 investigates whether the use of traditional NSAIDs with a different duration can affect the risk of active TB. The cumulative incidence of active TB for the non NSAID user (5.74%), is lower than either the 7-14 days of NSAID user (8.95%) or >14 days of NSAID user (9.00%). After fpDRS adjustment of multiple covariates, use of 7-14 days of NSAID ([ARR], 1.46; 95%CI, 1.34 – 1.59) or >14 days' use of traditional NSIADs ([ARR], 1.25; 95%CI, 1.04 – 1.49) was still associated with higher risk than the reference. However, no duration response effect was observed.

Discussion

In this population-based study based on one million national representative participants, we found that use of traditional NSAIDs was at increased risk of active TB. No duration response effect was observed in the 90-day risk period.

NSAIDs are one of the most widely used medications in the world. According to a French national healthcare insurance system study from 2009-2010, about 43.6% of participants have used some form of NSAID at least once [5]. Thus, it is vital for us to report the contribution of NSAIDs to TB burden. In our cohort, it was found that new user of traditional NSAIDs accounts for approximately 26% cases of active TB among patients taking these medications (Additional file 2). By defining greater than 7 days' prescription of NSAID as a user, we found that 9.4% of Taiwanese had used traditional NSAIDs and 2.1% had used Coxibs in the year 2011. Using the above percentages, we can conclude that use of traditional NSAID accounts for 3.2% cases of active TB among the entire Taiwan population (see Additional file 2 for the attributable risk/ population attributable risk fraction calculation). Therefore, the risk of TB associating with the use of traditional NSAIDs is quite high and cannot be ignored by the health policy makers in Taiwan.

In general, our study agreed with three clinical reports associating the use of NSAIDs with an increase in TB risk [12–14]. However, our crude and adjusted estimates were often found lower than the Chang's group, but in line with the Brassard group [11, 14]. Part of the disparity could be due to the significant differences in our study design. The Chang's study cohort consists of patients with psoriasis or psoriatic arthritis but we were looking at the general population. As a result, there would be significant differences in the baseline characteristics of participants. In fact, we observed that 39.2% of Chang's control is prescribed with corticosteroids as compared to 7.1% of our control. It is unknown how many NSAID users in Chang's study were prescribed with corticosteroids, but it is likely to be higher than ours. Immunosuppressive drugs such as corticosteroids have long been associated with the risk of tuberculosis and can definitely contribute to the higher risk observed in Chang's study [1, 14].

Results of our study should be interpreted in light of both strength and weakness. To the best of our knowledge, this is the biggest TB and NSAIDs study that has ever been carried out. In addition, we constructed a database specific DRS by comprehensively including a

Table 2 Crude and adjusted effect measure for the association between use of NSAIDs and risk of active TB

	Effect estimate matched on age group, gender, and year (RR, 95% confidence interval)	Confounder adjusted effect estimate (RR, 95% confidence interval)	Disease Risk Score adjusted effect estimate (RR, 95% confidence interval)	Fractional Polynomial Disease Risk Score adjusted effect estimate (RR, 95% confidence interval)
Use of Traditional NSAIDs	1.39 (1.24 – 1.57)[a]	1.31 (1.15 –1.49)[a]	1.30 (1.15– 1.47)[a]	1.19 (1.05 1.35)[a]
Use of Coxibs	1.40 (1.03 – 1.92)[a]	1.18 (0.85 – 1.63)	1.23 (0.89 – 1.70)	1.07 (0.78 – 1.48)

[a]Refers to result that is statistically significant
RR refers to rate ratio

Table 3 Relationship between number of days that participants are prescribed with traditional NSAIDs and risk of active TB

	Risk estimate by different duration category/ drug use	
Total number of days using traditional NSAIDs	Cumulative Incidence (case/person)	Fractional Polynomial Disease Risk Score adjusted RR (95% CI)
0-7days (reference)	5.74%	NA
7-14 days	8.95%	1.46 (1.34 – 1.59)[a]
>14 days	9.00%	1.25 (1.04 – 1.49)[a]

[a]Refers to result that is statistically significant
RR refers to rate ratio

large number of covariates (71) and allowed a nonlinear fractional polynomial term to enter the model, which we believed may greatly relieve the concerns of residual confounding in a claim database research. We chose not to construct a propensity score because the indications for Coxib use have changed greatly in the past 10 years. The DRS can balance the disease risk among multiple drug exposure groups independent of the changing indications for NSAIDs, and can adjust for several rare covariates in the subgroup analysis [23]. Despite the comprehensiveness of the DRS and a large number of covariates, we recognized that unmeasured confounding could still be an issue. Since we were using a claims database for our study, many lifestyle factors such as smoking, alcohol, and body mass index are missing. Smoking and excessive alcohol consumption can increase TB risk by 2-3 fold [1]. We attempted to adjust for these missing confounder by including related diseases such as chronic obstructive pulmonary disease, liver disease, coronary artery disease, malnutrition and alcohol related disorders.

In addition, the unknown number of over the counter use of NSAIDs in the control group might also affect our result. However, we believed that there are few incentives for ≧ 7 days use of over the counter NSAIDs. In Taiwan, the purchase of 7 days of over the counter Ibuprofen actually costs more than the reimbursed cost of medication and the physician visit. Thus, there is little incentive for patients to purchase over the counter traditional NSAIDs. However, if we were to account for the over the counter use of NSAID, the result will be likely biased towards the null due to nondifferential misclassification.

Another limitation inherent in our database study was that active TB disease was defined on the basis of ICD-9 codes with compatible anti-TB prescription history. Since microbiological data is lacking, there is potential for misclassification of TB users. However, we believed that there was little misclassification of TB users, as past linked survey data showed that the definition is highly accurate [19, 20].

Protopathic bias, interpreted as fever symptoms preceding active TB disease leading to the prescription of NSAIDs, is another possible cause for the observed association [24]. However, we try to limit protopathic bias for users of NSAIDs in several ways. First, we looked at long-term users of NSAIDs (>7 days) and exclude short-term NSAID users, who have a higher probability of protopathic bias. By restricting to traditional NSAID users having a drug prescription record ≧ 7 days, we found that most of the patients are associated with codes for arthritis and other rheumatic conditions, and there are relatively fewer patients associated with codes for fever. Second, use of NSAID was defined as having a drug prescription record ≧ 7 days that was filled between 31 and 90 days prior to the TB diagnosis. There is evidence showing that the mean delay between the first medical visits and the confirmed diagnosis of TB is less than 30 days. The mean intervals between patients' first medical visit to the definite diagnosis were reported to be < 1 day, 6.07 days and 25.53 days in outpatient clinics, the emergency department and hospitalization, respectively [25]. Thus, taking the study design and the medical landscape in Taiwan together, we think that protopathic bias could play a part, but could not contribute entirely to the increase in TB risk associated with NSAIDs.

Conclusion

In conclusion, using a large population-based database we have identified an association between traditional NSAID use and active TB. We did not find evidence for a causative mechanism between traditional NSAIDs and TB, and more research is required to verify whether the association between traditional NSAIDs and TB is causal, or simply reflects an increased use of anti-inflammatory drugs in the early phases of TB onset.

Abbreviation

CI: Confidence interval; COX-1: Cyclooxygenase-1; COX-2: Cyclooxygenase-2; Coxibs: COX-2 inhibitors; NSAIDs: Non-steroidal anti-inflammatory drugs; TB: *Mycobacterium tuberculosis*

Acknowledgement

We thank the staff of the Core Labs, the Department of Medical Research, and National Taiwan University Hospital for technical support, medical wisdom consulting group for technical assistance in statistical analysis, and National Taiwan University Hospital Health Economics and Outcome Research Group for advice on study design.

Disclaimer

The interpretation and conclusions contained herein do not represent those of Bureau of National Health Insurance, Department of Health or National Health Research Institutes.

Funding
This study is supported by the Taiwan National Science Foundation Grant NSC 102-2314-B-002 -131 -MY3; Taiwan National Ministry of Science and Technology Grants MOST 104-2314-B-002 -039 -MY3, and MOST 105-2811-B-002-031. No funding bodies had any role in the study design; data collection and analysis; decision to publish; or preparation of the manuscript.

Authors' contributions
C-WW analyzed the data, conducted statistical analysis, and wrote the first and final draft. J-YW analyzed the data, and conducted statistical analysis. M-TL and C-CL analyzed the data, and wrote the final draft. I-LW and Y-WT conducted statistical analysis. S-SC designed the study, analyzed the data, wrote the final draft and provided critical feedback. C-CL designed the study, obtained funding, analyzed the data and authorized the final manuscript. All authors read and approved the final manuscript.

Competing interests
The authors declare that they have no competing interest.

Consent for publication
Not applicable.

Transparency
The lead author (the manuscript's guarantor) affirms that the manuscript is an honest, accurate, and transparent account of the study being reported; that no important aspects of the study have been omitted; and that any discrepancies from the study as planned (and, if relevant, registered) have been explained.

Author details
[1]Department of Emergency Medicine, Chang Gung Memorial Hospital, Keelung, Taiwan and Chang Gung University College of Medicine, Taoyuan, Taiwan. [2]Department of Emergency Medicine, National Taiwan University Hospital, Number 7, Chung-Shan South Road, Taipei 100, Taiwan. [3]Department of Intensive Care Medicine, Chi Mei Medical Center, Liouying, Tainan, Taiwan. [4]Department of Emergency Medicine, Taoyuan Armed Forces General Hospital, Taoyuan, Taiwan. [5]Department of Family Medicine, Chang Gung Memorial Hospital, Keelung and Chang Gung University College of Medicine, Taoyuan, Taiwan. [6]Department of Family Medicine, Taipei Medical University Hospital and School of Medicine, Taipei Medical University, Taipei 110, Taiwan. [7]Department of Family Medicine, Taipei Medical University Hospital, No.252, Wuxing St, Xinyi District, Taipei, Taiwan.

References

1. Lawn SD, Zumla AI. Tuberculosis. Lancet. 2011;378(9785):57–72.
2. Tuberculosis (TB) [http://www.who.int/gho/tb/en/index.html].
3. Paulose-Ram R, Hirsch R, Dillon C, Losonczy K, Cooper M, Ostchega Y. Prescription and non-prescription analgesic use among the US adult population: results from the third National Health and Nutrition Examination Survey (NHANES III). Pharmacoepidemiol Drug Saf. 2003;12(4):315–26.
4. Tielemans MM, Eikendal T, Jansen JB, van Oijen MG. Identification of NSAID users at risk for gastrointestinal complications: a systematic review of current guidelines and consensus agreements. Drug Saf. 2010;33(6):443–53.
5. Duong M, Salvo F, Pariente A, Abouelfath A, Lassalle R, Droz C, Blin P, Moore N. Usage patterns of 'over-the-counter'vs. prescription-strength nonsteroidal anti-inflammatory drugs in France. Br J Clin Pharmacol. 2014;77(5):887–95.
6. Flower R, Gryglewski R, Herbaczynska-Cedro K, Vane JR. Effects of anti-inflammatory drugs on prostaglandin biosynthesis. Nat New Biol. 1972;238(82):104–6.
7. Ferreira SH, Moncada S, Vane JR. Prostaglandins and the mechanism of analgesia produced by aspirin-like drugs. Br J Pharmacol. 1973;49(1):86–97.
8. Vane JR. Inhibition of prostaglandin synthesis as a mechanism of action for aspirin-like drugs. Nature. 1971;231(25):232–5.
9. Bombardier C, Laine L, Reicin A, Shapiro D, Burgos-Vargas R, Davis B, Day R, Ferraz MB, Hawkey CJ, Hochberg MC, VIGOR Study Group, et al. Comparison of upper gastrointestinal toxicity of rofecoxib and naproxen in patients with rheumatoid arthritis. N Engl J Med. 2000;343(21):1520–8. 1522 p following 1528.
10. Silverstein FE, Faich G, Goldstein JL, Simon LS, Pincus T, Whelton A, Makuch R, Eisen G, Agrawal NM, Stenson WF, et al. Gastrointestinal toxicity with celecoxib vs nonsteroidal anti-inflammatory drugs for osteoarthritis and rheumatoid arthritis: the CLASS study: A randomized controlled trial Celecoxib Long-term Arthritis Safety Study. JAMA. 2000;284(10):1247–55.
11. Chang CH, Chen HC, Lin JW, Kuo CW, Shau WY, Lai MS. Risk of hospitalization for upper gastrointestinal adverse events associated with nonsteroidal anti-inflammatory drugs: a nationwide case-crossover study in Taiwan. Pharmacoepidemiol Drug Saf. 2011;20(7):763–71.
12. Chen YJ, Wu CY, Shen JL, Chen TT, Chang YT. Association between traditional systemic antipsoriatic drugs and tuberculosis risk in patients with psoriasis with or without psoriatic arthritis: results of a nationwide cohort study from Taiwan. J Am Acad Dermatol. 2013;69(1):25–33.
13. Tomasson H, Brennan M, Bass M. Tuberculosis and nonsteroidal anti-inflammatory drugs. Can Med Assoc J. 1984;130(3):275.
14. Brassard P, Lowe AM, Bernatsky S, Kezouh A, Suissa S. Rheumatoid arthritis, its treatments, and the risk of tuberculosis in Quebec, Canada. Arthritis Rheum. 2009;61(3):300–4.
15. Lu J-FR, Hsiao WC. Does universal health insurance make health care unaffordable? Lessons from Taiwan. Health Affairs. 2003;22(3):77–88.
16. Lee MS, Lin RY, Chang YT, Lai MS. The risk of developing non-melanoma skin cancer, lymphoma and melanoma in patients with psoriasis in Taiwan: a 10-year, population-based cohort study. Int J Dermatol. 2012;51(12):1454–60.
17. Chang CH, Lin JW, Wu LC, Lai MS, Chuang LM, Chan KA. Association of thiazolidinediones with liver cancer and colorectal cancer in type 2 diabetes mellitus. Hepatology. 2012;55(5):1462–72.
18. Ray WA. Evaluating medication effects outside of clinical trials: new-user designs. Am J Epidemiol. 2003;158(9):915–20.
19. Baker MA, Lin HH, Chang HY, Murray MB. The risk of tuberculosis disease among persons with diabetes mellitus: a prospective cohort study. Clin Infect Dis. 2012;54(6):818–25.
20. Lin HH, Ezzati M, Chang HY, Murray M. Association between tobacco smoking and active tuberculosis in Taiwan: prospective cohort study. Am J Respir Crit Care Med. 2009;180(5):475–80.
21. Gagne JJ, Glynn RJ, Avorn J, Levin R, Schneeweiss S. A combined comorbidity score predicted mortality in elderly patients better than existing scores. J Clin Epidemiol. 2011;64(7):749–59.
22. Lubin JH, Gail MH. Biased selection of controls for case-control analyses of cohort studies. Biometrics. 1984;40(1):63–75.
23. Glynn RJ, Gagne JJ, Schneeweiss S. Role of disease risk scores in comparative effectiveness research with emerging therapies. Pharmacoepidemiol Drug Saf. 2012;21 Suppl 2:138–47.
24. Horwitz RI, Feinstein AR. The problem of "protopathic bias" in case-control studies. Am J Med. 1980;68(2):255–8.
25. Wu Y-C, Hsu G-J, Chuang KY-C, Lin R-S. Intervals before tuberculosis diagnosis and isolation at a regional hospital in Taiwan. J Formos Med Assoc. 2007;106(12):1007–12.

15

Evaluation of gene xpert for routine diagnosis of HIV-associated tuberculosis in Nigeria

Maxwell Oluwole Akanbi[1,2*], Chad Achenbach[3], Babafemi Taiwo[3], John Idoko[2], Agatha Ani[4], Yetunde Isa[5], Oche Agbaji[2], Christiana Ukoli[2], Patrick Akande[6], Mamoudou Maiga[7] and Robert Leo Murphy[3]

Abstract

Background: Xpert MTB/Rif (Xpert) is described as a game changer in tuberculosis (TB) control. We evaluated the impact of Xpert on diagnosis, time to treatment, and treatment outcome among patients with HIV associated TB in Nigeria.

Methods: Adults with HIV being evaluated for pulmonary TB (PTB) were consecutively enrolled into the study cohort. At baseline, expectorated sputa were examined using Xpert and smear microscopy for *Mycobacterium tuberculosis* (MTB) and acid fast bacilli, respectively. Patients diagnosed with TB were followed-up until 6 months post TB diagnosis. TB was defined as sputum positive by smear microscopy, Xpert detection of MTB (bacteriologically confirmed case), or clinician diagnosed TB with initiation of full TB treatment (clinical diagnosis). Time to treatment was time from first clinic presentation for TB evaluation to initiation of TB treatment. We examined the proportion PTB patients with a positive Xpert result and compared time to TB treatment and outcome of TB treatment in patients based on sputum test results.

Results: A total of 310 adults with HIV were enrolled. The median CD4 cell count was 242 (interquartile range (IQR) 120–425) cells/mm^3 and 88.1% were receiving antiretroviral therapy (ART). PTB was diagnosed in 76 (24.5%) patients, with 71 (93.4%) being bacteriologically confirmed. Among patients with PTB, 56 (73.7%) were Xpert positive. Median time to treatment was 5 (IQR 2–8) days and 12 (IQR 5–35) days in patient with and without Xpert positive results, respectively; $p = 0.005$. Overall 73.1% had symptom free survival at 6 months post PTB treatment initiation with no significant differences observed based on TB test method. 10 (14.9%) died within 6 months of TB treatment initiation. In analysis adjusted for age, sex, and mode of diagnosis (Xpert positive or negative), only ART use independently predicted mortality (AOR 0.10; 95% CI 0.01–0.93).

Conclusion: The use of Xpert for routine care reduced time to PTB treatment, but did not improve survival in patients with HIV treated for susceptible PTB.

Keywords: Xpert, Tuberculosis, HIV, Nigeria, Africa, Outcomes research

* Correspondence: Maxwell_akanbi@yahoo.com
[1]Institute of Public Health and Medicine, Northwestern University, Chicago, IL, USA
[2]Department of Medicine, University of Jos, Jos, Nigeria
Full list of author information is available at the end of the article

Background

Despite antiretroviral therapy (ART), tuberculosis (TB) remains a major cause of morbidity and mortality among persons with human immunodeficiency virus (HIV) infection in Sub-Saharan Africa [1]. Prompt and accurate diagnosis of TB and timely initiation of appropriate treatment decreases TB transmission and mortality [2]. To aid prompt TB diagnosis, the World Health Organization (WHO) in 2010 endorsed the Cepheid Xpert® MTB/RIF (Xpert) as a first line tool for diagnosis of HIV-associated TB [3]. Xpert is a nucleic acid amplification test that simultaneously detects MTB and rifampicin resistance, and has demonstrated high sensitivity (79.7–100%) as well as shorter diagnostic turnaround time (<2 h) when compared to TB culture [4–6]. As at 2015, 60% of countries recommended Xpert as the initial TB test for persons with possible drug-resistant (DR) TB, and 69% recommended it as the initial diagnostic test in cases of presumptive HIV-associated TB [7].

Nigeria, a country with high TB burden, commenced roll-out of Xpert in 2012 [8]. Xpert roll-out has however been slow, and sputum smear microscopy (SM) for acid fast bacilli (AFB) remains the primary mode of diagnosing TB in Nigeria. SM has a sensitivity of about 35% in children and in persons with HIV-infection [9, 10]; populations most adversely affected by TB in sub-Saharan Africa [11]. In recognition of these challenges, the government of Nigeria has prioritized Xpert use for people with HIV, suspected DR-TB, and children. Since introduction of Xpert in Nigeria, the few available studies have focused on its diagnostic performance in non-HIV clinical settings [12, 13]. Understanding the role of Xpert in the diagnosis of HIV-associated TB, as well as its impact on treatment outcomes, is crucial given the high mortality associated with this condition.

Using prospectively collected data during routine clinic care, we evaluated the impact of Xpert on diagnosis, time to treatment, and outcome of HIV-associated pulmonary tuberculosis (PTB). Our primary hypothesis was that 70 (±10) % of patients treated for PTB will have a positive Xpert result. Our secondary hypothesis was that PTB patients with positive Xpert result will initiate treatment earlier than those diagnosed using SM or clinical diagnosis. Lastly we explored the impact of Xpert on outcome of PTB treatment.

Methods

Study design and participants

The Jos University Teaching Hospital (JUTH) HIV clinic acquired a four module Xpert machine in 2012, and by 2013 Xpert became the standard first-line tool for evaluation of HIV-associated PTB. We enrolled consecutive HIV positive adults (≥18 years), accessing care at the JUTH HIV clinic referred for PTB testing using Xpert between June 2013 and June 2015 into the study cohort. We excluded known TB patients being evaluated for DR-TB. Written informed consent was obtained from all study participants and the study was approved by the Ethics Review Boards of Northwestern University, Chicago, USA and Jos University Teaching Hospital, Nigeria.

Study setting

The JUTH HIV treatment program commenced with support from the Government of Nigeria and the Bill & Melinda Gates Foundation in 2002. Subsequent support from the United States President's Emergency Plan for AIDS Relief (PEPFAR) in 2004 expanded access to free antiretroviral therapy (ART). At the time of this study approximately 10,000 patients were receiving comprehensive HIV care, which included treatment of opportunistic infections such as TB.

HIV treatment and monitoring

HIV treatment was guided by the Nigerian National ART guidelines [14]. Patients with a CD4 count of <350 cells/mm^3, and those with TB, pregnancy, or Hepatitis B irrespective of CD4 count were commenced on ART. Routine follow-up of patients on ART occurred monthly or every other month for drug pick-up, adherence counseling, and targeted clinical assessment. HIV treatment response was monitored using CD4 T-cell count and HIV-1 RNA assayed on site with Partec CyFlow Counter and Roche PCR Amplicor Monitor version 1.5, respectively. These tests were performed at presentation, ART initiation, and every 6 months subsequently for CD4 T-cell count and yearly for HIV-1 RNA assay.

TB diagnosis and treatment

In line with the WHO TB treatment guideline adopted by Nigeria [15], all HIV positive individuals were screened for TB symptoms at all clinic encounters. Patients with symptoms suggestive of PTB (presumptive PTB cases) were referred to the in-house TB Directly Observed Treatment (DOT) center, where sputa were collected for SM and Xpert testing at the JUTH TB Laboratory. Two expectorated same-day sputa samples were obtained from each patient for testing. SM was carried out on un-concentrated sputum samples as previously described [16]. One Xpert test was carried out using combined samples from each patient and was reported as: (1) MTB detected rifampicin resistance detected, (2) MTB detected rifampicin resistance not detected, (3) MTB not detected, or (4) Indeterminate. Patients with indeterminate results had the test repeated using fresh samples, and results of the repeat Xpert test were documented as the final Xpert result. External quality control for SM was carried out by the National

TB Control program, while quality control for Xpert was carried out using the manufacturer's manual [17].

The JUTH TB laboratory was the only facility with Xpert capability in the state at the time of the study and received samples from other hospitals. In addition to the Xpert, the GenoType MTBDRplus assay [18], another molecular diagnostic tool, was available but mostly used for research purposes. JUTH also housed a free-standing regional TB laboratory that carried out TB culture using solid media, which was routinely done for patients with rifampicin resistance following Xpert as per protocol. Chest X-ray facilities were also available and were requested at the discretion of the treating physician.

Based on the WHO case definition, a patient was classified as having PTB if sputum sample was positive by SM or Xpert (bacteriologically confirmed case) or if SM and Xpert were negative but the treating physician made a diagnosis of PTB and initiated full TB treatment (clinical diagnosis) [15]. TB cases, without rifampicin resistance on Xpert were treated with quadruple anti-tubercular therapy for six months consisting of rifampicin (or rifabutin, if on a protease inhibitor), isoniazid, ethambutol, and pyrazinamide for the first two months, then rifampicin and isoniazid for the remaining four months. Patients with rifampicin resistant PTB were referred to designated DR-TB treatment facilities for specialized care.

The in-house TB DOT center routinely documented date of initiation of TB treatment and treatment outcome in a designated register. The register was provided and supervised by the Nigerian National TB control program. Based on WHO guidelines [15], TB treatment outcome was reported as:

(1) Cured: a PTB patient with bacteriologically confirmed TB at the beginning of treatment who was smear- or culture-negative in the last month of treatment and on at least one previous occasion.
(2) Completed treatment: a TB patient who completed treatment without evidence of failure but had no record to show that sputum smear or culture results in the last month of treatment, and on at least one previous occasion were negative, either because tests were not done or because results are unavailable.
(3) Treatment failure: a TB patient whose sputum smear or culture was positive at month 5 or later during treatment.
(4) Default: a TB patient who whose treatment was interrupted for 2 consecutive months or more
(5) Death: a TB patient who died for any reason during the course of treatment.

The sum of cured and treatment completed was reported as treatment success.

Data collection

During routine clinic visits, patient data were collected by health providers and transferred to an electronic database (File Maker Pro). Data from the laboratory (hematology, chemistry, and CD4 T-cell count) and pharmacy (medication history, pick-up dates, and percentage adherence) were entered on the same database and merged, to aid real time patient management.

At study baseline (day of first presentation for evaluation for presumptive PTB), in addition to routine sputum collection for SM and Xpert test, a structured interviewer-administered questionnaire was used to obtain demographic data, patient symptoms, and history of previous TB treatment. This questionnaire was updated at all patients' subsequent visits to the clinic, to capture date of TB diagnosis, date of initiation of TB treatment, and outcome of TB treatment. For patients without a diagnosis of TB, follow-up was terminated when a diagnosis of TB was excluded. For patients diagnosed with TB without rifampicin resistance, follow-up continued until outcome of TB treatment was determined. If Xpert indicated rifampicin resistance, follow-up terminated at point of diagnosis because patients were referred to the specialized DR-TB program. We extracted CD4 T cell counts (pre-ART and most recent-within 3 months of study baseline interview) from the electronic patients' records.

Variables

Patients with either bacteriologically confirmed PTB or clinical PTB were grouped together as PTB [15]. Time to treatment was computed as the number of days from the date of baseline visit to the date of initiation of TB treatment. The outcome of PTB treatment was documented at the end of the 6th month of TB treatment and corroborated using the DOTS TB register at the JUTH HIV clinic. For patients who did not complete 6 months of treatment, follow-up was terminated on the date of death (which is usually reported to the clinic and captured in the electronic patient records) or date of last clinic visit (loss to follow-up).

The main exposure was Xpert result indicating 'MTB detected'. In addition, PTB diagnosis was further categorized as: (1) both Xpert and SM positive (Xpert+/SM+), (2) positive Xpert and negative SM (Xpert+/SM-), (3) Xpert negative and SM positive (Xpert-/SM+), and (4) negative or indeterminate Xpert and negative SM (Xpert-/SM-). Other variables of interest were age, sex, number of TB symptoms, CD4 T-cell count at TB diagnosis, use of ART at time of TB diagnosis, and history of prior TB treatment.

Statistical analysis

The study population was characterized using descriptive statistics and the data of patients with and without

PTB were compared using chi square test, t-test, or Mann Whitney U tests as appropriate. The number of patients with PTB with positive Xpert or SM results was presented as proportions, and compared using chi square. Time to treatment was compared using Kaplan Meier analysis. The outcome of TB treatment was reported as a proportion. Predictors of treatment outcomes were determined using logistic regression models. In all regression models, factors were included in the multivariate model if they had a $p < 0.2$ in the univariate model or had been shown to predict outcome in previous studies. A $p < 0.05$ was considered statistically significant.

Statistical analyses were done using Stata version 14 (College Station, TX).

Results

A total of 310 HIV-positive adults were enrolled onto the study cohort. Of these, 195 were females (62.9%). The mean age (standard deviation (SD)) was 38.5 (10.6) years. Males were older than females; 41.6 (10.6) years, 36.6 (10.7) years, $p = 0.0001$. The median CD4 cell count at time of TB testing was 242 (Interquartile range (IQR) 120–425) cells/mm^3, and 88.1% of the participants were on ART. The study flow chart is shown in Fig. 1.

Tuberculosis diagnosis

A total of 76 (24.5%) patients had a diagnosis of PTB. Among PTB patients, 56 (73.7%) had MTB detected by Xpert, 18 (23.7%) had no MTB detected, and 2(2.6%) had persistent indeterminate results after a repeat Xpert. 5/56 (8.9%) had rifampicin resistance. Of the patients diagnosed with PTB, 57 (75%) were SM positive. Sixty three patients (82.9%) had bacteriologically confirmed PTB. Further analysis showed that 50 patients (65.8%) had Xpert+/SM+, 6 (7.9%) Xpert+/SM-, 7 (9.2) Xpert-/SM+, and 13 (17.1%) Xpert-/SM- sputum test results. Table 1 shows patients characteristics stratified by PTB diagnosis. Patients treated for PTB who had a positive Xpert results (irrespective of SM) were more likely to be male, report weight loss or night sweats, and have positive sputum SM results (Table 2).

Time to treatment

Time to initiation of TB treatment was analyzed in 67 patients who initiated TB treatment. The median time to treatment was 6 (IQR 2–12) days. Only three patients (4.2%) commenced TB treatment on the day of baseline visit. Cumulatively 47.2% commenced treatment within 5 days of baseline visit. Median time to treatment was 5 (IQR 2–8) days and 12 (IQR 5–35) in patient with and without Xpert positive results respectively; Mann Whitney U $p = 0.0045$. The median time to treatment was 5 (IQR 2–7) days for Xpert+/SM+, 6 (IQR 4–9) days for Xpert+/SM-, 8 (IQR 6–31) days for Xpert-/SM+, and 27 (IQR 5–35) days for Xpert-/SM- cases; Kruskal Wallis $p = 0.04$. Figure 2 shows differences in time to treatment based on TB sputum test results. Using Kaplan-Meier analysis, time to treatment was shortest in patients with Xpert+/SM+ and longest in Xpert-/SM-test results (Log rank $p = <0.001$ Fig. 2a and $p = 0.002$ Fig. 2b).

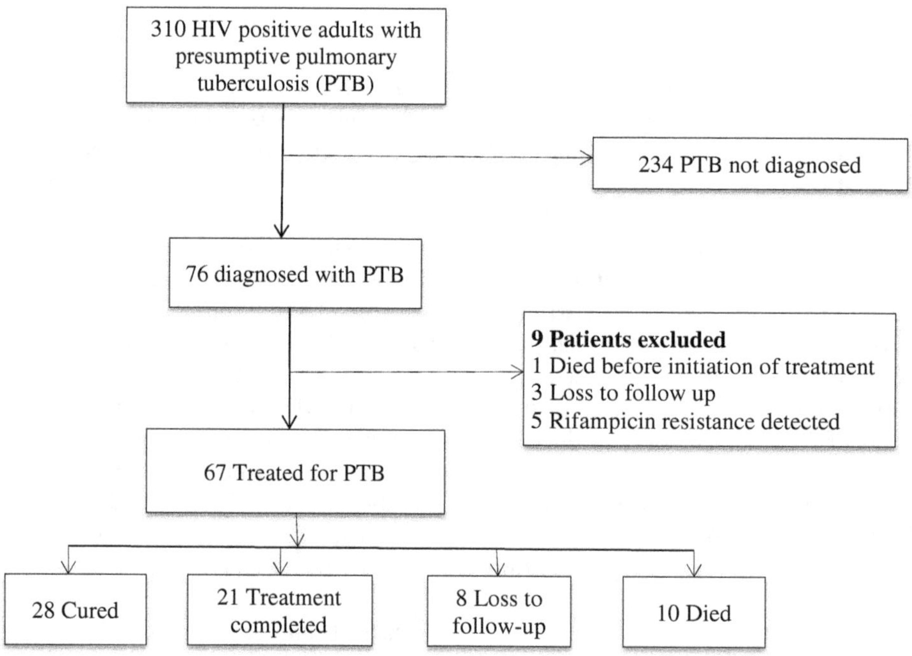

Fig. 1 Study Flow diagram showing patient enrolment, tuberculosis treatment and outcomes

Table 1 Characteristics of 310 adults with HIV evaluated for pulmonary tuberculosis, Nigeria (June 2013- June 2015)

Characteristics	Total Population ($n = 310$)	Treated for TB ($n = 76$)	No evidence of TB ($n = 234$)	*P*-value
Age,years, Mean (SD)	38.5 (10.6)	35.7 (9.6)	39.4 (10.7)	0.007
Sex				0.03
Male, n (%)	115 (37.1)	36 (47.4)	79 (33.8)	
Female, n (%)	195 (62.9)	40 (52.6)	155 (66.2)	
Body Mass Index	21.9 (3.9)	20.9 (3.8)	22.3 (3.9)	0.02
TB symptoms				
†Cough duration,Weeks, Median (IQR)	3 (2–6)	4 (2–8)	3 (2–5)	0.002
Fever, n (%)	227 (73.2)	62 (81.6)	165 (70.5)	0.06
Weight loss, n (%)	250 (80.6)	67 (88.2)	183 (78.2)	0.06
Night Sweat, n (%)	209 (67.4)	56 (73.7)	153 (65.4)	0.18
Cough > 2 weeks, n (%)	195 (62.9)	56 (73.7)	139 (59.4)	0.03
Previous TB treatment, n (%)	81 (26.1)	11 (14.5)	70 (29.9)	0.008
On ART, n (%)	273 (88.1)	63 (82.9)	210 (89.1)	0.34
†Latest CD4 Count, cells/mm^3, (Median, IQR)	242 (120–425)	224 (99–354)	259 (128–457)	0.11

SD Standard deviation, *IQR* Interquartile range, *TB* Tuberculosis, *ART* Antiretroviral Therapy, †Mann Whitney U test

Outcomes of TB treatment

Of the 67 patients who initiated PTB treatment, 49 patients (73.1%) achieved TB treatment success (28 cured, 21 completed treatment). Eight patients (11.9%) defaulted and 10 (14.9%) died within 6 months of initiating TB treatment. There was no association between Xpert result and successful TB treatment (Xpert MTB detected, 37/49 (75.5%) versus MTB not detected or indeterminate, 12/49 (25.5%) X^2 1.34; $p = 0.25$). Treatment success was recorded in 5/5 (100%), 32/43 (74.4%), 3/6 (50%) and 9/13 (69.2%) of patients diagnosed with Xpert +/SM -, Xpert+/SM+, Xpert-/SM+, and Xpert-/SM- PTB respectively (Chi square 3.61, $p = 0.31$).

A total of 10 deaths were documented within 6 months of initiation of TB therapy (analysis excluded 8 patients who defaulted). Deaths recorded based on diagnostic group were 0/5 (0%) Xpert+/SM-, 5/37 (13.5%) Xpert +/SM+, 1/4 (25%) Xpert-/SM+, and 4/13 (30.8%) Xpert-/SM- (Chi square 3.3, $p = 0.35$). By analysis in which the summation of death and default were

Table 2 Characteristic of 76 adults with HIV treated for pulmonary tuberculosis, Jos, Nigeria (June 2013– June 2015)

Characteristics	Xpert MTB Detected ($n = 56$)	Xpert No MTB Detected ($n = 20$)	*P*-value
Age, years,Mean (SD)	37.3 (13.2)	35.0 (12.3)	0.39
Sex			0.004
Male, n (%)	32 (57.1)	4 (20.0)	
Female, n (%)	24 (42.9)	16 (80)	
TB symptoms			
Cough > 2 weeks, n (%)	42 (75.0)	14 (70.0)	0.66
Fever, n (%)	48 (85.7)	14 (70.0)	0.12
Weight loss, n (%)	52 (92.9)	15 (75.0)	0.03
Night Sweat, n (%)	45 (80.4)	11 (55)	0.03
Previous TB treatment, n (%)	7 (12.5)	4 (20)	0.4
On ART, n (%)	48 (88.9)	15 (83.3)	0.54
Current CD4 ≤ 200 cells/mm^3,n (%)	38 (67.9)	10 (50.0)	0.16
[a]CD4 count at TB diagnosis, cells/mm^3, Median (IQR)	198 (68–354)	309 (123–507)	0.09
SM positive, n (%)	50 (89.3)	7 (35.0)	<0.001
Rifampicin Resistance, n (%)	5 (8.93)	-	-

SD Standard deviation, *IQR* Interquartile range, *TB* Tuberculosis, *MTB* Mycobacterium tuberculosis, *ART* Antiretroviral Therapy, *SM* Sputum smear microscopy for acid fast bacilli [a]Kruskal Wallis test

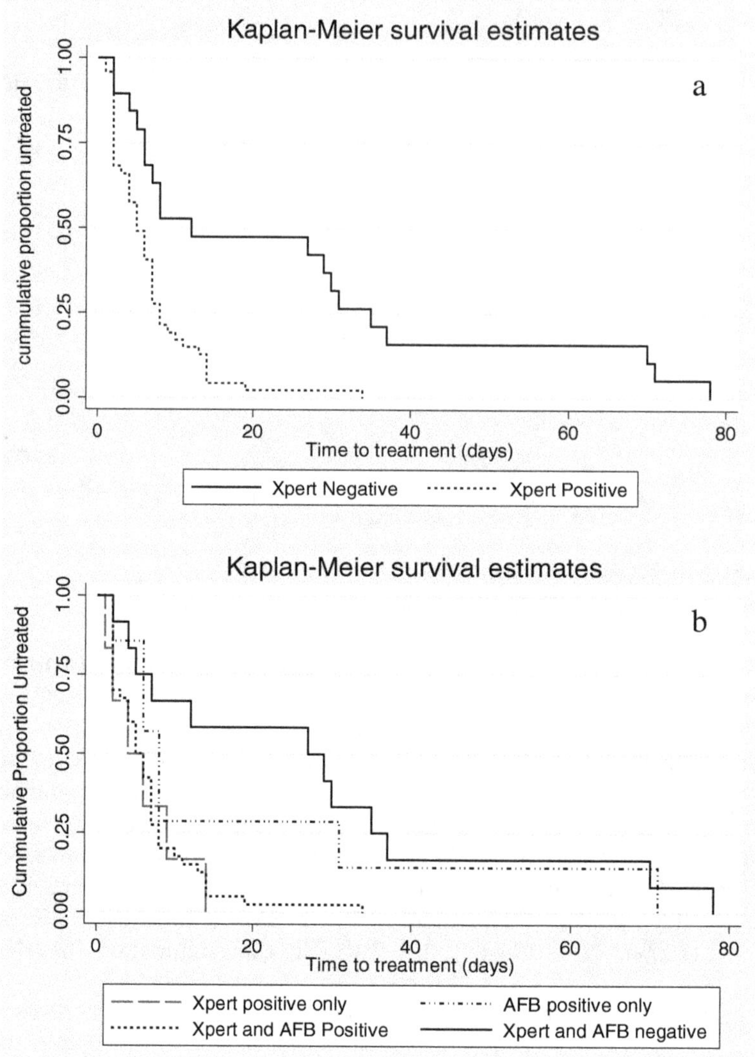

Fig. 2 Kaplan Meier curves of time to pulmonary tuberculosis treatment among 67 adults with HIV in Jos, Nigeria. Legend for fig. 2: Fig. 2a compares time to treatment in adults with HIV-associated tuberculosis with positive and negative Xpert. Time to treatment was significantly shorter in patients with positive Xpert results. In (**b**), four patient subgroups are defined using a combination of Xpert and Acid fast bacilli (AFB) result on smear microscopy. Similar to (**a**), Xpert positive adults with HIV-associated tuberculosis had shorter time to tuberculosis treatment, while the greatest treatment delay was in those with negative Xpert & AFB results

considered as a composite poor treatment outcome, 0/5 (0%) Xpert+/SM-, 11/43 (25.6%) Xpert+/SM+, 3/6 (50%) Xpert-/SM+, and 4/13 (30.8%) Xpert-/SM- had poor treatment outcomes (Chi square 3.6, $p = 0.31$). In univariate logistic regression analysis of age, sex, mode of diagnosis (Xpert positive versus negative or indeterminate) and use of ART (Yes/No), only ART reduced poor treatment outcome (OR 0.16; 95% CI 0.03–1.0; $p = 0.48$).

Predictors of mortality

Table 3 shows predictors of mortality in 59 patients treated for PTB (8 patients who were lost to follow-up were excluded). An Xpert positive result was not associated with lower mortality in bivariate or multivariate analysis. In analysis adjusted for age, sex, and mode of diagnosis (Xpert positive versus negative or indeterminate) odds for death during treatment were 90% lower in patients on ART at time of TB diagnosis (AOR 0.10; 95% CI 0.01–0.93).

Discussion

We evaluated the diagnosis, time to treatment, and outcome of HIV-associated PTB in a clinic cohort in Nigeria, following the implementation of Xpert as a first-line tool for TB diagnosis. A quarter of patients enrolled had a diagnosis of PTB. The majority of patients diagnosed with PTB (73.7%) had MTB detected using Xpert. Patients with Xpert positive results had

Table 3 Logistic regression analysis of predictors of mortality in 59 adults with HIV treated for pulmonary tuberculosis in Jos, Nigeria

	Unadjusted Analysis			Adjusted Analysis		
	OR	95% CI	*P*-value	AOR	95% CI	*P*-value
Xpert positive	0.32	0.08–1.32	0.12	0.67	0.11–4.05	0.66
Age, years	1.03	0.97–1.10	0.19	1.04	0.96–1.12	0.31
BMI < 18.5 Kg/m^2	1.90	0.41–8.82	0.41	-	-	-
Sex, Female	4.52	0.87–23.50	0.07	5.63	0.69–45.93	0.11
3 or more TB symptoms	0.66	0.11–3.81	0.65	-	-	-
Recent CD4 count <200 cells/mm^3	0.87	0.21–3.50	0.84	-	-	-
Recent CD4 count (cell/mm^3)	1.00	0.99–1.00	0.66	-	-	-
On ART	0.11	0.02–0.77	0.03	0.10	0.01–0.93	0.04
Time to treatment (days)	0.99	0.95–1.05	0.87	-	-	-

OR Odds ratio, *AOR* Adjusted odds ratio, *CI* Confidence interval, *BMI* Body mass index, *TB* tuberculosis, *ART* Antiretroviral therapy
Variables with $p < 0.2$ in the bivariate analysis were included in the adjusted model

significantly shorter time to treatment, but Xpert had no impact on survival.

The use of Xpert is expected to significantly improve the diagnosis of HIV-associated TB compared to microscopy, due to its increased sensitivity [6, 19–21]. However, we observed that among our cohort of patients with HIV-associated PTB, yield from Xpert was similar to microscopy (73.5% Xpert, 75% microscopy, 65.8% concordance). Similar to what we found, a retrospective analysis of data from 13 regions in Namibia showed that 77.1% of HIV patients with Xpert positive results were also positive by microscopy [22]. With this high level of concordance between Xpert and microscopy it is unlikely that Xpert significantly improved sensitivity of TB diagnosis in these populations. Likewise, in Uganda, Xpert did not significantly increase the number of patients starting TB treatment, compared to microscopy, when routinely collected TB program data were analyzed [23]. In contrast to these, Lawn et al. reported that Xpert increased TB diagnostic yield by 45% compared to microscopy in a clinical trial among ART naïve adults with HIV in South Africa [19]. A Cochrane review of 27 clinical trials also showed that Xpert increased TB detection by 23% (95% CI 15–32) when compared to microscopy [24]. It is unclear why the efficacy of Xpert reported in these trials are not being replicated during routine use in clinical settings. The level of immuno-competence of patients may be a contributing factor. Our patient population, in contrast to those in the Lawn study, was mostly on ART and had a higher CD4 count (242 (IQR 120–242 cells/mm^3 versus 171 (IQR 102–236) cells/mm^3). Advanced immunosuppression significantly reduces sensitivity of microscopy and use of Xpert may yield greater diagnostic benefit in patients with immunosuppression. A previous study also reported a high rate of microscopy positive PTB in our clinic population [16].

Another factor that could reduce the diagnostic benefit of Xpert during routine use is empirical TB treatment. In our cohort, 17.1% of patients treated for TB, had negative Xpert and microscopy results. TB diagnosis in these patients was likely made using symptoms and chest radiography (empirical therapy). Empirical therapy is widely used even in facilities where Xpert is available [25, 26]. It has been proposed that widespread empirical TB therapy could reduce the impact of Xpert in improving TB diagnosis at the population level [26]. Calling for cessation of empirical treatment, however is unethical since as many as 14–30% of Xpert negative samples end up being culture positive [24].

Rapid diagnosis of rifampicin resistance, a surrogate marker of multidrug resistance TB, facilitates prompt initiation of DR-TB treatment. Five patients, representing 8.9% of TB diagnosis, had rifampicin resistance and were referred to specialized DR-TB treatment facilities. Prompt diagnosis and treatment of DR-TB would reduce disease spread and could lead to better treatment outcomes. This may be a major benefit of Xpert in populations, such as ours, with high prevalence of DR-TB.

One of the limitations of microscopy is its inability to differentiate MTB from other smear positive organisms, particularly non-tuberculous mycobacteria (NTM). Because Xpert specifically detects MTB, smear positive/ Xpert negative samples should prompt further evaluation for NTM. This becomes more important in patients with immunosuppressive conditions like HIV, at high risk for NTM [27]. Diagnosis of NTM remains a challenge in resource limited settings because it requires culture of relevant biological samples [28]. Facilities for culture are scarce in these settings. Seven patients (9.2%) in our cohort of patients treated for PTB had Xpert negative/SM positive results, suggesting these may be cases of NTM, and this group had the worse treatment outcome (50% mortality). A high prevalence of NTM has been reported among patients evaluated for TB in this region of Nigeria. A recent study reported that 15% of individuals with culture positive TB had NTM; this proportion rose to 38% in those with HIV [29]. Although not all patients in whom NTM is isolated require treatment, when treatment is indicated, drugs used to treat NTM differ from those for MTB [30]. Patients with NTM treated with conventional TB drugs are unlikely to respond to this treatment and may have poorer treatment outcomes.

The capacity of Xpert to diagnose TB within two hours suggests that patients with symptoms of TB could get a diagnosis and commence treatment during one clinic visit. With smear microscopy, patients have to make at least one more clinic trip to get test results and commence treatment. Some patients never return for the visit to complete sputum collection or commence treatment [31, 32]. We observed significant differences in time to treatment, ranging from a median of 5 days in Xpert positive/smear positive patients to 27 days in Xpert negative/smear negative patients. While Xpert positive cases had shorter time to treatment, only 3 patients (4.2%) commenced treatment during a single clinic visit, which is the presumed norm if Xpert is used. Cumulatively 47.2% commenced treatment within 5 days of baseline visit. Delay in initiating TB treatment despite implementation of Xpert is not unique to our population [26, 33, 34], and we need to better understand factors contributing to this delay. We observed that the four-cartridge Xpert machine at the study site not only served the clinic but the whole state with a population of 3.2 million with an estimated 40,000 cases of TB/HIV co-infection in 2012 [35]. At full capacity, only 12–16 specimens can be processed in a day using a four-module Xpert machine [36], meaning processing of additional specimen will spill into a second day. While deployment of more Xpert machines may be a viable solution, delay in initiation of treatment has also been observed after making test results available to patients during their first visit [26]. Patient contribution to delays in TB treatment remains a challenge which Xpert may not completely eliminate. In a study of the Zambian TB program, patient factors were found to be the major contributor to TB treatment delay [37].

Few studies have evaluated the impact of Xpert on outcomes of TB treatment. Similar to previous studies [33, 38], Xpert result did not predict mortality. Use of ART however independently reduced mortality by 90%. Some factors may attenuate the impact of Xpert on TB outcomes. The first is a prevailing practice of empiric treatment [39]. Irrespective of TB test results, when suspicion for TB is strong, treating physicians are likely to initiate TB therapy, which is reasonable given the sensitivity of Xpert in persons with HIV. Another reason is that recent studies, including ours, did not consider the treatment benefits for patients diagnosed with rifampicin resistance. Improved outcomes for patients with DR-TB, may be one of the main benefits of Xpert.

This study has limitations. The study was carried out at a single site which may limit its generalizability. TB management at the site however followed WHO guidelines, which is widely used in many low- and middle-income countries with high prevalence of TB and HIV. Another limitation was that cultures were not available to confirm PTB diagnosis. While this may be considered a limitation, the goal of the study was not to determine the test characteristics of Xpert or microscopy. Our aim to evaluate the contribution of Xpert to diagnosis and its impact on treatment of HIV-associated TB, during routine use. Moreover, our study setting is similar to health facilities in other low- and middle-income countries where TB culture is not available and Xpert is being rolled out as the first line for diagnosis of HIV associated TB. One other limitation was that sample size for outcome analysis may be underpowered to identify small effect sizes in subgroup analysis. Our outcome analysis also excluded patients with rifampicin resistance.

Conclusions

We have demonstrated the utility of Xpert in routine clinical evaluation of patients with HIV-associated TB in a middle-income country with high TB and HIV burden. While Xpert did not significantly increase microbiological confirmation of TB among treated cases or outcome of treatment, it did aid rapid diagnosis of rifampicin resistance and resulted in shorter time to treatment. Larger studies incorporating benefits attributable to early diagnosis and treatment of DR-TB will be needed to fully elucidate the impact of Xpert in TB patients. As Xpert is rolled out, its contribution to TB treatment may be modest, due to delays in TB treatment initiation as well as the wide use of empiric treatment. TB programs need to find innovative ways to aid prompt initiation of treatment in patients with Xpert positive TB. Furthermore, other rapid diagnostic tools are also urgently needed to address the 14–30% of culture positive TB patients with negative Xpert results, as well as cases of NTM. Finally, where resources are constrained, ART needs to be prioritized as it was the only factor we identified that independently improved survival during TB treatment.

Abbreviations

AFB: Acid fast bacilli; ART: Antiretroviral therapy; DOT: Directly observed treatment; DR-TB: Drug resistant tuberculosis; HIV: Human immunodeficiency virus; IQR: Interquartile range; JUTH: Jos University Teaching Hospital;

PEPFAR: The United States President's Emergency Plan for AIDS Relief; PTB: Pulmonary tuberculosis; SD: Standard deviation; SM: Smear microscopy; TB: Tuberculosis

Acknowledgements
The authors are grateful to all staff and patients of the Jos University Teaching Hospital, HIV Clinic, Nigeria, for their valuable contributions. We also acknowledge the contributions of Tope Ashi-Sulaiman towards the success of the study. We thank Dr Brian Pool for his contribution towards data collection. Lastly, we appreciate Elizabeth Christian and Natalie Sheneman for their editorial review of the manuscript.

Funding
MOA was supported by the NIH through the Fogarty International Center grants 1D43TW009575 and D43TWOO7995 (R.L.M as PI). The funding agencies had no role in the design of the study, data collection or analysis, interpretation of data, or in writing the manuscript. The contents of this article are solely the responsibility of the authors and do not necessarily represent the official views of the Fogarty International Center or the National Institutes of Health.

Authors' contributions
MOA has full access to all study data and takes responsibility for the accuracy of the data. Study concept and design was by MOA, CA, BT, OA, CU and RLM. Data acquisition was by MOA, AA, YI, JI, PA and CA. Data analysis and interpretation was by MOA, CA, BT, RLM, CU, and MM. Initial draft of the manuscript was done by M.O.A. All authors contributed to the initial draft, reviewed the manuscript, approved the final version, and agree to be accountable for all aspects of the work.

Competing interests
The authors declare that they have no competing interests.

Consent for publication
Not applicable.

Author details
[1]Institute of Public Health and Medicine, Northwestern University, Chicago, IL, USA. [2]Department of Medicine, University of Jos, Jos, Nigeria. [3]Department of Medicine, Northwestern University, Chicago, IL, USA. [4]Department of Medical Microbiology, University of Jos, Jos, PL, Nigeria. [5]AIDS Prevention Initiative in Nigeria (APIN) Center, Jos University Teaching Hospital, Jos, PL, Nigeria. [6]AIDS Prevention Initiative in Nigeria (APIN), Abuja, Nigeria. [7]Department of Biomedical Engineering, Northwestern University, Evanston, IL, USA.

References

1. Cox JA, Lukande RL, Lucas S, Nelson AM, Van Marck E, Colebunders R. Autopsy causes of death in HIV-positive individuals in sub-Saharan Africa and correlation with clinical diagnoses. AIDS Rev. 2010;12(4):183–94.
2. Lienhardt C, Rowley J, Manneh K, Lahai G, Needham D, Milligan P, McAdam KPWJ. Factors affecting time delay to treatment in a tuberculosis control programme in a sub-Saharan African country: the experience of The Gambia. Int J Tuberc Lung Dis. 2001;5(3):233–9.
3. World Health Organization. Rapid implementation of the Xpert MTB/RIF diagnostic test: technical and operational 'How-to'; practical considerations. Geneva: World Health Organization; 2011.
4. Rie AV, Page-Shipp L, Scott L, Sanne I, Stevens W. Xpert® MTB/RIF for point-of-care diagnosis of TB in high-HIV burden, resource-limited countries: hype or hope? Expert Rev Mol Diagn. 2010;10(7):937–46.
5. Helb D, Jones M, Story E, Boehme C, Wallace E, Ho K, Kop J, Owens MR, Rodgers R, Banada P, et al. Rapid detection of mycobacterium tuberculosis and rifampin resistance by use of on-demand. Near-Patient Technol J Clin Microbiol. 2010;48(1):229–37.
6. Boehme CC, Nabeta P, Hillemann D, Nicol MP, Shenai S, Krapp F, Allen J, Tahirli R, Blakemore R, Rustomjee R, et al. Rapid molecular detection of tuberculosis and rifampin resistance. N Engl J Med. 2010;363(11):1005–15.
7. World Health Organization. Global tuberculosis report. 2015. 20th ed. Geneva: World Health Organization; 2015.
8. Abdurrahman ST, Emenyonu N, Obasanya OJ, Lawson L, Dacombe R, Muhammad M, Oladimeji O, Cuevas LE. The hidden costs of installing xpert machines in a tuberculosis high-burden country: experiences from Nigeria. Pan Afr Med J. 2014;18:277.
9. Corbett EL, Watt CJ, Walker N, Maher D, Williams BG, Raviglione MC, Dye C. The growing burden of tuberculosis: global trends and interactions with the HIV epidemic. Arch Intern Med. 2003;163(9):1009–21.
10. Mathew P, Kuo YH, Vazirani B, Eng RH, Weinstein MP. Are three sputum acid-fast bacillus smears necessary for discontinuing tuberculosis isolation? J Clin Microbiol. 2002;40(9):3482–4.
11. Bassett IV, Wang B, Chetty S, Giddy J, Losina E, Mazibuko M, Bearnot B, Allen J, Walensky RP, Freedberg KA. Intensive tuberculosis screening for HIV-infected patients starting antiretroviral therapy in Durban, South Africa. Clin Infect Dis. 2010;51(7):823–9.
12. John S, Gidado M, Dahiru T, Fanning A, Codlin AJ, Creswell J. Tuberculosis among nomads in Adamawa, Nigeria: outcomes from two years of active case finding. Int J Tuberc Lung Dis. 2015;19(4):463–8.
13. Abdurrahman ST, Mbanaso O, Lawson L, Oladimeji O, Blakiston M, Obasanya J, Dacombe R, Adams ER, Emenyonu N, Sahu S, et al. Testing pooled sputum with Xpert MTB/RIF for diagnosis of pulmonary tuberculosis To increase affordability in low-income countries. J Clin Microbiol. 2015;53(8):2502–8.
14. Federal Ministry of Health Nigeria: National Guidelines For HIV And AIDs Treatment And Care In Adolescents And Adults. Nigeria; 2010. http://www.who.int/hiv/pub/guidelines/nigeria_art.pdf. Accessed 2 Feb 2017.
15. World Health Organization. Stop TB Dept.: treatment of tuberculosis: guidelines. 4th ed. Geneva: World Health Organization; 2010.
16. Ani A, Isah Y, Pwol R, Lekuk C, Ashi-Sulaiman T, Akindgh M, Akanbi M, Akande P, Agbaji O. Detection of Mycobacterium tuberculosis by rapid molecular methods augments acid fast bacilli (AFB) smear microscopy in a non-culture tuberculosis laboratory. Afr J Microbiol Res. 2015;9(13):960–4.
17. GeneXpert® Quality Control Features for All Cepheid Xpert® Assays. http://www.swacm.org/workshops/4XpertAssayControl%20Info%20Sheet.pdf. Accessed 8 May 2017.
18. Dinic L, Akande P, Idigbe EO, Ani A, Onwujekwe D, Agbaji O, Akanbi M, Nwosu R, Adeniyi B, Wahab M, et al. Genetic determinants of drug-resistant tuberculosis among HIV-infected patients in Nigeria. J Clin Microbiol. 2012; 50(9):2905–9.
19. Lawn SD, Brooks SV, Kranzer K, Nicol MP, Whitelaw A, Vogt M, Bekker LG, Wood R. Screening for HIV-associated tuberculosis and rifampicin resistance before antiretroviral therapy using the Xpert MTB/RIF assay: a prospective study. PLoS Med. 2011;8(7):e1001067.
20. Sharma SK, Kohli M, Yadav RN, Chaubey J, Bhasin D, Sreenivas V, Sharma R, Singh BK. Evaluating the diagnostic accuracy of Xpert MTB/RIF assay in pulmonary tuberculosis. PLoS One. 2015;10(10):e0141011.
21. Kaur R, Kachroo K, Sharma JK, Vatturi SM, Dang A. Diagnostic accuracy of xpert test in tuberculosis detection: A systematic review and meta-analysis. J Global Infect Dis. 2016;8(1):32–40.
22. Mavenyengwa RT, Shaduka E, Maposa I. Evaluation of the Xpert(R) MTB/RIF assay and microscopy for the diagnosis of Mycobacterium tuberculosis in Namibia. Infect Dis Poverty. 2017;6(1):13.
23. Hanrahan CF, Haguma P, Ochom E, Kinera I, Cobelens F, Cattamanchi A, Davis L, Katamba A, Dowdy D. Implementation of xpert MTB/RIF in Uganda: missed opportunities to improve diagnosis of tuberculosis. Open forum Infect Dis. 2016;3(2):ofw068.
24. Steingart KR, Sohn H, Schiller I, Kloda LA, Boehme CC, Pai M, Dendukuri N. Xpert(R) MTB/RIF assay for pulmonary tuberculosis and rifampicin resistance in adults. Cochrane Database Syst Rev. 2013;1:CD009593.
25. Nakiyingi L, Bwanika JM, Kirenga B, Nakanjako D, Katabira C, Lubega G, Sempa J, Nyesiga B, Albert H, Manabe YC. Clinical predictors and accuracy

of empiric tuberculosis treatment among sputum smear-negative HIV-infected adult TB suspects in Uganda. PLoS One. 2013;8(9):e74023.
26. Theron G, Zijenah L, Chanda D, Clowes P, Rachow A, Lesosky M, Bara W, Mungofa S, Pai M, Hoelscher M, et al. Feasibility, accuracy, and clinical effect of point-of-care Xpert MTB/RIF testing for tuberculosis in primary-care settings in Africa: a multicentre, randomised, controlled trial. Lancet. 2014; 383(9915):424–35.
27. Lan R, Yang C, Lan L, Ou J, Qiao K, Liu F, Gao Q. Mycobacterium tuberculosis and non-tuberculous mycobacteria isolates from HIV-infected patients in Guangxi, China. Int J Tuberc Lung Dis. 2011;15(12):1669–75.
28. Ryu YJ, Koh W-J, Daley CL. Diagnosis and treatment of nontuberculous mycobacterial lung disease: clinicians' perspectives. Tuberc Respir Dis (Seoul). 2016;79(2):74–84.
29. Aliyu G, El-Kamary SS, Abimiku A, Brown C, Tracy K, Hungerford L, Blattner W. Prevalence of non-tuberculous mycobacterial infections among tuberculosis suspects in Nigeria. PLoS One. 2013;8(5):e63170.
30. Griffith DE, Aksamit T, Brown-Elliott BA, Catanzaro A, Daley C, Gordin F, Holland SM, Horsburgh R, Huitt G, Iademarco MF, et al. An official ATS/IDSA statement: diagnosis, treatment, and prevention of nontuberculous mycobacterial diseases. Am J Respir Crit Care Med. 2007;175(4):367–416.
31. Rawat J, Biswas D, Sindhwani G, Kesharwani V, Masih V, Chauhan BS. Diagnostic defaulters: an overlooked aspect in the Indian Revised National Tuberculosis Control Program. J Infect Dev Ctries. 2012;6(1):20–2.
32. Afutu FK, Zachariah R, Hinderaker SG, Ntoah-Boadi H, Obeng EA, Bonsu FA, Harries AD. High initial default in patients with smear-positive pulmonary tuberculosis at a regional hospital in Accra, Ghana. Trans R Soc Trop Med Hyg. 2012;106(8):511–3.
33. Mupfumi L, Makamure B, Chirehwa M, Sagonda T, Zinyowera S, Mason P, Metcalfe JZ, Mutetwa R. Impact of Xpert MTB/RIF on antiretroviral therapy-associated tuberculosis and mortality: A pragmatic randomized controlled trial. Open Forum Infect Dis. 2014;1(1):038.
34. Cohen GM, Drain PK, Noubary F, Cloete C, Bassett IV. Diagnostic delays and clinical decision-making with centralized Xpert MTB/RIF testing in Durban, South Africa. J Acquir Immune Defic Syndr. 2014;67(3):e88–93.
35. National Agency for the control of AIDS (NACA) Nigeria: Plateau State HIV and AIDS Epidemiology and Impact. http://naca.gov.ng/test/sites/default/files/Plateau%20State%20profile%20ppt_0.pdf. Aaccessed 9 Feb 2017.
36. Xpert MTB/RIF Implementation Manual: Technical and Operational 'How-To'; Practical Considerations. edn. Geneva; 2014: 7.
37. Takarinda KC, Harries AD, Nyathi B, Ngwenya M, Mutasa-Apollo T, Sandy C. Tuberculosis treatment delays and associated factors within the Zimbabwe national tuberculosis programme. BMC Public Health. 2015;15:29. doi:10.1186/s12889-015-1437-7.
38. Yoon C, Cattamanchi A, Davis JL, Worodria W, den Boon S, Kalema N, Katagira W, Kaswabuli S, Miller C, Andama A, et al. Impact of Xpert MTB/RIF testing on tuberculosis management and outcomes in hospitalized patients in Uganda. PLoS One. 2012;7(11):e48599.
39. Theron G, Peter J, Dowdy D, Langley I, Squire SB, Dheda K. Do high rates of empirical treatment undermine the potential effect of new diagnostic tests for tuberculosis in high-burden settings? Lancet Infect Dis. 2014;14(6):527–32.

Elevated *Aspergillus*-specific antibody levels among HIV infected Ugandans with pulmonary tuberculosis

Richard Kwizera[1*], Rosalind Parkes-Ratanshi[1,2], Iain D. Page[3,4], Christine Sekaggya-Wiltshire[1], Joseph Musaazi[1], Jan Fehr[5], Barbara Castelnuovo[1], Andrew Kambugu[1] and David W. Denning[3,4]

Abstract

Background: The incidence of tuberculosis (TB) is high among human immunodeficiency virus (HIV) infected Ugandans. Recent evidence suggests that Chronic Pulmonary Aspergillosis and *Aspergillus* sensitisation might be responsible for significant mortality in patients treated for tuberculosis in Uganda.

Methods: We retrieved and tested paired serum aliquots for 101 HIV-TB co-infected patients at the beginning and week 24 of TB treatment. We tested samples for *Aspergillus*-specific immunoglobulin G (IgG) and immunoglobulin E (IgE) using ImmunoCAP®; and *Aspergillus*-specific IgG and total serum IgE using Immulite® immunoassays. We compared antibody levels between baseline and week 24, relating them to selected baseline characteristics.

Results: 10% of the patients had elevated *Aspergillus*-specific IgE (*Aspergillus* sensitization) and *Aspergillus*-specific IgG antibodies were elevated in 9% of the patients at the end of TB treatment. There was a significant fall in the *Aspergillus*-specific IgG antibody levels between baseline and week 24 ($P = 0.02$). Patients with cluster of differentiation 4 (CD4) T-cell count <100 cells/μl and those who were not on anti-retroviral therapy at baseline had more elevated *Aspergillus*-specific IgG antibodies ($P = 0.01$, $P = 0.03$). The ImmunoCAP® *Aspergillus*-specific IgG antibody titres were higher at week 24 than baseline with more positives at week 24; even though the difference in means was small. However, this difference was statistically significant ($P = 0.02$). Pulmonary infiltrates were the commonest x-ray abnormality and only 5% of the patients had pulmonary cavities on chest x-ray at week 24.

Conclusion: These results suggest that *Aspergillus* infection may complicate active pulmonary TB and further studies including fungal culture and thoracic imaging may now be indicated to measure the prevalence of pulmonary aspergillosis complicating tuberculosis.

Keywords: Aspergillosis, HIV, Tuberculosis, Fungal diagnostics; serology

Background

Tuberculosis (TB) remains one of the major causes of morbidity and mortality worldwide with the highest burden found in Africa and Asia, mainly linked to the human immunodeficiency virus (HIV) epidemic [1]. The 2016 World Health Organization (WHO) report on TB revealed that there were an estimated 10 million new cases of TB in the year 2015 worldwide, with 11% having HIV. An estimated 1.8 million people died due to TB in 2015, including 0.4 million deaths due to HIV/TB co-infection. The incidence of TB among HIV patients in Uganda was estimated at 202 new cases per 100,000 population [2].

Due to the limited published data on fungal disease epidemiology in sub-Saharan Africa, a recent review attempted to estimate the burden of fungal infections in Uganda using specific populations [3]. In this review, chronic pulmonary aspergillosis (CPA) was estimated at 12–22% in TB patients with cavities and 1–4% in those

* Correspondence: kwizerarichard@ymail.com
[1]Infectious Diseases Institute, College of Health Sciences, Makerere University, P.O.BOX 22418 Kampala, Uganda
Full list of author information is available at the end of the article

without cavities. Considering post-TB data in Uganda, asymptomatic CPA was estimated at 7% with an additional 1.7% having detectable *Aspergillus*-specific immunoglobulin G (IgG) antibodies with cavitation.

Recent work done in Northern Uganda has validated some of these estimates, with a CPA prevalence of 8.2%, and 6.7% having cavities among patients who had been successfully treated for pulmonary TB within the last 7 years [4, 5]. More results from this work showed *Aspergillus*-specific IgG antibody levels were raised in 26% of patients with "smear negative TB" and suggested that previously unrecognized CPA might be responsible for significant mortality in patients treated for TB in Uganda [6–8]. Beyond this limited data, little is known about the epidemiology of fungal colonisation and sensitisation, and their contribution to TB disease progress and treatment outcomes in Uganda where pulmonary TB is very common, in part driven by the high prevalence of HIV [9].

We hypothesized that patients with pulmonary TB may get colonized with *Aspergillus* during and in the post treatment period leading to a chronic lung infection and/or allergic fungal disease if the patient was pre-sensitized to *Aspergillus* antigens. Pulmonary cavitation is a pre-disposing factor for CPA [10] and may or may not present together with *Aspergillus* sensitization. We therefore aimed to establish and compare *Aspergillus*-specific antibody levels among HIV-infected Ugandans with TB, at the beginning and end of TB treatment; using ImmunoCAP® and Immulite® immunoassays.

Methods

Study design and population

This was a nested cohort study under the "Study on Outcomes related to Tuberculosis and HIV drug concentrations in Uganda" (SOUTH) (ClinicalTrials.gov: NCT01782950). SOUTH was a prospective study investigating the correlation of anti-tuberculosis drug concentrations and TB treatment outcomes in HIV-infected individuals with pulmonary TB at the Infectious Diseases Institute, Kampala, Uganda [11]. All participants were HIV-TB co-infected patients above 18 years with a diagnosis of their first episode of pulmonary TB i.e. proven or highly suspected TB considered for TB treatment qualifying for 6 months (24 weeks) anti-TB drugs regimen (2 months HRZE [isoniazid (H), rifampicin (R), pyrazinamide (Z) and ethambutol (E)] and 4 months HR [isoniazid (H) and rifampicin (R)]). Patients with multi-drug resistant TB were excluded. Only 32% of the participants already had an HIV diagnosis with an average time since diagnosis of 53 days. The rest of the participants were diagnosed at TB screening. Each participant was followed up for 24 weeks.

Study samples

Samples used for this study were stored serum samples from the SOUTH study population (stored at −80°c). We cross checked the sample storage inventories to look out for participants that had a sample stored at beginning (baseline) and end of TB treatment (week 24). We included all patients with two aliquots i.e. one at baseline and one at week 24. Samples were then shipped and tested at the Mycology Reference Centre Manchester and Christie Hospital, Manchester, United Kingdom (UK).

Study assays

Testing was initially done using the ImmunoCAP® machine (ThermoFisher®, previously Phadia) to check for levels of *Aspergillus*-specific IgG (Asp IgG) at baseline and week 24. Also, using ImmunoCAP *Aspergillus*-specific IgE (Asp IgE) antibody levels were checked at week 24 only. Further testing for total serum IgE (TIgE) levels at both baseline and week 24 was undertaken on the Immulite 2000® machine (Siemens). Remaining serum was re-tested for *Aspergillus*-specific IgG levels using the Immulite machine (Additional file 1).

Assay cut-offs

We used a cut-off of 40 mg/l for the ImmunoCAP *Aspergillus*-specific IgG levels as recommended by manufacturer, and a cut-off of 20 mg/l for the Immulite *Aspergillus*-specific IgG levels based on preliminary results of a cross-sectional survey in Uganda [4]. Variations in the cut-off for total serum IgE have been reported ranging from 150 to 1000 UI/ml [12]. However, a cut-off of 1000 UI/ml is recommended for diagnosis of allergic bronchopulmonary aspergillosis (ABPA) [13]. Therefore, for our study, we used a cut-off of 170 UI/ml to check for general allergy and a cut-off of 1000 UI/ml as a screen for evidence of ABPA. A cut-off of 0.35 kU/l was used for *Aspergillus*-specific IgE levels as recommended by the manufacturer.

Data analysis

Data were analyzed using STATA® version 13 (STATA, College Station, Texas). Our primary data analysis aimed at comparing the *Aspergillus*-specific IgG antibody levels at baseline compared with week 24, and relating them to baseline demographics and clinical parameters (Additional file 1) at a 95% confidence interval.

Results

Study population characteristics

Of 268 patients in the SOUTH study, we selected all participants ($n = 101$) with a pre and post treatment serum sample; that were enrolled into the SOUTH study between March 2013 and July 2014. Of participants, 56%

(56/101) were men and the median age of all participants at TB diagnosis was 33 years (interquartile range (IQR), 27–38). All participants were HIV-infected adults with a median baseline CD4 T cell count of 155 cells/μl (IQR, 31–269, $n = 98$). Only 31% (31/101) of the participants were receiving anti-retroviral therapy (ART) at TB diagnosis. At baseline, 41% (41/101) had chest pain, 27% (27/101) had difficulty in breathing, 94% (95/101) had a cough and 89% (90/101) had sputum production with a median cough duration of 4 weeks (IQR, 3–12, $n = 95$) (Table 1).

TB was diagnosed by direct microscopy (smear), genexpert-MTB/RIF®, Mycobacteria growth indicator tube (MGIT) and Löwenstein–Jensen (LJ) culture. Only 47% (46/97) of the participants had positive sputum smears at TB diagnosis and 73% (24/33) had positive sputum genexpert MTB/RIF results. 68% (64/94) of the participants had positive MGIT while 60% (55/92) had positive LJ cultures. For participants who had chest x-rays done at baseline, 91% (80/88) had abnormal x-rays. The commonest chest x-ray abnormalities registered were pulmonary infiltrates (91% [73/80]) followed by pleural effusion (19% [15/80]) and cavities (6% [5/80]) (Table 1).

Aspergillus-specific IgG antibody levels using ImmunoCAP®

Using the ImmunoCAP immunoassay, the baseline median *Aspergillus*-specific IgG antibody levels were 4.43 mg/l (IQR, 2.07–7.17) with 4% (3/76) of the patients having elevated levels (>40 mg/l); while at week 24, the median *Aspergillus*-specific IgG antibody levels were 4.9 mg/l (IQR, 2.13–9.14) with 2% (2/94) having elevated levels (Table 2). All three patients who were positive for *Aspergillus*-specific IgG at baseline had become sero-negative by week 24 without antifungal treatment. Their x-rays had also improved with a normal picture at week 24.

Seven patients were negative for all the TB diagnostics (i.e. smear, genexpert, MGIT, LJ) but with abnormal chest x-rays. For these patients, a presumptive diagnosis of TB was made based on the abnormal chest x-ray. However, on comparing the baseline and week 24 x-rays, they all showed marked improvement, but only two had normal week 24 x-rays. These seven patients had *Aspergillus*–specific IgG antibodies in the range of <2 to 7.22 mg/l at baseline and <2 to 21.8 mg/l at week 24. The higher titers at week 24 than baseline could suggest that there is an

Table 1 Characteristics of the study population at TB diagnosis

Descriptions	N	Statistics
Baseline Demographics		
Males, n (%)	101	56 (56)
Age at TB diagnosis, mean (SD)/ median (IQR)	101	34 (8)/ 33 (27, 38)
On ART at TB diagnosis, n (%)	101	31 (31)
CD4 (cells/μL) at TB diagnosis, median (IQR)[a]	98	155 (31, 269)
Respiratory symptoms at TB diagnosis		
Cough, n (%)	101	95 (94)
Cough duration in weeks, median (IQR)[a]	95	4 (3, 12)
Chest pain, n (%)	101	41 (41)
Difficulty in breathing, n (%)	101	27 (27)
TB diagnostics		
Positive Sputum smear, n (%)[a]	97	46 (47)
Abnormal Chest X-ray, n (%)[a]	88	80 (91)
Pulmonary Infiltrates on chest x-ray, n (%)[a]	80	73 (91)
Pleural Effusion on chest x-ray, n (%)[a]	80	15 (19)
Cavities on chest x-ray, n (%)[a]	80	5 (6)
Positive Genexpert, n (%)[a]	33	24 (73)
Positive MGIT, n(%)[a]	94	64 (68)
Positive LJ culture, n(%)[a]	92	55 (60)

Data presented are percentages (%), standard deviations (SD) and interquartile ranges (IQR)
EH ethambutol and Isoniazid, *RH* rifampicin and Isoniazid, *MGIT* Mycobacteria growth indicator tube, *LJ* Löwenstein–Jensen
[a]Some parameters have $N < 101$ due to missing data

Table 2 Summary of *Aspergillus*-specific antibody titers and total serum IgE in HIV/TB patients in relation to selected baseline characteristics

Test/ Assay/ Cut-off	Factor at TB diagnosis	BASELINE			WEEK 24			Overall P value[$]
		N	Median (IQR)	P value*	N	Median (IQR)	P value*	
Aspergillus IgG ImmunoCAP® cut-off = 40 mg/L	Overall	76	4.4 (2.1,7.2)	NA	94	4.9 (2.1, 9.1)	NA	0.02
	Not on ART	52	4.3 (2.1,7.3)	0.85	65	4.9 (2.7,10.4)	0.35	
	On ART	24	4.8 (2.0,6.9)		28	2.8 (2.0,7.5)		
	CD4 < 100/μL	26	6.2 (2.7,8.7)	0.01	31	5.3 (2.1,12.7)	0.47	
	CD4 ≥ 100/μL	47	3.2 (2.0,6.0)		59	4.8 (2.1,7.5)		
	Coughed for <3 weeks	27	5.2 (2.1,8.5)	0.50	29	4.9 (2.3,10.4)	0.96	
	Coughed for ≥3 weeks	49	4.3 (2.0,7.1)		64	4.9 (2.1,9.0)		
	No Chest pain	41	5.4 (2.7,8.2)	0.03	55	4.8 (2.1,8.8)	0.95	
	Chest pain	35	2.9 (2.0,6.2)		38	5.1 (2.4,10.1)		
	Abnormal Chest X-Ray	59	4.3 (2.0,7.1)	0.79	75	4.9 (2.1,8.8)	0.88	
	Normal Chest X-Ray	6	3.9 (2.6,8.7)		6	3.1 (2.1,10.9)		
Aspergillus IgG Immulite® cut-off = 20 mg/L	Overall	75	7.5 (6.1, 10.3)	NA	87	7.2 (6.1, 9.96)	NA	0.66
	Not on ART	52	8.0 (6.7,10.6)	0.03	61	7.6 (6.2,10.5)	0.27	
	On ART	23	6.6 (5.8,8.2)		26	6.9 (6.1,8.8)		
	CD4 < 100/μL	25	7.9 (5.9,9.1)	0.94	29	7.8 (6.0,11.3)	0.60	
	CD4 ≥ 100/μL	47	7.5 (6.1,10.4)		56	7.0 (6.1,9.5)		
	Coughed for <3 weeks	26	7.3 (6.0,8.8)	0.37	28	7.6 (5.9,10.5)	0.98	
	Coughed for ≥3 weeks	49	7.5 (6.4,10.7)		59	7.2 (6.2,8.8)		
	No Chest pain	40	7.5 (6.4,10.8)	0.54	51	7.5 (6.1,9.7)	0.92	
	Chest pain	35	7.9 (6.0,9,3)		36	7.2 (6.1,10.8)		
	Abnormal Chest X-Ray	58	7.5 (6.1,9.1)	0.30	69	7.0 (6.1,10.1)	0.80	
	Normal Chest X-Ray	6	6.8 (5.0,8.2)		6	8.2 (7.5,8.7)		
Total IgE Immulite® cut-off = 1000 IU/mL	Overall	76	379 (129, 908)	NA	85	251 (64, 794)	NA	<0.01
	Not on ART	52	371 (122,1059)	0.82	59	297 (55,1021)	0.53	
	On ART	24	382 (175,837)		26	231 (77,777)		
	CD4 < 100/μL	26	462 (149,1440)	0.11	29	595 (113,1272)	0.03	
	CD4 ≥ 100/μL	47	355 (114,634)		54	185 (57,532)		
	Coughed for <3 weeks	27	207 (48,489)	0.02	26	213 (39,821)	0.49	
	Coughed for ≥3 weeks	49	493 (172,1200)		59	359 (71,794)		
	No Chest pain	41	355 (149,605)	0.40	49	183 (55,570)	0.06	
	Chest pain	35	489 (121,1221)		36	460 (72,1192)		
	Abnormal Chest X-Ray	59	457 (149,1055)	0.53	68	332 (66,835)	0.54	
	Normal Chest X-Ray	6	401 (322,1487)		6	153 (73,292)		
						NORMAL (≤0.35), n(%)	HIGH (>0.35), n(%)	*P*-VALUE
Aspergillus IgE	Overall, *N* = 93	NOT APPLICABLE				84 (90.3)	9 (9.7)	

Table 2 Summary of *Aspergillus*-specific antibody titers and total serum IgE in HIV/TB patients in relation to selected baseline characteristics *(Continued)*

Test/ Assay/ Cut-off	Factor at TB diagnosis	BASELINE			WEEK 24			Overall P value$
		N	Median (IQR)	P value*	N	Median (IQR)	P value*	
ImmunoCAP® cut-off = 0.35 kU/L	Not on ART					59(90.8)	6(9.2)	0.99
	On ART					25(89.3)	3(10.7)	
	CD4 < 100/μL					26 (83.9)	5 (16.1)	0.26
	CD4 ≥ 100/μL					56 (93.3)	4 (6.7)	
	Coughed for <3 weeks					25(86.2)	4(13.8)	0.45
	Coughed for ≥3 weeks					59(92.2)	5(7.8)	
	No Chest pain					51(92.7)	4(7.3)	0.48
	Chest pain					33(86.8)	5(13.2)	
	Abnormal Chest X-Ray					67(89.3)	8(10.7)	0.99
	Normal Chest X-Ray					6(100.0)	0 (0.0)	

Data presented are diagnostic cut-offs, antibody median (interquartile ranges) and *P*-values comparing antibody titers between selected parameters, baseline and end of TB treatment (wk24)
NA not applicable
*P-values were obtained using Kruskal-Wallis equality-of-populations rank test. $ *P*-values were obtained using Wilcoxon matched-pairs sign-rank test because of skewed data

increase in the aspergillus colonization due to the increasing pulmonary abnormalities especially cavities caused by TB. However, for these seven patients, both titers were below the diagnostic cut-off and not significantly different ($P > 0.05$).

There was a significant difference in the *Aspergillus*-specific IgG antibody levels between baseline and week 24 ($P = 0.02$) (Fig 1a). Patients with a baseline CD4 T-cell count <100 cells/μl had significantly higher median baseline *Aspergillus*-specific IgG titers ($n = 26$, median = 6.2 mg/l, IQR = 2.7 to 8.7) than those with a baseline CD4 T-cell count of ≥100 cells/μl ($n = 47$, median = 3.2 mg/l, IQR = 2.0 to 6.0) ($P = 0.01$). Patients with chest

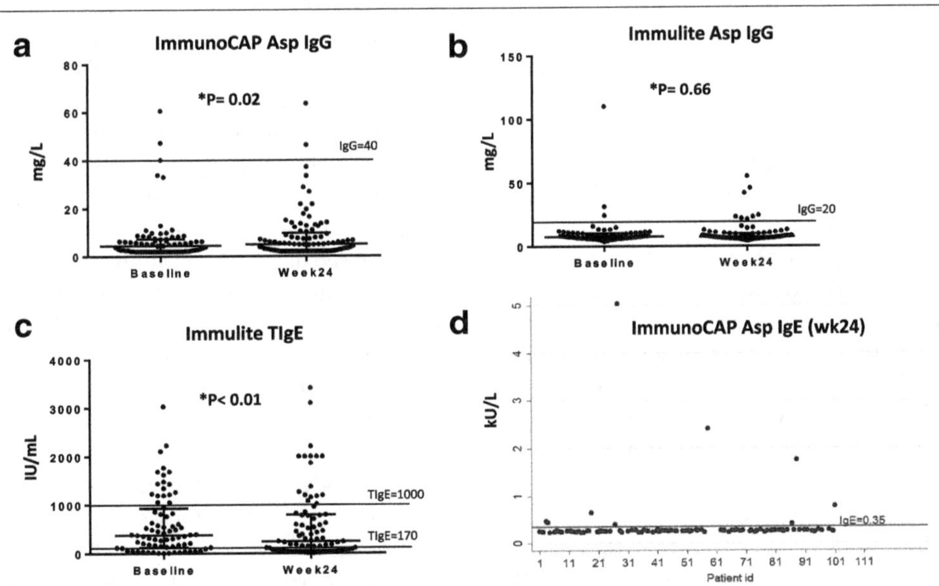

Fig. 1 Scatter plots of antibody levels at baseline and week 24. **a** Shows a significant difference in *Aspergillus*-specific IgG levels between baseline and week 24 using ImmunoCAP. **b** Shows no significant difference in *Aspergillus*-specific IgG levels between baseline and week 24 using Immulite. **c** Shows a significant difference in total serum IgE levels between baseline and week 24 using Immulite. **d** Shows distribution of *Aspergillus*-specific IgE levels at week 24

pain at baseline had significantly lower median *Aspergillus*-specific IgG titers ($n = 35$, median = 2.9 mg/l, IQR = 2.0 to 6.2) than those without chest pain ($n = 41$, median = 5.4 mg/l, IQR = 2.7 to 8.2) ($P = 0.03$) (Table 2). Chest pain is not a specific symptom. Out of the 41/101 patients who had chest pain, only one had elevated IgG levels. Out of the 60/101 patients without chest pain, only two had elevated IgG levels. The observed outcome could be explained by other factors related to TB but not CPA.

Aspergillus-specific IgG antibody levels using Immulite 2000®

Using the Immulite immunoassay, the median *Aspergillus*-specific IgG antibody levels were 7.52 mg/l (IQR, 6.08–10.3) with 4% (3/75) of the patients having elevated titers at baseline; while at end of week 24, the median *Aspergillus*-specific IgG antibody levels were 7.21 mg/l (IQR, 6.08–9.96) with 9.2% (8/87) having elevated levels (Table 2). Only three patients (different from the 3 in ImmunoCAP) were positive at baseline and two of them remained positive at week 24, but with lower antibody titers. Seven patients were negative for all the TB diagnostics (i.e. smear, genexpert, MGIT, LJ) but with abnormal chest x-rays. These seven patients had *aspergillus* IgG antibodies in the range of 4.26 to 8.23 mg/l at baseline and 4.31 to 14.9 mg/l at week 24.

There was no significant difference in the *Aspergillus*-specific IgG antibody levels between baseline and week 24 ($p = 0.66$) (Fig 1b). Patients who were not on antiretroviral therapy at TB diagnosis had significantly higher median *Aspergillus*-specific IgG titers ($n = 52$, median = 8.0 mg/l, IQR = 6.7 to 10.6) than those who were already taking antiretroviral therapy at TB diagnosis ($n = 23$, median = 6.6 mg/l, IQR = 5.8 to 8.2) ($P = 0.03$) (Table 2).

Total serum IgE using Immulite 2000®

Total serum IgE was measured using Immulite assay with a cut-off of 170 IU/ml. The median total serum IgE levels were 379 IU/ml (IQR, 129–908) with 71% (54/76) of the patients having elevated titers at baseline; while at week 24, the median total serum IgE levels were 251 IU/ml (IQR, 64–794) with 58% (49/85) of patients having elevated levels (Table 2). We then analyzed results using a cut-off to 1000 IU/ml. Only 24% (18/76) of the patients had total serum IgE greater than 1000 IU/mL at baseline and 21% (18/85) at week 24. There was a significant difference in the total serum IgE antibody levels between baseline and week 24 ($p < 0.01$) (Fig 1c).

Patients who had coughed for more than three weeks at TB diagnosis had significantly higher median total serum IgE titers ($n = 49$, median = 493 IU/ml, IQR = 172 to 1200) than those who had coughed for less than three weeks at TB diagnosis ($n = 27$, median = 207 IU/ml, IQR = 48 to 489) ($P = 0.02$). Patients with a CD4 T-cell count <100 cells/μl at week 24, had significantly higher median total serum IgE titers ($n = 29$, median = 595 IU/ml, IQR = 113 to 1272) than those with a baseline CD4 T-cell count of ≥100 cells/μl ($n = 54$, median = 185 IU/ml, IQR = 57 to 532) ($P = 0.03$) (Table 2).

Aspergillus-specific IgE antibody levels using ImmunoCAP®

Aspergillus-specific IgE antibody levels were measured at end of TB treatment only (Fig 1d), and were elevated in 9.7% (9/93) of the patients using a diagnostic cut-off of <0.35kU/l (Table 2). There was no significant relationship between *Aspergillus* sensitization (Asp IgE) and baseline characteristics or respiratory symptoms.

Discussion

The study demonstrated that *Aspergillus*-specific IgG antibodies were elevated in 4% of HIV-infected Ugandan adults at the start of TB treatment and in 9% at the end of TB treatment. Using ImmunoCAP, participants with CD4 T-cell counts <100 cell/μl had more elevated *Aspergillus*-specific IgG antibodies ($P = 0.01$). The increased level of immunosuppression could have increased their susceptibility to the opportunistic fungal infection. Hyper IgG levels are common in acquired immune deficiency syndrome (AIDS) patients and represent an unrestrained B-cell response in the absence of T-cells [14]. The ImmunoCAP *Aspergillus*-specific IgG antibody titers were higher with more positives at end of TB treatment than baseline, even though the difference in means was small. However, this difference was statistically significant ($P = 0.02$). Initiation of antiretroviral therapy and anti-TB medication could have improved the patients' ability to mount a good immune response at week 24 than baseline.

Patients who were not on antiretroviral therapy at TB diagnosis (68%) had significantly higher *Aspergillus*-specific IgG titers ($P = 0.03$) using Immulite, and 45% (14/31) of them had CD4 T-cell counts less than 200 cells/μl. Increased level of immunosuppression could still be the contributing factor to this increased susceptibility to the opportunistic fungal infection. There was no significant difference in the Immulite *Aspergillus*-specific IgG antibody levels ($P = 0.66$) between baseline and end of TB treatment.

We observed a discrepancy in the *Aspergillus*-specific IgG antibody levels between the ImmunoCAP and Immulite. Previous studies comparing the ImmunoCAP and Immulite have shown that the values for both tests are highly correlated with antibody levels measured by Immulite having a mean of 3 times higher than when measured by ImmunoCAP. However, this correlation is lost at high ImmunoCAP values [15]. This ratio may change based on the specific antibody in question. In our current study, this ratio was approximately 1.6 on average.

About 10% (9/93) of the participants had evidence of *Aspergillus* sensitization at the end of TB treatment. This was an expected outcome in this population since persistence of pulmonary cavities after successful pulmonary TB treatment is very common [16] and these cavities are thought to harbour mould spores leading to fungal colonisation. Besides, ABPA can be misdiagnosed as pulmonary TB, with some similar clinical features [10, 17]. However, ABPA is rarely described outside chronic obstructive pulmonary disease (COPD), asthma and cystic fibrosis. There was no record of these three conditions in our participants, and therefore we argue that *Aspergillus* sensitisation is the explanation for these high IgE results, which could represent a strong T-helper 2 (Th2) response. The association between ABPA and pulmonary TB has been weakly described before mainly in case reports [18–20].

In a recent review, CPA in Uganda was estimated to affect up to 22% of TB patients with cavities and 4% in those without cavities [3]. However, in the current population, pulmonary infiltrates were the most common chest x-ray abnormality both at baseline (91%) and week 24 (41%). Only 5% of our participants had pulmonary cavities on chest x-ray at week 24. This did not change much from the 6% cavities registered at baseline. All the five patients with cavities at week 24 had a good treatment outcome (cured) but 3/5 had been diagnosed with smear negative TB at baseline. This result supports previous work indicating persistence of pulmonary cavities after successful pulmonary TB treatment [16].

At week 24, 95% (95/100) of the chest x-rays showed marked improvement from the baseline chest x-rays and only 52% (52/100) were abnormal. Using ImmunoCAP, all patients with normal and abnormal chest x-rays at week 24 were negative for *Aspergillus*-specific IgG (range: <2 to 9). However, using Immulite, there were five positives among those with normal chest x-ray (median 7 [IQR: 5.9, 9.2]) and three positives among those with abnormal chest x-rays (median 7.6 [IQR: 6.3, 10.3]). We were unable to do computed tomography (CT) scans of the chest, which might have provided better definition of any residual abnormalities.

Total serum IgE is a test for general allergic disease and parasitic infections. It is commonly used together with fungal-allergy diagnostics. Using a cut-off of 170 IU/ml for total serum IgE antibodies, 71% of participants had evidence of allergic disease. This reduced to 58% (49/85) at the end of TB treatment. Of these 49 participants with elevated total serum IgE antibodies at the end of TB treatment, 12% (6/49) had elevated *Aspergillus*-specific IgE antibody titers in the range of 0.41 to 2.4, and *Aspergillus*-specific IgG antibody titers in the range of 6.7 to 55.2.

The implication of the raised total serum IgE levels in this population was not obvious. However, there is evidence that total serum IgE levels tend to be more elevated in non-asthmatic Africans than asthmatic Africans [21]. Most scholars attribute this paradox to parasitic infestations in the African population [21, 22]. This paradox therefore calls for the need to re-evaluate the role of total serum IgE levels in asthma in areas with a high gut parasite prevalence. Recent evidence from genotyping ancestry informative markers indicated that African ancestry is a risk factor for elevated total serum IgE levels in African admixed population [23]. Intestinal helminths are also known to raise total serum IgE levels in HIV patients even without a fully functional CD4 T-cell repertoire [24–26].

Raising the cut-off for total serum IgE to 1000 IU/mL reduced the positivity rate to more than 50%. Only 18 participants had total serum IgE greater than 1000 IU/mL at the end of TB treatment. Of these, 28% (5/18) had elevated *Aspergillus*-specific IgE antibody titers in the range of 0.41 to 2.4, and only two of these (2/5) had elevated *Aspergillus*-specific IgG antibody titers (Immulite). Long term coughing for more than three weeks at baseline was also significantly related to increased total serum IgE titers ($P = 0.02$). It is possible that some participants had both TB and some form of allergy at baseline; which would explain the prolonged cough durations.

53% (51/97) of the patients had negative sputum smears. Smear-negative tuberculosis was registered in 13 to 21% of our participants at baseline. Among smear negative patients ($n = 51$), there were 16 positive genexperts, 20 positive MGIT and 13 positive LJ cultures. Seven patients were negative for all the TB diagnostics (i.e. smear, genexpert, MGIT, LJ) but with abnormal chest x-rays. These seven patients were negative for *Aspergillus* IgG antibodies with very low titers at both baseline and week 24. CPA associated with TB constitutes a significant unrecognized public health problem, which is probably being incorrectly identified as 'smear-negative tuberculosis' especially in Africa.

Based on data from India, reduced pulmonary function is associated with *Aspergillus* sensitisation, which unfortunately we were unable to measure. Post-tuberculous sequelae include CPA, bronchiectasis [10] and to this we add *Aspergillus* sensitisation. Reduced pulmonary function persists in patients cured of TB [27], and *Aspergillus* sensitisation could be one of the explanations, through poorly understood mechanisms. The prevalence of pulmonary Aspergillosis in HIV patients is underestimated in Africa because of difficulty in accurate diagnosis. We have only had a few epidemiological studies in Uganda [4, 6, 8]. However, in collaboration with The Global Action Fund for Fungal Infections (GAFFI) and the University of Manchester, efforts are being put in place to train more mycologist and build laboratory capacity in Uganda. We hope that this might solve the problem in the near future.

Study limitations

The major limitation to the study was that we failed to access control samples for comparison of these antibody titers. This would possibly give more useful information. So we agreed to move on without the controls since the primary goal of this study was not to define diagnostic cut-offs for assays that might subsequently be used in a prevalence study in Uganda. Due to the limited published data on fungal disease epidemiology in sub-Saharan Africa, we found a major challenge in defining which diagnostic cut-offs to use for Aspergillus-specific IgG antibodies in both ImmunoCAP and Immulite. Previously published cut-offs range in 10 to 50 mg/l in similar populations. We were unable to do computed tomography (CT) scans of the chest, which might have provided better definition of any residual abnormalities. Similarly, we did not add other tests like culture since we used stored serum samples. Intestinal helminths are known to raise total serum IgE levels in HIV patients even without a fully functional CD4 T-cell repertoire [24–26]. So the implication of the raised total serum IgE levels in this population was not obvious. We observed a discrepancy in the *Aspergillus*-specific IgG antibody levels between the ImmunoCAP and Immulite similar to what has been described before [15]. Cavities are known to be the major predisposing factor to CPA in TB. However, in our population, cavities were seen in only 5% of the participants.

Conclusion

In conclusion, *Aspergillus*-specific antibody levels were significantly raised in patients being managed for pulmonary tuberculosis. This colonization and/or sensitization by *Aspergillus* antigens may complicate disease progression and treatment outcomes among TB patients. Detection of *Aspergillus* antibodies is an indispensable tool in the diagnosis and management of the patients with pulmonary aspergillosis. However, the detection of Aspergillus-specific antibodies does not imply that the patient has an active fungal disease; further diagnostic tests would be needed to ascertain the presence of pulmonary aspergillosis. More epidemiological studies are needed to explore and expand the utility of *Aspergillus* antibody testing in resource limited setting.

Abbreviations

ABPA: Allergic bronchopulmonary aspergillosis; ART: Antiretroviral therapy; CD4: Cluster of differentiation 4; COPD: Chronic obstructive pulmonary disease; CPA: Chronic Pulmonary Aspergillosis; CT: Computerized Tomography; Fig: Fig.; HIV: Human immunodeficiency virus; HR: Isoniazid and Rifampicin; HRZE: Isoniazid, Rifampicin, Pyrazinamide and Ethambutol; IDI: Infectious Diseases Institute; IgE: Immunoglobulin E; IgG: Immunoglobulin G; IQR: Interquartile range; ISID: International Society for Infectious Diseases; LJ: Löwenstein–Jensen; MGIT: Mycobacteria growth indicator tube; SD: Standard deviation, n- sample size; SOUTH: Study on Outcomes related to Tuberculosis and HIV drug concentrations In Uganda; TB: Tuberculosis; Th2: T Helper Type 2 Cell; UK: United Kingdom; WHO: World Health Organisation

Acknowledgements

We would like to acknowledge all our participants and their families. We especially thank the team of the TB/HIV clinic at the IDI in Kampala for patient care. We also thank Mr. Allan Buzibye for laboratory support during retrieving and shipping samples.

Funding

This study was funded by the collaboration between the Infectious Diseases Institute (IDI) Makerere University and the University of Zurich (supported by Abbvie, Bristol Myers Squibb, Gilead Sciences, Janssen, Lunge Zurich, Merck, Shimadzu, Swiss HIV Cohort Study, ViiV Healthcare) and a grant from the International Society for Infectious Diseases (ISID) to Richard Kwizera. Siemens ® Company donated to us the Immulite test kits and the Laboratory at Christie Hospital, Manchester allowed us to use their Immulite 2000 machine for free. Richard Kwizera is also currently supported by a THRiVE-2 PhD fellowship (THRiVE is being supported through the DELTAS Africa Initiative [107,742/Z/15/Z]). The funders had no role in study design, data collection and analysis, decision to publish, or preparation of the manuscript.

Authors' contributions

RK, RPR, DWD conceived and designed concept. RK, IP performed experiments. RK, JM, IP analysed data. RK, IP, DWD contributed reagents/materials/analysis tools. RK, JM, IP, CS participated in initial manuscript drafting. RK, CS, JF, BC, AK, IP, RPR, DWD participated in critical revisions for intellectual content. RK, RPR, DWD, BC, AK, JF participated in obtaining funding. CS, AK, RPR participated in administrative, technical, or material support. All authors have read and approved the manuscript.

Consent for publication

Not applicable.

Competing interests

The authors declare that they have no competing interests.

Author details

[1]Infectious Diseases Institute, College of Health Sciences, Makerere University, P.O.BOX 22418 Kampala, Uganda. [2]Cambridge Institute of Public Health, University of Cambridge, Cambridge, UK. [3]The University of Manchester, Manchester, UK. [4]National Aspergillosis Centre, University Hospital of South Manchester, Manchester, UK. [5]Infectious Diseases and Hospital Hygiene, University Hospital, Zurich, Switzerland.

References

1. Keeler E, Perkins MD, Small P, Hanson C, Reed S, Cunningham J, Aledort JE, Hillborne L, Rafael ME, Girosi F. Reducing the global burden of tuberculosis: the contribution of improved diagnostics. Nature. 2006;444:49–57.
2. GLOBAL TUBERCULOSIS REPORT 2016. http://www.who.int/tb/publications/global_report/en/.
3. Parkes-Ratanshi R, Achan B, Kwizera R, Kambugu A, Meya D, Denning D. Cryptococcal disease and the burden of other fungal diseases in Uganda;

where are the knowledge gaps and how can we fill them? Mycoses. 2015; 58(S5):85–93.
4. Page I, Onyachi N, Opira C, Opwonya J, Odongo-Aginya E, Mockridge A, Byrne G, Richardson M, Denning D. Chronic pulmonary aspergillosis (CPA) is likely to be a common complication of pulmonary tuberculosis: initial results of a cross-sectional survey. In: 19th Congress of the International Society for Human and Animal Mycology; 2015. abstract No: EV0971.
5. Page I, Worodria W, Andama A, Ayakaka I, Kwizera R, Davis L, Huang L, Richardson M, Denning D. Onset of chronic pulmonary Aspergillosis (Cpa) may occur during active pulmonary tuberculosis. In: 7th advances against Aspergillosis conference. Manchester; 2016. abstract No: 100. http://www.aspergillus.org.uk/content/onset-chronic-pulmonary-aspergillosis-cpa-may-occur-duringactive-pulmonary-tuberculosis-0.
6. Page ID, Worodria W, Andama A, Ayakaka I, Davis L, Huang L, Richardson M, Denning DW. Pulmonary aspergillosis may be common in AIDS with smear negative tuberculosis. In: Conference on retrovirus and opportunistic infections. Boston; 2016. POSTER NUMBER 764. http://www.croiconference.org/sites/default/files/posters-2016/764.pdf.
7. Page I, Kwizera R, Richardson M, Denning D. Comparative efficacy of five Aspergillus-specific IgG ELISAs for the diagnosis of chronic pulmonary aspergillosis (CPA). In: 25th EUROPEAN CONGRESS OF CLINICAL MICROBIOLOGY AND INFECTIOUS DISEASES. Denmark; 2015. abstract No: P1099. http://www.aspergillus.org.uk/content/comparative-efficacy-five-aspergillus-specific-igg-elisas-diagnosischronic-pulmonary.
8. Page I. Pulmonary aspergillosis in association with tuberculosis and HIV in Uganda. PhD Research thesis. research.manchester.ac.uk: The University of Manchester; 2015. https://www.research.manchester.ac.uk/portal/files/54577119/FULL_TEXT.PDF.
9. Shafer LA, Biraro S, Nakiyingi-Miiro J, Kamali A, Ssematimba D, Ouma J, Ojwiya A, Hughes P, Van der Paal L, Whitworth J. HIV prevalence and incidence are no longer falling in southwest Uganda: evidence from a rural population cohort 1989–2005. AIDS (London, England). 2008;22(13):1641–9.
10. Dhooria S, Kumar P, Saikia B, Aggarwal A, Gupta D, Behera D, Chakrabarti A, Agarwal R. Prevalence of Aspergillus sensitisation in pulmonary tuberculosis-related fibrocavitary disease. Int J Tuberc Lung Dis. 2014;18(7):850–5.
11. Sekaggya-Wiltshire C, von Braun A, Scherrer A, Manabe Y, Buzibye A, Muller D, Ledergerber B, Gutteck U, Corti N, Kambugu A. Anti-TB drug concentrations and drug-associated toxicities among TB/HIV-coinfected patients. J Antimicrob Chemother. 2017;72(4):1172–7.
12. Laurent J, Noirot C, Ansquer J, Laurent G, Kestenbaum S, Lagrue G. How to define the normal level of serum IgE in adults? In: Annales de medecine interne, vol. 1984; 1984. p. 419–22.
13. Tillie-Leblond I, Tonnel AB. Allergic bronchopulmonary aspergillosis. Allergy. 2005;60(8):1004–13.
14. Kaushik K, Khurana S, Wanchu A, Malla N. Serum immunoglobulin G, M and a response to Cryptosporidium Parvum in cryptosporidium-HIV co-infected patients. BMC Infect Dis. 2009;9:179.
15. Graham F, Begin P, Paradis L, Lacombe-Barrios J, Paradis J, Des Roches A. Comparison of ImmunoCAP and Immulite serum specific IgE assays for the assessment of egg allergy. Allergy, Asthma Clin Immunol. 2016;12:29.
16. Denning DW, Riniotis K, Dobrashian R, Sambatakou H. Chronic cavitary and Fibrosing pulmonary and pleural aspergillosis: case series, proposed nomenclature change, and review. Clin Infect Dis. 2003;37:S265–80.
17. Kant S. Allergic bronchopulmonary aspergillosis mimicking as pulmonary tuberculosis. Lung India. 2007;24(4):142.
18. Agarwal R, Singh N, Aggarwal A. An unusual association between mycobacterium tuberculosis and Aspergillus fumigatus. Monaldi Arch Chest Dis. 2016;69(1):32–4.
19. Min KH, Park SJ, Kim SR, Lee MH, Chung CR, Han HJ, Choi KH, Chung MJ, Lee YC, Jin GY. Coexistence of allergic bronchopulmonary aspergillosis and active pulmonary tuberculosis. Am J Respir Crit Care Med. 2011;183(1):137–9.
20. Gupta M, Roshan R, Chhabra SK. Allergic bronchopulmonary aspergillosis without asthma complicating pulmonary tuberculosis. Lung India. 2012; 29(3):286–8.
21. Scrivener S, Britton J. Immunoglobulin E and allergic disease in Africa. Clin Exp Allergy. 2000;30(3):304.
22. Houba V, Rowe D. A comparison of African and European serum levels of immunoglobulin E. Bull World Health Organ. 1973;49(6):539.
23. Vergara C, Murray T, Rafaels N, Lewis R, Campbell M, Foster C, Gao L, Faruque M, Oliveira RR, Carvalho E. African ancestry is a risk factor for asthma and high total IgE levels in African admixed populations. Genet Epidemiol. 2013;37(4):393–401.
24. Kassu A, Mohammad A, Fujimaki Y, Moges F, Elias D, Mekonnen F, Mengistu G, Yamato M, Wondmikun Y, Ota F. Serum IgE levels of tuberculosis patients in a tropical setup with high prevalence of HIV and intestinal parasitoses. Clin Exp Immunol. 2004;138(1):122–7.
25. Marth K, Wollmann E, Gallerano D, Ndlovu P, Makupe I, Valenta R, Sibanda E. Persistence of IgE-associated allergy and allergen-specific IgE despite CD4+ T cell loss in AIDS. PLoS One. 2014;9(6):e97893.
26. Mulu A, Anagaw B, Gelaw A, Ota F, Kassu A, Yifru S. Effect of deworming on Th2 immune response during HIV-helminths co-infection. J Transl Med. 2015;13(1):236.
27. Pasipanodya JG, Miller TL, Vecino M, Munguia G, Bae S, Drewyer G, Weis SE. Using the St. George respiratory questionnaire to ascertain health quality in persons with treated pulmonary tuberculosis. CHEST Journal. 2007;132(5):1591–8.

17

Diagnostic value of interleukins for tuberculous pleural effusion

Ni Zeng, Chun Wan, Jiangyu Qin, Yanqiu Wu, Ting Yang, Yongchun Shen*, Fuqiang Wen and Lei Chen*

Abstract

Background: The ability of interleukins (ILs) to differentiate tuberculous pleural effusion from other types of effusion is controversial. The aim of our study was to summarize the evidence for its use of ruling out or in tuberculous pleural effusion.

Methods: Two investigators independently searched PubMed, EMBASE, Web of Knowledge, CNKI, WANFANG, and WEIPU databases to identify studies assessing diagnostic role of ILs for tuberculous pleural effusion published up to January, 2017. Study quality was assessed using Quality Assessment of Diagnostic Accuracy Studies-2. The pooled diagnostic sensitivity and specificity of ILs were calculated by using Review Manager 5.3. Area under the summary receiver operating characteristic curve (AUC) was used to summarize the overall diagnostic performance of individual markers.

Results: Thirty-eight studies met our inclusion criteria. Pooled sensitivity, specificity and AUC for chosen ILs were as follows: IL-2, 0.67,0.76 and 0.86; IL-6, 0.86, 0.84 and 0.90; IL-12, 0.78, 0.83 and 0.86; IL-12p40, 0.82,0.65 and 0.76; IL-18, 0.87, 0.92 and 0.95; IL-27, 0.93, 0.95 and 0.95; and IL-33, 0.84, 0.80 and 0.88.

Conclusions: Some of these ILs may assist in diagnosing tuberculous pleural effusion, though no single IL is likely to show adequate sensitivity or specificity on its own. Further studies on a large scale with better study design should be performed to assess the diagnostic potential of ILs.

Keywords: Interleukin, Tuberculous pleural effusion, Diagnosis, Meta-analysis

Background

Tuberculosis remains a leading cause of morbidity and mortality, especially in Asia and Africa with high tuberculosis burden. In China, the prevalence of active pulmonary tuberculosis in 2010 among those older than 15 years was 459/100,000, and the prevalence of smear-positive pulmonary tuberculosis was 66/100,000. [1] Up to 30% of patients with tuberculosis have tuberculous pleural effusion (TPE), in which extrapulmonary involvement causes pleural effusions [2]. Properly treating pleural effusions requires determining whether the effusions are TPEs or another type of effusion.

* Correspondence: shen_yongchun@126.com; lchens@126.com
Ni Zeng and Chun Wan share joint first authorship.
Ni Zeng and Chun Wan contributed equally to this work.
Department of Respiratory and Critical Care Medicine, West China Hospital of Sichuan University and Division of Pulmonary Diseases, State Key Laboratory of Biotherapy of China, Chengdu 610041, China

The gold standard for diagnosing TPE is the isolation of *Mycobacterium tuberculosis (M. tuberculosis)* from samples of either pleural effusion or pleural biopsy. This culturing offers 100% diagnostic specificity, but it usually takes several weeks, delaying diagnosis and increasing the risk that patients are lost to follow-up. In addition, pleural biopsy is invasive and technically difficult to some extent, particularly in children, such that success can depend strongly on the individual performing the biopsy. [3] Detecting granulomas in pleural biopsies can diagnose TPE with approximately 95% specificity, [2–4] but the sensitivity of culture- or granuloma-based methods is limited. [5] Although image-guided biopsies and local anesthetic thoracoscopic (LAT) biopsies can highly evaluated the sensitivity compared to blind pleural biopsy, both those techniques are not recommended as the first procedure for patients presenting with pleural effusions. Thus, this highlights the need for alternative less invasive diagnostic strategies.

TPE is largely the result of pathological immune reactions associated with an increase in cytokines, including interleukins (ILs). [6] ILs are secreted proteins that bind to specific receptors and help mediate communication among leukocytes. For example, IL-12 is essential for initially activating inrerferon(INF)-γ-mediated T cell responses to primary *M. tuberculosis* infection. [7, 8] ILs can promote various types of inflammatory responses, playing a role in activation-induced death of skin keratinocytes, mucosal epithelial cells, and T cells. [9] Evidence that pleural levels of some ILs are elevated in patients with TPE has led investigators to explore their potential for differentiating TPE from other types of pleural effusion. Most studies have looked at only one or a few ILs, and some studies looking at the same ILs have arrived at different conclusions. This led us to systematically review the literature and meta-analyze available data to gain a more comprehensive understanding of the potential of ILs for diagnosing TPE.

Methods

Search strategy and study selection

The systematic review was conducted following the PRISMA (Preferred Reporting Items for Systematic Reviews and Meta-Analysis) guidelines. [10] Two investigators independently searched PubMed, EMBASE, Web of Knowledge, CNKI, WANFANG, and WEIPU databases to identify studies assessing the role of ILs in diagnosing TPE published up to January, 2017. Before the full search, we performed a preliminary search to decide on the ILs to include in the review. The following search terms were used: "interleukins *or* IL" *and* "IL-2 *or* IL-6 *or* IL-12 *or* IL-12p40 *or* IL-18 *or* IL-27 *or* IL-33" *and* "tuberculosis" *and* "pleural effusion/pleural fluid" *and* "sensitivity or specificity or accuracy". Reference lists in retrieved studies and review articles were examined manually to identify additional studies.

Two authors (NZ and CW) independently assessed each study for eligibility; disagreements were resolved by consensus. Studies were included if they fulfilled all the following criteria: (1) the work was an original research article published in English or Chinese, (2) human samples were analyzed, (3) standard methods were used to definitively diagnose the type of effusion as TPE or other type, and (4) data sufficient for calculating specificity and sensitivity were reported. Conference proceedings, letters to the editor, and studies including fewer than 10 patients with TPE were excluded.

Quality assessment and data extraction

The same two authors (NZ and CW) assessed the quality of included studies using the Quality Assessment of Diagnostic Accuracy Studies-2 tool (QUADAS-2). [11] For each criterion, a response of "yes" was assigned if it was fulfilled; "unclear", if doubt existed whether it was fulfilled; or "no" if it was not fulfilled. The following data were retrieved from each study: authors, country, publication year, population characteristics, testing methods, cut-off value, methodological quality, and 2-by-2 tables showing rates of true positives (TPs), true negatives (TNs), false positives (FPs) and false negative (FNs).

Statistical analysis

Data were compiled in Excel, then transferred to Review Manager 5.3 (The Cochrane Collaboration, Copenhagen, Denmark) and STATA Version 12.0 (Stata Corp., College Station, TX) for statistical analysis. For each study, sensitivity, specificity, positive likelihood ratio (PLR), negative likelihood ratio (NLR), and diagnostic odds ratio (DOR) were calculated, together with 95% confidence intervals (CIs). A summary ROC (SROC) curve was generated for each IL in each study, [12] from which a single test threshold value was determined and used to calculate sensitivity and specificity. [13] Overall diagnostic performance for that IL was assessed as the area under the SROC curve (AUC).

The Q test and inconsistency index (I^2) were used to detect potential heterogeneity in the natural logarithm of DOR (lnDOR) meta-analyzed across studies. [14] Presence of implicit cut-off point effects and correlation between sensitivity and specificity were assessed for each IL by calculating the Spearman rank correlation coefficient for each IL. Deeks' funnel plot and Egger's test were used to detect publication bias [15]. All statistical tests were two-sided, with $P < 0.05$ taken as the threshold of significance.

Results

Our systematic review included 38 studies examining the ability of pleural concentrations of IL-2, IL-6, IL-12, IL-12p40, IL-18, IL-27, and IL-33 to diagnose TPE. [16–53] Other ILs in the Table 1 were excluded for meta-analysis because relevant data were available from fewer than 3 studies [54–58] (Fig. 1). Two authors (NZ and CW) assessed studies for possible overlap in the populations analyzed. Data were pooled from overlapping populations as long as the different studies reported on different ILs or IL combinations. Otherwise, if studies with overlapping populations reported on the same IL or IL combination, only the data from the largest study were used.

Study characteristics

Table 1 summarizes clinical characteristics of patients in the 38 studies that used for quantitative meta-analysis [16–53]. Average sample size was 98 (range, 43 to 431) for each IL (Table 2). 23 studies stated that the pleural effusion samples were collected before any drug treatment [16–38], while the rest 15 studies didn't report such

Table 1 Clinical summary of all studies

Interleukins	Author	Country(incidence)	Year	Cut-off (pg/ml)	Index test	Design
IL-27	Wu et al. [16]	China (high)	2013	900.8	ELISA	P
	Liu et al. [42]	China (high)	2015	1012	ELISA	R
	Luo et al. [27]	China (high)	2015	353.47	ELISA	R
	Skouras et al. [46]	Greece (low)	2015	391	ELISA	NA
	Sun et al. [29]	China (high)	2014	838	ELISA	R
	Valdes et al. [31]	Spain (low)	2014	550	ELISA	P
	Yang et al. [50]	China (high)	2012	1007	ELISA	P
	Niu et al. [38]	China (high)	2012	846	ELISA	R
IL-18	Chen et al. [17]	China (high)	2011	843.7	ELISA	R
	Dai et al. [18]	China (high)	2015	503.58	ELISA	R
	Ding et al. [19]	China (high)	2008	640	ELISA	R
	Hu et al. [21]	China (high)	2009	365	ELISA	R
	Jiang et al. [22]	China (high)	2009	503.88	ELISA	R
	Klimiuk et al. [39]	Poland (low)	2014	327.7	ELISA	P
	Liu et al. [43]	China (high)	2015	438.86	ELISA	R
	Okamoto et al. [44]	Japan (low)	2005	992.7	ELISA	NA
	Wang et al. [47]	China (high)	2008	358	ELISA	R
	Wu et al. [33]	China (high)	2006	150	ELISA	R
	Xiong et al. [34]	China (high)	2007	358	ELISA	R
	Yu et al. [51]	China (high)	2003	150	ELISA	NA
IL-6	Kiropoulos et al. [24]	Greece (low)	2007	17,215	ELISA	P
	Wang et al. [32]	China (high)	2005	1950	ELISA	R
	Wong et al. [48]	China (high)	2003	4000	ELISA	P
	Wu et al. [49]	China (high)	2005	550	ELISA	R
	Zan et al. [35]	China (high)	2014	277	RIA	NA
	Yang et al. [37]	China (high)	2006	220	RIA	R
IL-33	Lee et al. [26]	Korea (low)	2013	10	ELISA	R
	Li et al. [40]	China (high)	2015	68.3	ELISA	R
	Liu et al. [42]	China (high)	2015	19.31	ELISA	R
	Xuan et al. [36]	China (high)	2014	19.86	ELISA	R
IL-12	Chen et al. [17]	China (high)	2011	785.6	ELISA	R
	Gu et al. [20]	China (high)	2002	300	ELISA	NA
	Jiang et al. [23]	China (high)	2010	87.41	ELISA	R
	Okamoto et al. [44]	Japan (low)	2005	129	ELISA	NA
	Tian et al. [28]	China (high)	2004	73.5	ELISA	R
	Zhou et al. [53]	China (high)	2012	90	ELISA	R
IL-2	Liu et al. [43]	China (high)	2015	67.17	ELISA	R
	Liu et al. [42]	China (high)	2015	99.08	ELISA	R
	Ren et al. [25]	China (high)	2014	41.91	ELISA	R
	Wu et al. [49]	China (high)	2005	250	ELISA	R
	Zhang et al. [52]	China (high)	1998	400	RIA	R
IL-12p40	Fernández et al. [41]	Venezuela (low)	2011	89	ELISA	NA
	Klimiuk et al. [39]	Poland (low)	2014	296	ELISA	P
	Tural Önür et al. [45]	Turkey (low)	2015	210	ELISA	NA

Table 1 Clinical summary of all studies *(Continued)*

Interleukins	Author	Country(incidence)	Year	Cut-off (pg/ml)	Index test	Design
	Valdes et al. [30]	Spain (low)	2009	550	ELISA	P
IL-8	Yamada et al. [57]	Japan (low)	2001	228	ELISA	R
	Yang et al. [56]	China (high)	2001	1000	ELISA	R
IL-10	Wu et al. [49]	China (high)	2005	50	ELISA	R
IL-22	Jin et al. [58]	China (high)	2011	49	ELISA	R
	Yuan et al. [55]	China (high)	2014	186.6	ELISA	R
IL-23	Klimiuk et al. [39]	Poland (low)	2014	0.7	ELISA	P
IL-31	Gao et al. [54]	China (high)	2015	67.5	ELISA	R

Abbreviations: *IL* interleukin, *ELISA* enzyme-linked immunosorbent assay, *RIA* radioimmunoassay, *NA* not available, *P* prospective, *R* retrospective

information [39–53]. Diagnosis of TPE or other type of pleural effusion was based only on clinical course in 5 studies, [22, 23, 28, 35, 41] i.e. on clinical presentation, pleural fluid analysis, radiology and responsiveness to anti-tuberculosis chemotherapy. Diagnosis was based on bacteriology, histology or both (gold standard) in 11 studies. In the remaining 21 studies, some patients were diagnosed with TPE based on clinical course and others based on the gold standard. One study [51] did not report the diagnostic standard for TPE. All but 3 studies [35, 37, 52] measured IL levels using enzyme-linked immunosorbent assays (ELISA), with the remaining 3 studies using radioimmunoassays.

Determination of statistical pooling model

Diagnostic studies are typically meta-analyzed using an SROC-based fixed-effects model, [59] a random-effects model using a bivariate normal approximation, [60] or a hierarchical SROC (HSROC)-based full Bayesian [61] or empirical Bayes method [62]. In our study, lnDOR heterogeneity was statistically significant and associated with high I^2 values for most ILs (Table 3). These indications of substantial heterogeneity in lnDOR made the use of a SROC-based fixed-effects model inappropriate [63].

The possible presence of implicit cut-off point effects was examined for each included IL, using the Spearman rank correlation between sensitivity and specificity (Table 3). A negative correlation was found for most ILs, indicating no detectable implicit cut-point effect. Therefore, we used a random-effects model to estimate the mean sensitivity and specificity and associated CIs.

Diagnostic accuracy

These data were meta-analyzed using a random-effects model (Table 3). Fig. 2 summarizes the sensitivities and

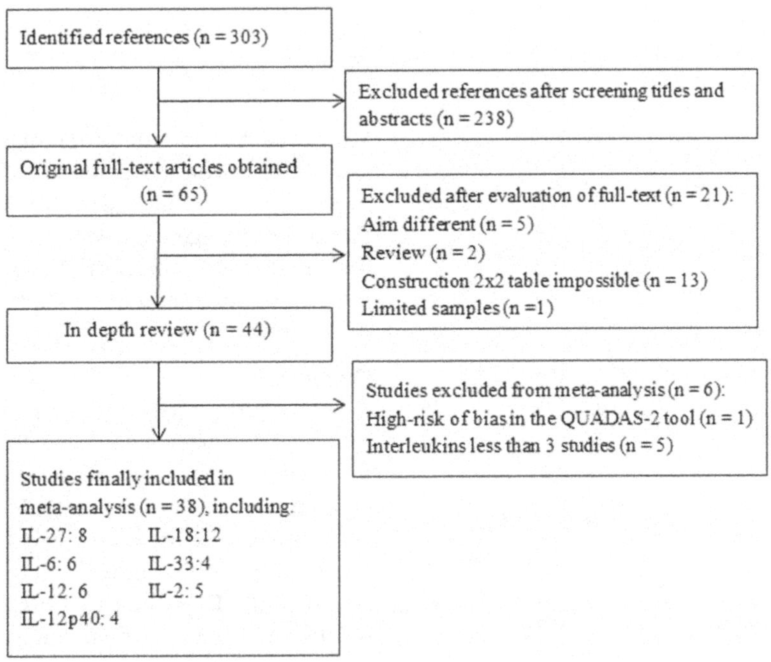

Fig. 1 Flow diagram of study selection. QUADAS: Quality Assessment of Diagnostic Accuracy Studies

Table 2 Diagnostic performance of interleukins from individual studies

Interleukins	Author	Subjects	TP	FP	FN	TN
IL-27	Wu et al. [16]	81	38	1	2	40
	Liu et al. [42]	147	88	3	7	49
	Luo et al. [27]	62	32	1	2	27
	Skouras et al. [46]	121	8	10	2	101
	Sun et al. [29]	76	38	1	2	35
	Valdes et al. [31]	431	64	54	6	307
	Yang et al. [50]	174	63	1	5	105
	Niu et al. [38]	44	23	1	0	20
IL-18	Chen et al. [17]	64	28	4	6	26
	Dai et al. [18]	52	21	2	2	27
	Ding et al. [19]	72	33	2	1	36
	Hu et al. [21]	102	48	3	4	47
	Jiang et al. [22]	60	26	2	4	28
	Klimiuk et al. [39]	203	27	20	17	139
	Liu et al. [43]	80	36	3	4	37
	Okamoto et al. [44]	43	4	1	7	31
	Wang et al. [47]	44	17	2	2	23
	Wu et al. [33]	48	20	2	4	22
	Xiong et al. [34]	86	41	3	5	37
	Yu et al. [51]	52	30	0	2	20
IL-6	Kiropoulos et al. [24]	97	22	17	3	55
	Wang et al. [32]	71	33	2	1	35
	Wong et al. [48]	66	29	8	3	26
	Wu et al. [49]	109	31	9	25	44
	Zan et al. [35]	56	30	5	12	9
	Yang et al. [37]	54	20	2	2	30
IL-33	Lee et al. [26]	220	47	56	13	104
	Li et al. [40]	87	27	16	5	39
	Liu et al. [42]	147	82	5	13	47
	Xuan et al. [36]	44	20	2	3	19
IL-12	Chen et al. [17]	64	30	5	4	25
	Gu et al. [20]	52	27	5	5	25
	Jiang et al. [23]	60	22	3	8	27
	Okamoto et al. [44]	43	6	1	5	31
	Tian et al. [28]	190	120	17	21	32
	Zhou et al. [53]	73	31	8	14	20
IL-2	Liu et al. [43]	80	25	6	15	34
	Liu et al. [42]	147	53	18	42	34
	Ren et al. [25]	88	39	4	3	42
	Wu et al. [49]	109	34	21	22	32
	Zhang et al. [52]	69	23	6	4	36
IL-12p40	Fernández et al. [41]	60	11	20	9	20
	Klimiuk et al. [39]	203	38	44	6	115

Table 2 Diagnostic performance of interleukins from individual studies *(Continued)*

Interleukins	Author	Subjects	TP	FP	FN	TN
	Tural Önür et al. [45]	120	42	27	10	41
	Valdes et al. [30]	96	36	17	3	40
IL-8	Yamada et al. [57]	70	17	14	4	35
	Yang et al. [56]	64	38	4	2	20
IL-10	Wu et al. [49]	109	46	7	20	36
IL-22	Jin et al. [58]	56	23	1	5	27
	Yuan et al. [55]	87	47	7	5	28
IL-23	Klimiuk et al. [39]	203	13	66	31	93
IL-31	Gao et al. [54]	71	33	0	7	31

Abbreviations: *IL* interleukin, *TP* true-positive, *FP* false-positive, *FN* false-negative, *TN* true-negative

specificities for IL-27 and IL-18 reported by each study. (Results for the other ILs are reported in Additional file 1: Figure S1.) Sensitivity of IL-27 ranged from 0.80 to 1.00, and the pooled value was 0.93 (95%CI 0.90–0.95). Sensitivity of IL-18 ranged from 0.44 to 0.97, and the pooled value was 0.87 (95%CI 0.79–0.92). Specificity of IL-27 varied from 0.85 to 0.99, and the pooled value was 0.95 (95%CI 0.90–0.98). Specificity of IL-18 varied from 0.82 to 1.00, and the pooled value was 0.92 (95% CI 0.88–0.95). The pooled parameters for all included ILs are shown in Table 4.

Unlike a traditional ROC plot, each data point on an SROC curve represents a separate study, allowing the curve to provide an overall assessment of diagnostic performance. Plotting the rate of TP against the rate of FP gave curves showing AUCs of 0.95 for IL-18 and IL-27 (Fig. 3). Among all ILs, IL-27 showed the highest overall accuracy, with a sensitivity of 93% and specificity of 95%.

Study quality and publication bias

QUADAS-2 assessment of included studies showed that most studies had low risk of bias (Fig. 4). Both Egger's and Deeks' tests suggest no evidence of bias among the studies for any ILs meta-analyzed (Table 3). Funnel plots indicate low risk of publication bias (Additional file 1: Figure S2).

Discussion

Assaying pleural levels of ILs may be a cost-effective and minimally invasive alternative to traditional tests for differentiating TPE from other types of pleural effusion. Our meta-analysis of the available evidence suggests that IL-27 and IL-18 show relatively high diagnostic accuracy for TPE, while five other well-studied ILs do not (IL-2, IL-12, IL-27, IL-33 and IL-12p40). Even IL-27 and IL-18 do not appear to have adequate diagnostic potential on their own, so they would need to be used in conjunction with other methods or conventional markers.

Table 3 Statistical measures of heterogeneity, cut-off effect, and publication bias for each interleukin

interleukins	I^2 for heterogeneity in lnDOR(%)	Spearman's coefficient	Egger test *P* value	Deeks test *P* value
IL-27	53.5	−0.467	0.101	0.57
IL-18	61.7	−0.511	0.5	0.73
IL-6	77.8	−0.657	0.532	0.66
IL-33	77.7	−1.00	0.359	0.54
IL-12	34.3	0.493	0.029	0.23
IL-2	88.4	−0.900	0.17	0.18
IL-12p40	83.2	−0.800	0.9	0.34

Our meta-analysis showed that IL-2, despite being centrally involved in the regulation of immune tolerance and activation, [64] is associated with quite low sensitivity and specificity. This may reflect the fact that IL-2 data were available from only 5 studies, all of which were conducted in China. Future work, preferably in Caucasians and other groups of Asians, should investigate the diagnostic potential of this IL.

DOR combines sensitivity and specificity into a single indicator of test performance. [65] Higher DOR indicates better discriminatory test performance. Mean DOR was 64.12 for IL-18 and 227.9 for IL-27, indicating high overall accuracy. Potentially more clinically meaningful than DOR are likelihood ratios. [66] A likelihood ratio > 10 or <0.1 suggests a 10-fold difference between the pre- and post-test probability that a condition is present. Of the ILs meta-analyzed here, only IL-18 and IL-27 had PLRs >10, suggesting that a positive test result for these ILs indicates a relatively high probability of TPE. In addition, IL-27 was associated with an NLR of 0.08, indicating an 8% probability that a negative IL-27 test result is a false negative for TPE. This may be sufficient for ruling out TPE in the clinic.

Pleural levels of a number of biomarkers have been proposed as aids in the diagnosis of TPE, including adenosine deaminase (ADA) and interferon-γ(INF-γ), both of which are present in patients with TPE at significantly higher concentrations than in patients with other types of pleural effusion. The diagnostic performance determined here for IL-18 and IL-27 compares favorably with that of ADA and INF-γ. Meta-analyses [67, 68] indicate that these latter two assays on their own are associated with the following diagnostic indices: sensitivity, 0.89 (95%CI 0.87–0.91) and 0.92 (95%CI 0.90–0.93); specificity, 0.97 (95%CI 0.96–0.98) and 0.90 (95%CI 0.89–0.91); PLR, 23.45 (95%CI 17.31–31.78) and 9.03 (95%CI 7.19–

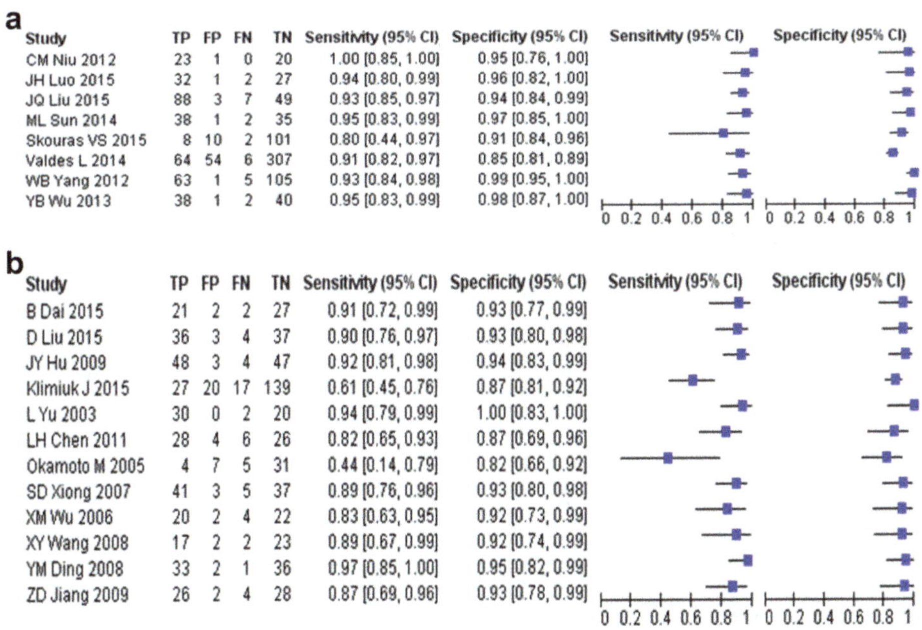

Fig. 2 Forest plot of the sensitivities and specificities. **a**. interleukin-27, **b**. interleukin-18. The calculated pooled mean with corresponding confidence interval is also reported

Table 4 Pooled means of sensitivity and specificity, diagnostic odds ratio(DOR), area under the curve(AUC), and calculated likelihood ratios for each interleukin

Interleukins	sensitivity(95%CI)	specificity(95%CI)	DOR	AUC	PLR	NLR
IL-27	0.93(0.90–0.95)	0.95(0.90–0.98)	264	0.95	19.5(9.4–40.5)	0.07(0.05–0.11)
IL-18	0.87(0.79–0.92)	0.92 (0.88–0.95)	76	0.95	10.8 (7.2–16.3)	0.14(0.09–0.23)
IL-6	0.86(0.70–0.94)	0.84(0.74–0.90)	30	0.90	5.2(3.0–9.1)	0.17(0.07–0.41)
IL-33	0.84(0.77–0.89)	0.80(0.65–0.89)	20	0.88	4.2(2.21–7.9)	0.20(0.13–0.32)
IL-12	0.78(0.69–0.84)	0.83(0.72–0.91)	17	0.86	4.6(2.8–7.8)	0.27(0.20–0.37)
IL-2	0.67(0.61–0.73)	0.76(0.70–0.82)	11	0.86	3.4(1.7–6.8)	0.36(0.20–0.66)
IL-12p40	0.82(0.66–0.91)	0.65(0.54–0.74)	8	0.76	2.3(1.6–3.4)	0.28(0.13–0.61)

Abbreviations: *IL* interleukin, *DOR* diagnostic odds ratio, *AUC* area under the curve, *PLR* positive likelihood ratio, *NLR* negative likelihood ratio

11.35); NLR, 0.11 (95%CI 0.07–0.16) and 0.10 (95%CI 0.07–0.14); and DOR, 272.7 (147.5–504.2) and 110.08 (95%CI 69.96–173.20). Although the available evidence suggests that IL-18 and IL-27 seem to have higher accuracy than ADA, the higher-cost and more complicated determination of IL-27 and IL-18 may limit their practical applicability. [69, 70] In addition, it has been reported that the combination of positive IL-27 with positive ADA values [16, 31, 46], can reach a sensitivity of 100% for the identification of TBP, Our meta-analysis, combined with previous ones, suggests that combining IL-18 and IL-27 with INF-γ and ADA may strengthen TPE diagnosis. We also suggest further studies should be carried out to determine the diagnostic accuracy of IL-27 and IL-18 combination or their combination with ADA or INF-γ.

Our meta-analysis suggests an association between elevated levels of at least certain pleural ILs and TPE. TPE has been characterized as a hypersensitive T cell reaction to mycobacteria or antigens in the pleural space, leading to the accumulation of protein-rich fluid. [6] ILs are divided into different families based on sequence homology, receptor chains or functional properties. IL-18 and IL-33 belong to the IL-1 family, [71] which contains

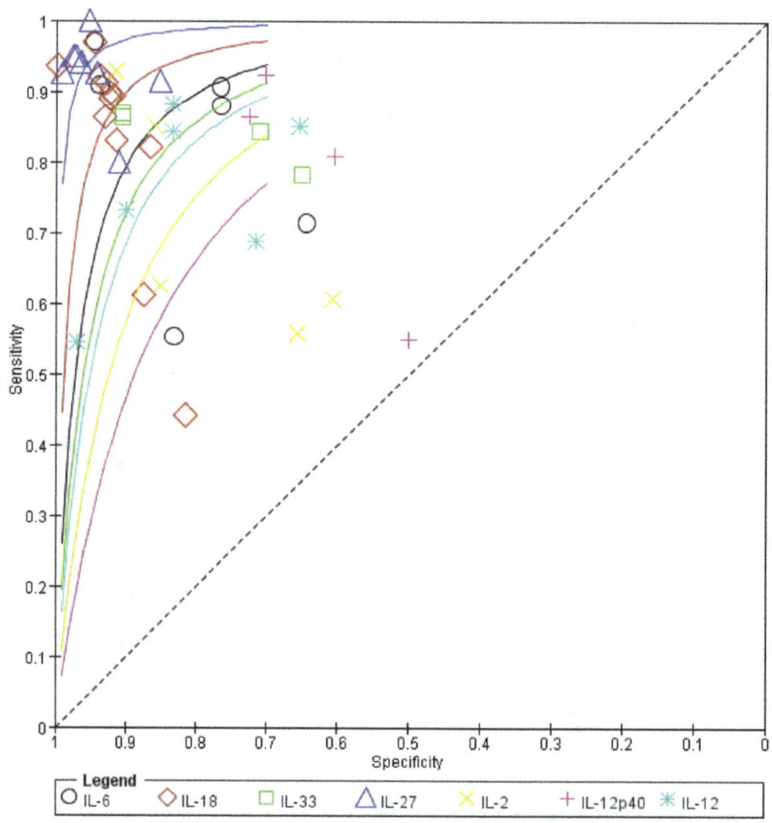

Fig. 3 Summary receiver operating characteristic (SROC) curve for all the interleukins included

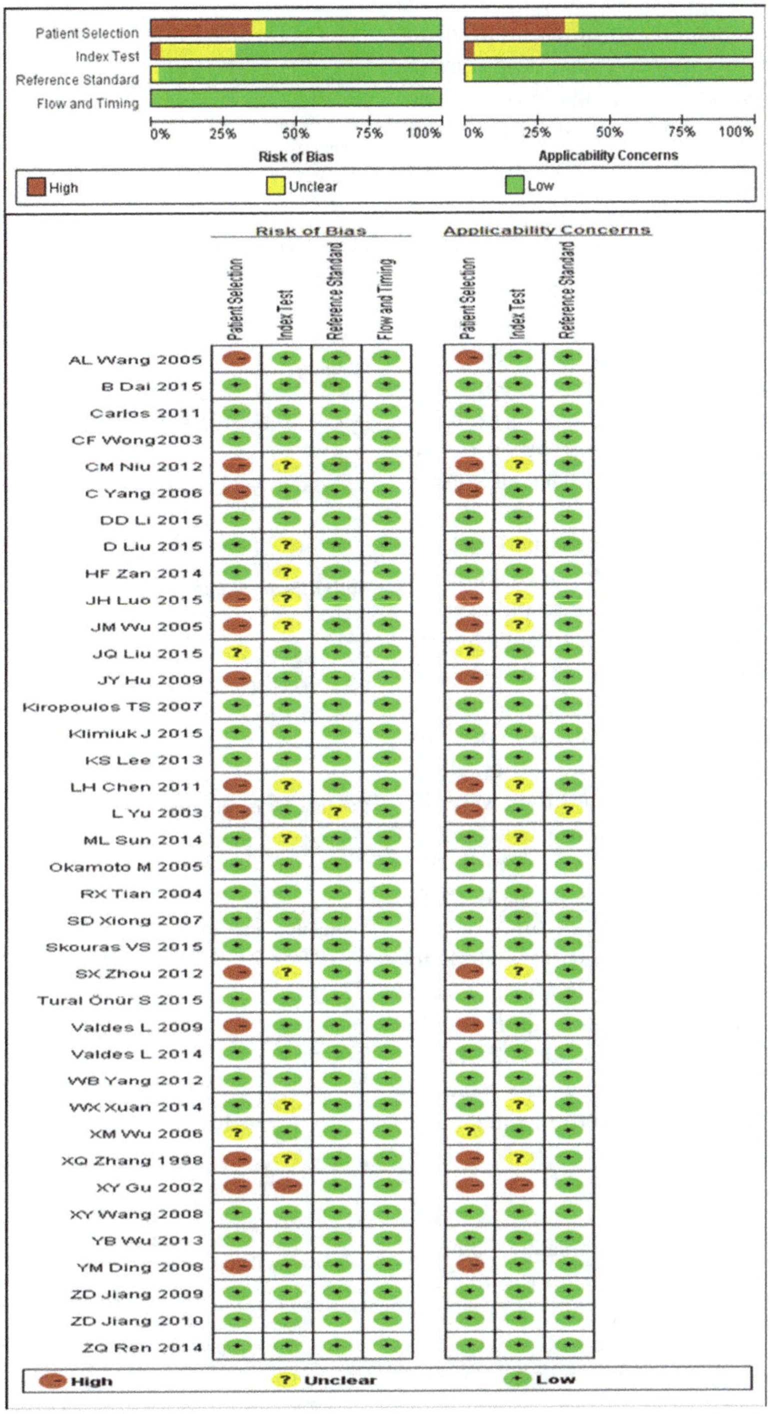

Fig. 4 Summary of QUADAS-2 assessments of included studies. QUADAS-2: Quality Assessment of Diagnostic Accuracy Studies-2. Patient Selection: Describe methods of patient selection; Index Text: Describe the index test and how it was conducted and interpreted; Reference Standard: Describe the reference standard and how it was conducted and interpreted; Flow and Timing: Describe any patients who did not receive the index tests or reference standard or who were excluded from the 2 × 2 table, and describe the interval and any interventions between index tests and the reference standard

inflammatory mediators playing a major role in early innate immune responses. IL-6, which belongs to a cytokine family of the same name, is a multifunctional, pleiotropic regulator of immune responses, acute-phase responses, hematopoiesis, and inflammation. [72] IL-2, a member of the γ-chain cytokine family, is produced mainly by CD4+ and CD8+ T cells and is essential for Treg cell development. [73] Although both blood and pleural fluid samples can be processed for all ILs, these assays are limited by their inability to differentiate drug resistant TB, consequently, cannot replace appropriate microbiological and molecular investigations. Future work is needed to examine how ILs may affect onset and/or progression of TPE and the probable association between ILs and drug sensitivity of TB.

To ensure reliable results, we meta-analyzed only ILs for which sensitivity and specificity data were available from at least 3 studies. As a result, we did not analyze several ILs for which levels appear to be elevated in tuberculosis [74], including IL-8 [57] and IL-22 [58]. Further work should examine the diagnostic potential of these ILs. In addition, more work should also examine the diagnostic performance of these and other ILs in combination, which we could not do for lack of studies including such combinations.

Our meta-analysis has additional limitations. First, exclusion of conference abstracts, letters to journal editors and unpublished data may have given rise to publication bias, such that our results overestimate actual diagnostic performance. Second, patients were diagnosed with TPE based on both bacteriological and histological assessment in only a few studies; in most studies, patients were diagnosed on the basis of one or the other, alone or in combination with clinical course, and they were diagnosed based solely on clinical course in a few studies. This increases risk of misclassification bias. Third, description of methodology was incomplete in many studies, leading to a QUADAS-2 assessment of "unclear". In addition, we did not perform meta-regression analysis to determine the source of heterogeneity, because of the limited numbers of the studies included. Our results highlight the need for more rigorous studies of ILs in the diagnosis of TPE. Future work should also examine the diagnostic potential of IL levels in serum, since most studies have focused on pleural levels.

Conclusion

The available evidence suggests that assaying pleural levels of certain ILs may aid in the diagnosis of TPE when used in combination with other biomarkers and approaches. By confirming such diagnosis, ILs may help avoid the need for more invasive diagnostic procedures.

Additional files

Additional file 1: Figure S1. Forest plot of the sensitivities and specificities reported by each interleukin. The Forest plots of the sensitivities and specificities reported by A. interleukin-6; B.interleukin-33; C interleukin-12; D interleukin-2; E interleukin-12p40. **Figure S2.** Funnel graph for the assessment of potential publication bias in each interleukin. The Funnel graphs for the assessment of potential publication bias in each interleukin: A for IL-27; B for IL-18;C for IL-6; D for IL-33; E for IL-12; F for IL-2; G for IL-12p40.

Abbreviations

ADA: Adenosine deaminaselNF-γlnterferon-γ; AUC: The area under the SROC curve; DOR: Diagnostic odds ratio; FN: False negative; FP: False positive; IL: Interleukins; NLR: Negative likelihood ratio; PLR: Positive likelihood ratio; QUADAS-2: Quality Assessment of Diagnostic Accuracy Studies-2; SROC: Summary ROC; TN: True negative; TP: True positive; TPE: Tuberculous pleural effusion

Acknowledgments

Not applicable

Funding

This work was supported by grants from the National Natural Science Foundation of China (81300032) and Science Foundation for Young Scholars of Sichuan University (2015SCU11999-10). The funders had no role in study design, data collection and analysis, decision to publish, or preparation of the manuscript.

Authors' contributions

NZ and CW: conceived the article and contributed the systematic review, meta-analysis, and manuscript writing. JQ, YQW, TY, and FQW: contributed to the systematic review and manuscript writing. YCS and LC: contributed to the conception and design and been involved in the revision. All authors read and approved the final manuscript.

Consent for publication

Not applicable

Competing interests

The authors declare that they have no competing interests.

References

1. Technical guidance group of the fifth national TB epidemiological survey. The fifth national tuberculosis epidemiological survey in 2010 [in Chinese]. Chin J Antituberc. 2012;34(08):485–508.
2. Qiu L, Teeter LD, Liu Z, Ma X, Musser JM, Ea G. Diagnostic associations between pleural and pulmonary tuberculosis. J Inf Secur. 2006;53(6):377–86.
3. Trajman A, Pai M, Dheda K, Smit R, Zyl V, Zwerling AA, Joshi R, Kalantri S, Daley P, Menzies D. Novel tests for diagnosing tuberculous pleural effusion: what works and what does not? Eur Respir J. 2008;31(5):1098–106.
4. Light RW. Update on tuberculous pleural effusion. Respirology. 2010;15(3):451¯8.
5. Mcgrath EE, Anderson PB. Diagnostic tests for tuberculous pleural effusion. Eur J Clin Microbiol Infect Dis. 2010;29(10):1187–93.
6. Sharma SK, Mitra DK, Balamurugan A, Pandey RM, Mehra NK. Cytokine polarization in Miliary and pleural tuberculosis. J Clin Immunol. 2002;22(6): 345–52.
7. Cooper AM. Cell-mediated immune responses in tuberculosis. Annu Rev Immunol. 2009;27(1):393–422.
8. Reddy VM, Andersen BR. Immunology of tuberculosis. Annu Rev Immunol. 2001;19(4):70–4.
9. Burgler S, Ouaked N, Bassin C, Basinski TM, Mantel PY, Siegmund K, Meyer N, Akdis CA, Schmidt-Weber CB. Differentiation and functional analysis of human T(H)17 cells. J Allergy Clin Immunol. 2009;123(3):1–7.
10. Moher D, Shamseer L, Clarke M, Ghersi D, Liberati A, Petticrew M, Shekelle P, Stewart LA. Preferred reporting items for systematic review and meta-analysis protocols (PRISMA-P) 2015 statement. Syst Rev. 2015;4(1):1–9.

11. Whiting PF, Rutjes AW, Westwood ME, Mallett S, Deeks JJ, Reitsma JB, Leeflang MM, Sterne JA, Bossuyt PM, Group Q. QUADAS-2: a revised tool for the quality assessment of diagnostic accuracy studies. Ann Intern Med. 2011;155(8):529–36.
12. Moses LE, Shapiro D, Littenberg B. Combining independent studies of a diagnostic test into a summary ROC curve: data-analytic approaches and some additional considerations. Stat Med. 1993;12(14):1293–316.
13. Lau J, Ioannidis JPA, Balk EM, Milch C, Terrin N, Chew PW, Salem D. Diagnosing acute cardiac ischemia in the emergency department: a systematic review of the accuracy and clinical effect of current technologies. Ann Emerg Med. 2001;37(5):453–60.
14. Fleiss JL. The statistical basis of meta-analysis. Stat Methods Med Res. 1993; 2(2):121–45.
15. Deeks JJ, Macaskill P, Irwig L. The performance of tests of publication bias and other sample size effects in systematic reviews of diagnostic test accuracy was assessed. J Clin Epidemiol. 2005;58(9):882–93.
16. Wu YB, Ye ZJ, Qin SM, Wu C, Chen YQ, Shi HZ. Combined detections of interleukin27, interferon-γ, and adenosine deaminase in pleural effusion for diagnosis of tuberculous pleurisy. Chin Med J. 2013;126(17):3215–21.
17. Chen L, Jiang H, Lin C. Detections of interferon-γ, IL18, IL12 and sIL2R for diagnosis of tuberculosis pleural effusion and malignant pleural effusions [in Chinese]. Chin J Clinicians (Electrionc Edition). 2011;05(12):3602–4.
18. Dai B, Xu X. Diagnostic value of interleukin-18 on tuberculous and malignant pleural effusion [in Chinese]. J Clin Pulm Med. 2015;20(2):228–30.
19. Ding YM. Combined detections of interleukin 18, interferon-γ, and adenosine deaminase in pleural effusion for diagnosis of tuberculous pleurisy and malignant pleurisy [in Chinese]. China: Zhejiang University; 2008.
20. Gu XY, Li DY, Wang SY, Zhao WG, Li RY, Li XH. Diagnostic significance of Interleukin-12 in tuberculous pleurisy [in Chinese]. Chin J Antitubercul. 2002;24(4):240.
21. Hu J, Wang Y, Chen J, Yang M, Jiang L. Significance of interleukin-18 (IL-18) and vascular endothelial growth factor (VEGF) in differentiating tuberculous pleural effusion from malignant pleural effusions (in Chinese). Clinical Misdiagnosis&Mistherapy. 2009;22(3):1–3.
22. Jiang ZD, Wang WR, Liu X. Diagnostic significance of interleukin-18 in tuberculous and malignant pleurisy [in Chinese]. Chin Prac Med. 2009;4(35):83–4.
23. Jiang ZD, Wang WR, Liu X. Diagnostic value of interleukin-12 in tuberculous pleurisy [in Chinese]. Chin Prac Med. 2010;5(1):50–1.
24. Kiropoulos TS, Kostikas K, Oikonomidi S, Tsilioni I, Nikoulis D, Germenis A, Gourgoulianis KI. Acute phase markers for the differentiation of infectious and malignant pleural effusions. Respir Med. 2007;101(5):910–8.
25. Ren ZQ, Xing WC, Sun Y, Liu F, Lin CZ. The differential diagnostic value of interferon-γ, interleukin-2, tumor necrosis factor α and adenosine deaminase in tuberculous and malignant pleural effusion. Prog Modern Biomed. 2014; 14(23):4471–4.
26. Lee KS, Kim HR, Kwak S, Choi KH, Cho JH, Lee YJ, Lee MK, Lee JH, Park SD, Park DS. Association between elevated pleural interleukin-33 levels and tuberculous pleurisy. Ann Lab Med. 2013;33(1):45–51.
27. Luo JH, Wu N. Diagnostic value of IL-27, ADA and INF-γ in Tuberculous pleural effusion and malignant pleural effusion [in Chinese]. Hebei Med J. 2015;37(4):512–4.
28. Tian RX. Clinical investigation of the diagnostic value of interferon-γ, interlukin-12 and adenosine deaminase isoenzyme in tuberculous pleurisy. Chin J Tubere Respir Dis. 2004;27(7):435–8.
29. Sun M, Yan D, Jiang S, Gu X, Ma W. Diagnostic value of interleukin-27 in tuberculous pleural effusion [in Chinese]. Natl Med J China. 2014;94(34):2641–4.
30. Valdes L, San-Jose ED, Jm AD, Golpe A, Valle J, Penela P, Gonzalez-Barcala F. Diagnostic value of interleukin-12 p40 in tuberculous pleural effusions. Eur Respir J. 2009;33(33):816–20.
31. Valdés L, San JE, Ferreiro L, Golpe A, Gude F, Á-D JM, Pereyra MF, Toubes ME, González-Barcala FJ. Interleukin 27 could be useful in the diagnosis of tuberculous pleural effusions. Respir Care. 2014;59(3):399–405.
32. Wang A. Diagnostic significance of adenosine deaminase activity, interferon-γ andilnterleukin-6 in tuberculous pleural effusions [in Chinese]. J Hubei Med Univ. 2005;26(1):117–20.
33. Wu XM. Level of interlukin 18 and its significance in tuberculous pleural effusion and malignant pleural effusion [in Chinese]. Chin J Mod Med. 2006; 16(15):2356–60.
34. Xiong DS, Xu GP, Xiong WN, Gao YP, Ni W, Chen SX. Combined detections of interleukin 18 and adenosine deaminase for diagnosis of tuberculous pleural effusion and malignant pleural effusion [in Chinese]. Zhonghua Jie He He Hu Xi Za Zhi. 2007;30(10):779–80.
35. Zan H, Xie W, Tao S. Diagnostic significance of adenosine deaminase activity and interleukin-6 in tuberculous pleural effusions [in Chinese]. Sichuan Med J. 2014;35(5):588–91.
36. Xuan WX, Zhang JC, Zhou Q, Yang WB, Li-Jun MA. IL-33 levels differentiate tuberculous pleurisy from malignant pleural effusions. Oncol Lett. 2014;8(1):449–53.
37. Yang C. Level of IL-6, IL-8 and its significance in tuberculous pleural effusion and malignant pleural effusion [in Chinese]. China: Dalian Medical University; 2006.
38. Niu CM. Interlukin-27 in tuberculous and malignant pleural effusion [in Chinese]. China: Huazhong University of Science and Technology; 2012.
39. Klimiuk J, Krenke R, Safianowska A, Korczynski P, Chazan R. Diagnostic performance of different pleural fluid biomarkers in tuberculous pleurisy. Adv Exp Med Biol. 2014;852:21–30.
40. Li D, Shen Y, Fu X, Li M, Wang T, Wen F. Combined detections of interleukin-33 and adenosine deaminase for diagnosis of tuberculous pleural effusion. Int J Clin Exp Pathol. 2015;8(1):888–93.
41. Fernández dLC, Duplat A, Giampietro F, de Waard JH, Luna J, Singh M, Araujo Z. Diagnostic accuracy of immunological methods in patients with tuberculous pleural effusion from Venezuela. Investig Clin. 2011;52(1):23–34.
42. Liu J, Zhang L, Feng S, Zhang L, Sun H, Liu G, Xiao H, Wu M, Du Y, Liu S. Evaluating the value of detecting cytokines for diagnosis of tuberculous pleural effusion by liquid array technology [in Chinese]. Chin J Lab Med. 2015;38(8):562–6.
43. Liu D, Xu XL. Diagnostic value of CD1c, IL-2, IL-18 in tuberculous pleural effusion and malignant pleural effusion [in Chinese]. World Latest Medicine Information. 2015;15(54):159–60.
44. Okamoto M, Kawabe T, Iwasaki Y, Hara T, Hashimoto N, Imaizumi K, Hasegawa Y, Shimokata K. Evaluation of interferon-γ, interferon-γ-inducing cytokines, and interferon-γ–inducible chemokines in tuberculous pleural effusions. J Lab Clin Med. 2005;145(2):88–93.
45. Önür ST, Sökücü SN, Dalar L, Seyh EC, Akbaş A, Alti S. Are soluble IL-2 receptor and IL-12p40 levels useful markers for diagnosis of tuberculous pleurisy? Infect Dis (Lond). 2015;47(3):1–6.
46. Skouras VS, Magkouta SF, Psallidas I, Tsilioni I, Maragozidis P, Gourgoulianis KI, Kalomenidis I. Interleukin-27 improves the ability of adenosine deaminase to rule out tuberculous pleural effusion regardless of pleural tuberculosis prevalence. Infect Dis (Lond). 2015;47(7):1–7.
47. Wang XY, Han L, Yang ZH. Combined detections of interleukin 18 and adenosine deaminase in pleural effusion for diagnosis of tuberculous pleural effusion and malignant pleural effusion [in Chinese]. Chin J Gerontol. 2008;28(21):2125–7.
48. Wong C, Yew W, Leung S, Chan C. Assay of pleural fluid interleukin-6, tumour necrosis factor-alpha and interferon-gamma in the diagnosis and outcome correlation of tuberculous effusion. Respir Med. 2003; 97(12):1289–95.
49. Wu J, Li Y, Jiang S. Diagnostic value of combined determination of serum and chest fluid adenosine deaminase(ADA), IL-2, IL-6, IL-10 contents for differentiation of tuberculous from malignant pleural effusion. J of Radioimmunology. 2005;18(2):97–9.
50. Yang WB, Liang QL, Ye ZJ, Niu CM, Ma WL, Xiong XZ, Du RH, Zhou Q, Zhang JC, Shi HZ. Cell origins and diagnostic accuracy of interleukin 27 in pleural effusions. PLoS One. 2012;7(7):e40450.
51. Yu L, Wang M, Ma X, Zhang Y, Zuo L. Diagnostic value of IL-18 and INF-gama levels in tuberculous and malignant pleural effusions [in Chinese]. Shanghai J of Med Lab Sci. 2003;18(1):39.
52. Zhang XQ, Hua ZX, Lu DM, Liu HS, Lv XY, Chen LH. The differential diagnostic value of interleukin-2 in tuberculous pleural or ascitic effusion [in Chinese]. J Chengde Med Coll. 1998;15(2):108–9.
53. Zhou SX, Tan J, Xiao XP. Comparison of clinical values of adenosine deaminase,tumor necrosis factor-α and interleukin-12 in diagnosing tuberculous pleural effusion [in Chinese]. Lab Med Clin. 2012;9(12):1436–7.
54. Gao Y, Ou Q, Wu J, Zhang B, Wen X, Zhang W, Shao L. Expressions and diagnostic value of interleukin-31 in tuberculous pleural effusion [in Chinese]. Chin J Infect Dis. 2015;33(6):323–6.
55. Yuan YM, Wang ZY, Wang XJ, Cheng XX, Hui-Ru AN, Zhai SH, Zhang LL, Shuang-Mei L. The application of Mtb-antigen-specific Interleukin-22 in the differential diagnosis of Tuberculous pleurisy [in Chinese]. Modern Instruments & Medical Treatment. 2014;20(3):1–3.
56. Yang J, Liu W. Role of combination of CA50、TSA、CEA、SF and IL-8 assays in differentiation of benign from malignant pleural effusion [in Chinese]. Chin Med J Metall Industry. 2001;18(5):264–6.

57. Yamada Y, Nakamura A, Hosoda M, Kato T, Asano T, Tonegawa K, Itoh M. Cytokines in pleural liquid for diagnosis of tuberculous pleurisy. Respir Med. 2001;95(7):577–81.
58. Jin D, Chen Y, Wang Z, Wang S, Bunjhoo H, Zhu J, Cao Y, Xiong W, Xiong S, Xu Y. Diagnostic value of interleukin 22 and carcinoembryonic antigen in tuberculous and malignant pleural effusions. Exp Ther Med. 2011;2(6):1205–9.
59. Littenberg B, Moses LE. Estimating diagnostic accuracy from multiple conflicting reports a new meta-analytic method. Med Decis Mak. 1993; 13(13):313–21.
60. Reitsma JB, Glas AS, Rutjes AWS, Scholten RJPM, Bossuyt PM, Zwinderman AH. Bivariate analysis of sensitivity and specificity produces informative summary measures in diagnostic reviews. J Clin Epidemiol. 2005;58(10):982–90.
61. Rutter CM, Gatsonis CA. A hierarchical regression approach to meta-analysis of diagnostic test accuracy evaluations. Stat Med. 2001;20(19):2865–84.
62. Macaskill P. Empirical Bayes estimates generated in a hierarchical summary ROC analysis agreed closely with those of a full Bayesian analysis. J Clin Epidemiol. 2004;57(9):925–32.
63. Chappell FM, Raab GM, Wardlaw JM. When are summary ROC curves appropriate for diagnostic meta-analyses? Stat Med. 2009;28(21):2653–68.
64. Boyman O, Kolios AG, Raeber ME. Modulation of T cell responses by IL-2 and IL-2 complexes. Clin Exp Rheumatol. 2015;33(4):S54–7.
65. Glas AS, Lijmer JG, Prins MH, Bonsel GJ, Bossuyt PMM. The diagnostic odds ratio: a single indicator of test performance. J Clin Epidemiol. 2003;56(11):1129–35.
66. Deeks JJ. Systematic reviews in health care: systematic reviews of evaluations of diagnostic and screening tests. BMJ. 2001;323(7322):1188.
67. Jiang J, Shi HZ, Liang QL, Qin SM, Qin XJ. Diagnostic value of interferon-γ in tuberculous pleurisy : a meta-analysis. Chest. 2007;131(4):1133–41.
68. Liang QL, Shi HZ, Ke W, Qin SM, Qin XJ. Diagnostic accuracy of adenosine deaminase in tuberculous pleurisy: a meta-analysis. Respir Med. 2008;102(5):744–54.
69. Wallis RS, Kim P, Cole S, Hanna D, Andrade BB, Maeurer M, Schito M, Zumla A. Tuberculosis biomarkers discovery: developments, needs, and challenges. Lancet Infect Dis. 2013;13(4):362–72.
70. Porcel JM. Advances in the diagnosis of tuberculous pleuritis. Ann Transl Med. 2016;4(15):282.
71. Palomo J, Dietrich D, Martin P, Palmer G, Gabay C. The interleukin (IL)-1 cytokine family–balance between agonists and antagonists in inflammatory diseases. Cytokine. 2015;76(1):25–37.
72. Hurst SM, Wilkinson TS, Mcloughlin RM, Jones S, Horiuchi S, Yamamoto N, Rose-John S, Fuller GM, Topley N, Jones SA. IL-6 and its soluble receptor orchestrate a temporal switch in the pattern of leukocyte recruitment seen during acute inflammation. Immunity. 2001;14(14):705–14.
73. Malek TR. The biology of interleukin-2. Annu Rev Immunol. 2008;26(1):453–79.
74. Chomej P, Bauer K, Bitterlich N, Hui DSC, Chan KS, Gosse H, Schauer J, Hoheisel G, Sack U. Differential diagnosis of pleural effusions by fuzzy-logic-based analysis of cytokines. Respir Med. 2004;98(4):308–17.

18

Delay in diagnosis of pulmonary tuberculosis in low-and middle-income settings

Fentabil Getnet[1*], Meaza Demissie[2], Nega Assefa[3], Bizatu Mengistie[3] and Alemayehu Worku[4]

Abstract

Background: Assessment of delays in seeking care and diagnosis of tuberculosis is essential to evaluate effectiveness of tuberculosis control programs, and identify programmatic impediments. Thus, this review of studies aimed to examine the extent of patient, health system, and total delays in diagnosis of pulmonary tuberculosis in low- and middle- income countries.

Methods: It was done following the Preferred Reporting Items for Systematic Reviews and Meta-Analyses. Electronic databases were searched to retrieve studies published from 2007 to 2015 including *Pubmed central, Springer link, Hinari* and *Google scholar*. Searching terms were *pulmonary tuberculosis, health care seeking, health care seeking behavior, patient delay, diagnostic delay, health system delay, provider delay, and doctor delay*. Retrieved studies were systematically reviewed and summarized using Comprehensive Meta-analysis software.

Results: Forty studies involving 18,975 patients qualified for systematic review, and 14 of them qualified for meta-analysis. The median diagnostic delay ranged from 30 to 366.5 days [IQR = 44–77.8], with a 4–199 days [IQR = 15–50] and 2–128.5 days [IQR = 12–34] due to patient and health system delays, respectively. The meta-analysis showed 42% of pulmonary tuberculosis patients delayed seeking care by a month or more; uneducated patients [pooled OR = 1.5, 95%CI = 1.1–1.9] and those who sought initial care from informal providers [pooled OR = 3, 95%CI = 2.3–3.9] had higher odds of patient delay.

Conclusion: Delay in diagnosis is still a major challenge of tuberculosis control and prevention programs in low- and middle- income settings. Efforts to develop new strategies for better case-finding using the existing systems and improving patients' care seeking behavior need to be intensified.

Keywords: Patient delay, Health system, Diagnosis delay, Pulmonary tuberculosis

Background

Tuberculosis (TB) causes an estimated 10.4 million cases and 1.7 million deaths globally, with the heaviest toll in Low- and Middle-Income countries (LMICs) [1]. The main strategies to control TB are early diagnosis and prompt treatment initiation [2]. Passive case-finding is the main approach currently applied by most national TB control programs (NTPs) [3]. The term "passive" implies that TB case detection entirely relies on people with TB symptoms presenting themselves to the health facilities [2]. Successful case detection also relies on health systems capacity to promptly diagnose and commence treatment [4].

However, this passive process has not been as effective as it should be in many LMICs [5]. The effectiveness of the passive case-finding system is influenced by many factors including patient health seeking behavior, the efficiency and competence of healthcare workers, and the quality of laboratory facilities [6, 7]. Failure to timely detect and treat TB could worsen illness severity,

* Correspondence: b.infen4ever@gmail.com
[1]Department of Public Health, College of Medicine and Health Sciences, Jigjiga University, PO Box = 1020, Jigjiga, Ethiopia
Full list of author information is available at the end of the article

prolongs patient suffering, increases the risk of patient death, and facilitates the transmission of the disease (if smear positive pulmonary TB) to close contacts [8–10].

Delay in diagnosis and treatment initiation of TB has remained unacceptably high especially among high burden countries [6, 7]. Related systematic reviews were reported on the subject matter in 2008 [6] and 2010 particularly from Sub-Saharan Africa [11]. These reviews included all studies done on delay in diagnosis and treatment of TB regardless of the disease type. However, most NTPs promote healthcare seeking for presumptive cases with pulmonary symptoms [12]. Plus, pulmonary tuberculosis (PTB) patients are responsible for disease transmission (specially smear positive patients), and longer delays facilitate the spreading to close contacts [13]. On the other side, extra-pulmonary TB (EPTB) forms are not easily detectable using clinical and laboratory examinations. As a result, delay will inflate if EPTB patients are included [2].

More importantly, massive efforts were implemented during the era of Stop TB Strategy (2006–2015) to substantially reduce the global burden of TB by 2015 through universal access to diagnosis and treatment regardless of socio-economic barriers [14]. A periodic conduct of systematic review is warranted to incorporate lessons learned from such massive and dynamic TB control programs to improve the practice of early detection and initiation of treatment. Therefore, this systematic review and meta-analysis was conducted to summarize the extent of delays and identify factors that influenced prompt detection and treatment of PTB in LMICs where access or utilization of TB services has not been optimal as required. We have also examined the median delay differences between Sub-Saharan Africa and Other LMICs.

Methods

We systematically reviewed studies reported from LMICs to summarize delays in diagnosis of PTB patients and to identify factors contributing to high extents of delay. We thought such a specific study on delay in diagnosis of PTB patients would be more beneficial from programmatic and interventional perspectives. Meta-analysis principles were applied to combine numeric data on delays and affecting factors. We followed the Preferred Reporting Items for Systematic Reviews and Meta-Analyses (PRISMA) [15] as a standard guideline.

Search strategy

Various electronic databases were searched to retrieve relevant published studies using Boolean searching technique [16]. We used 'AND' and 'OR'to connect key search terms to retrieve studies from *Pubmed*. The search terms we used include *pulmonary tuberculosis, diagnosis delay, patient delay, health system delay, provider delay, doctor delay, delayed consultation, health care seeking, and health care seeking behavior* (Table 1). In addition, we searched other web-based sources including *Springer link, Hinari,* and *Google scholar,* though not standard sources, to retrieve studies that are not indexed in *Pubmed.*

We searched each source twice. The first author (FG) conducted the primary searching of studies from sources listed above and then the co-author (NA) independently and blindly conducted it again using similar searching technique, databases and terms. All the potential studies identified by both authors were set for screening and selection process. We contacted 5 authors via email for unpublished studies and raw data but none responded to our requests.

Table 1 Pudmed search strategies

S. No.	Search terms or strategies	Remarks
1.	Pulmonary tuberculosis AND diagnosis Delay*	**Example of search detail (1)**: *("tuberculosis, pulmonary"[MeSH Terms] OR ("tuberculosis"[All Fields] AND "pulmonary"[All Fields]) OR "pulmonary tuberculosis"[All Fields] OR ("pulmonary"[All Fields] AND "tuberculosis"[All Fields])) AND (("diagnosis"[Subheading] OR "diagnosis"[All Fields] OR "diagnosis"[MeSH Terms]) AND delay[All Fields])* *indicates truncation
2.	Pulmonary tuberculosis AND delayed consultation*	
3.	Pulmonary tuberculosis AND patient delay*	
4.	Pulmonary tuberculosis AND healthcare seeking	
5.	Pulmonary tuberculosis AND healthcare seeking behavior	
6.	Pulmonary tuberculosis AND health system delay*	
7.	Pulmonary tuberculosis AND provider delay*	
8.	Pulmonary Tuberculosis AND doctor delay*	
9.	Patient delay OR health system delay*	
10.	Patient delay OR provider delay*	
11	Patient delay OR doctor delay*	
12.	Tuberculosis AND Diagnosis delay OR delayed consultation OR patient delay OR health system delay OR provider delay OR doctor delay	

Inclusion/exclusion criteria

We included studies that were reported in English, conducted in low and middle income countries, published between 2007 and 2015 (era of Stop TB strategy), with any observational study design (cross-sectional, case-control, or cohort studies), and those which fully or partially measured diagnosis delays (patient delay/health system delay/total diagnosis delay). With respect to the study participants, we included studies on pulmonary TB patients who sought healthcare themselves and above 15 years old regardless of smear type (positive/negative/unknown) and treatment category (new/retreatment). Studies done on PTB and EPTB patients were considered when data were presented for PTB patients separately. However, we excluded studies that were on presumptive TB cases (formerly called '*suspects*') and special groups (e.g. HIV, MDR), qualitative in design, and community based studies which applied active case-finding strategies.

Further inclusion criteria were used for Meta-analysis from eligible studies for systematic review. These included studies that categorized patient delay using 15, 21 or 30 days as cut-off points and reported cross tabulations and/or odds ratio/relative risk of explanatory variables.

Selection of studies

Eligible studies were selected using the pre-specified inclusion/exclusion criteria. Initially, the studies were searched and potential articles were identified using the title and then abstract by two reviewers (FG and NA) independently. Following identification of potential studies, FG made the final selection through thorough review of full articles including the study design, participants, outcome variable studied (delay), and publication year. Co-authors (NA and BM) closely supervised the selection process.

Quality assessment

All included studies were assessed for their scientific quality usingquality assessment tools developed by the National Collaborating Center for Environmental Health [17] and National Institute of Health (NIH) National Heart, Lung and Blood Institute [18].

The quality of each study was assessed using 4 parameters: 1) defined study population, 2) representativeness of participants and low non-response rate, 3) comparability of analysis groups and outcome ascertainment, and 4) adjusted analysis to control confounding. Each parameter was rated as 1 if 'Yes' and 0 if 'No'. Then the scores were added and the quality of each studywas leveled as good (if 3 or 4 'yes's), fair (2 'yes's) and poor (if 0 or 1 yes). Fair and good quality studies were considered as satisfying quality (Table 2). The quality of all included

Table 2 quality assessment result of the studies included in the systematic review and meta-analysis

Study	Study Design	A	B	C	D	Total score
Alavi et al. 2015 [45]	CS	1	0	1	1	3
Asefa et al. 2014 [27]	CS	1	1	1	1	4
Aye et al. 2010 [46]	RC	1	0	1	1	4
Basnet et al. 2009 [47]	CS	1	1	1	1	4
Behera et al. 2013 [48]	CS	1	1	1	1	4
Belkina et al. 2014 [44]	CS	1	1	1	1	4
Biya et al. 2010 [49]	CS	1	0	1	1	3
Buregyeya et al. 2014 [50]	CS	1	0	1	1	3
Cambanis et al 2007 [51]	CS	1	1	1	1	4
Deponti et al. 2013 [52]	CS	1	0	1	1	3
Ekinci et al. 2014 [22]	CS	1	0	1	1	3
Ford et al. 2009 [21]	CS	1	0	1	1	3
Gebeyehu et al. 2014 [34]	CS	1	0	1	1	3
Gosoniu et al. 2008 [19]	CS	1	0	1	1	3
Gosoniu et al. 2008 [19]	CS	1	0	1	1	3
Gosoniu et al. 2008 [19]	CS	1	0	1	1	3
Huong et al. 2007 [30]	CS	1	1	1	1	4
Hussen et al. 2012 [35]	CS	1	0	1	1	3
Jurcev-Savicevic et al. 2013 [53]	CS	1	1	1	1	4
Kansiime et al. 2013 [54]	CS	1	1	1	1	4
Li et al. 2012 [55]	CS	1	1	1	1	4
Maamari et al. 2008 [25]	CS	1	1	1	1	4
Maciel et al. 2010 [56]	CS	1	1	1	1	4
Maior et al. 2012 [57]	CS	1	1	1	1	4
Makwakwa et al. 2014 [58]	CS	1	1	1	1	4
Mesfin et al. 2009 [29]	CS	1	1	1	1	4
Mfinanga et al. 2008 [59]	CS	1	1	1	1	4
Mohamed et al. 2013 [36]	CS	1	1	1	1	4
Nasehi et al. 2012 [60]	CS	1	1	1	1	4
Ngadaya et al. 2009 [61]	CS	1	1	1	1	4
Ngangro et al. 2012 [62]	CS	1	1	1	1	4
Pradhan et al. 2010 [43]	CS	1	1	1	1	4
Rabin et al. 2013 [63]	CS	1	1	1	1	4
Sabawoon et al. 2011 [31]	CS	1	0	1	1	3
Saifodine et al. 2013 [37]	CS	1	1	1	1	4
Sendagire et al. 2010 [64]	CS	1	1	1	1	4
Takarinda et al. 2015 [32]	CS	1	1	1	1	4
Tamhane et al. 2012 [23]	CS	1	0	1	1	3
Ukwaja et al. 2013 [24]	CS	1	1	1	1	4
Woith et al. 2014 [65]	CS	1	0	1	1	3
Yimer et al. 2015 [66]	CS	1	1	1	1	4

CS; refers to cross-sectional and RC; refers to retrospective cohort. The columns: A. Study population defined; B. representativeness of participants and low non-response rate; C. Comparability of analysis groups and outcome ascertainment; D. analysis to control confounding
Rating: (0 = No and 1 = Yes). This format was adapted from a similar review done in China [67]

Table 4 The median delay (days) in diagnosis of pulmonary tuberculosis in low and middle income countries other than Sub-Saharan Africa, 2007 to 2015 ($n = 22$)

First Author	Country	Publication Year	Design	Setting	Sample size	Patient Delay	Health System Delay	Total Delay	Ref. No
Huong	Vietnam	2007	CS	TB units	2087	21	7	30	[30]
Maamari	Syria	2008	CS	TB centers	800	31 ($\bar{X} = 52.7$)	11.7 ($\bar{X} = 24.8$)	55 ($\bar{X} = 77.6$)	[25]
Gosoniu	Bangladesh	2008	CS	Clinics, HC	102	*	*	60	[19]
Gosoniu	India	2008	CS	Health centers, Clinics	127	*	*	74	[19]
Basnet	Nepal	2009	CS	Hospital &HC	307	50	18	60	[47]
Ford	Peru	2009	CS	Hospital & Health post	108	61	*	*	[21]
Maciel	Brazil	2010	CS	Primary PHF	304	76	30	110	[56]
Aye	Tajikistan	2010	RC	Hospital, HC, clinics	204	21.5	16	53	[46]
Pradhan	India	2010	CS	DOTs centers	266	6 ($\bar{X} = 30$)	31 ($\bar{X} = 61$)	37 ($\bar{X} = 91$)	[43]
Sabawoon	Afghanistan	2011	CS	Hospital & clinic	122	199 ($\bar{X} = 205.2$)	128.5 ($\bar{X} = 150$)	366.5 ($\bar{X} = 356$)	[31]
Li	China	2012	CS	TB clinics	323	10 ($\bar{X} = 31$)	*	*	[55]
Nasehi	Iran	2012	CS	Hospital, clinics	5702	*	*	59	[60]
Tamhane	India	2012	CS	Health center	150	15	31	*	[23]
Behera	India	2013	CS	Tertiary hospital	204	16 ($\bar{X} = 32.97$)	39 ($\bar{X} = 60.46$)	43 ($\bar{X} = 75.7$)	[48]
Rabin	Georgia	2013	CS	TB diagnostic centers	247	23.5 ($\bar{X} = 56.2$)	14($\bar{X} = 33.7$)	59.5 ($\bar{X} = 89$)	[63]
Deponti	Brazil	2013	CS	Tertiary hospital	153	30	18	60	[52]
Jurcev-Savicevic	Croatia	2013	CS	Hospital	241	*	15	*	[53]
Woith	Russia	2014	CS	TB clinics	105	30	*	*	[65]
Ekinci	Turkey	2014	CS	Referral hospital	136	12 ($\bar{X} = 30.5$)	29 ($\bar{X} = 48.7$)	54 ($\bar{X} = 82.2$)	[22]
Alavi	Iran	2015	CS	Health Center	139	*	*	48 ($\bar{X} = 73$)	[45]
Belkina	Uzbekistan	2014	CS	Hospitall	538	27	7	50	[44]
Maior	Brazil	2012	CS	TB clinic	199	56	14	70	[57]

Key: * Value not obtainable
X: Mean value
CS: Cross-sectional
HC: Health center
PHF: Public health facility
RC: Retrospective cohort

Table 3 The median delay (days) in diagnosis of pulmonary tuberculosis in Sub-Saharan Africa, 2007 to 2015 ($n = 19$)

First Author	Country	Publication Year	Design	Setting	Sample Size	Patient Delay	Health System Delay	Total Delay	Ref. No
Cambanis	Cameroon	2007	CS	Hospital	243	15	*	*	[51]
Mfinanga	Tanzania	2008	CS	Hospital, HC& dispensaries	639	14 ($\bar{X} = 37.4$)	*	*	[59]
Gosoniu	Malawi	2008	CS	Health centers, clinics	100	*	*	33.5	[19]
Mesfin	Ethiopia	2009	CS	Hospital & HC	924	30	*	*	[29]
Ngadaya	Tanzania	2009	CS	Hospital, HC,TB dispensary	206	62	*	90 ($\bar{X} = 125.5$)	[61]
Biya	Nigeria	2010	CS	Hospital	160	30	*	*	[49]
Sendagire	Uganda	2010	CS	Public health facility	253	28	28	56	[64]
Hussen	Ethiopia	2012	CS	Hospital & HC	129	63	34	97	[35]
Ngangro	Chad	2012	CS	Hospital	286	15	36	57.5	[62]
Ukwaja	Nigeria	2013	CS	Hospital	450	56	21	77	[24]
Kansiime	Uganda	2013	CS	Referral hospital	266	*	9	*	[54]
Saifodine	Mozambique	2013	CS	Hospital and HC	622	61	62	150	[37]
Mohamed	Sudan	2013	CS	TB management unit	292	4 ($\bar{X} = 27.2$)	*	*	[36]
Makwakwa	Malawi	2014	CS	Hospital	588	14	59	80	[58]
Gebeyehu	Ethiopia	2014	CS	Hospital &HC	153	28	*	*	[34]
Asefa	Ethiopia	2014	CS	Health center	328	30	7	37	[27]
Buregyeya	Uganda	2014	CS	Hospital and HC	158	30	77	112	[50]
Yimer	Ethiopia	2015	CS	Hospital &HC	231	21	*	*	[66]
Takarinda	Zimbabwe	2015	CS	Hospitals, clinics, PHF	383	28	2	30	[32]

Key: * indicates data not available

studies was assessed by first author (FG), followed by immediate and independent crosschecking by two co--authors (NA and BM). Discrepancies were solved through mutual understanding.

Data extraction

Excel spreadsheet was used to extract available data on the name of first author, country where the study was conducted, publication year, type of health-care facility (study setting), study design, sample size, and median and/or mean delays (patient, health system and total) in days. Data from a study by Gosoniu et al. that involved 3 countries (Bangladesh, India and Malawi) was extracted separately for each country [19]. Delays reported in weeks were transformed into days by a multiple of 7 (Tables 3 and 4). The predictor variables that have statistically significant association with patient, health system and total diagnosis delay were also extracted (Table 5).

Further data were extracted on the event (delay) among exposure categories and/or odds ratio for meta-analysis. Health system and total delays were not considered for meta-analysis because of lack of clear cutoff values. The studies we reviewed did not use standard cutoff value to categorize patient delays. Therefore, we used the WHO recommended cutoff points (15 and 21 days) [20] and the commonly used 30 days by numerous studies. There was also considerable variability in the way studies categorized explanatory variables, thus variables categorized in the same way were considered for meta-analysis. The final explanatory variables we came up with, therefore, were sex, residence, educational status, first care seeking from informal healthcare provider, and HIV status.

Definition of terms

The definitions of terms in included studies were critically reviewed. Different studies used different terms to describe patient, health system, and diagnosis delays. For instance, some studies described patient delay as TB test delay or TB test seeking delay [21] and patients' application interval [22]. Health system delay is also referred to as doctor delay or provider delay [22–24]. Most studies used the term 'total delay' as the time until the diagnosis while some until treatment. In such a case, we took the delay until diagnosis [25–29]. Accordingly, delay terms have been defined as follows:

Table 5 Summary of risk factors for delay in diagnosis in low and middle income countries, 2007 to 2015

Patient delay	Health System Delay	Total Delay
Socio-demographic: Poor literacy [21, 24, 28, 29, 35, 62], Rural residence [29, 34, 35], Urban residence [24, 36, 37], Older age [24], long distance to the nearest HF [24, 30–32, 35, 59], Being female [30, 32, 36, 59, 63], Being male [21, 50] Socio-economic: Average monthly working days > 24 [55], Unemployment [36, 59], Being main income earner [51], Low economic status [36, 61]	Socio-demographic: Older age [24, 60], Long distance to nearest HF [24, 25, 44], Being female [19, 60, 63, 68], Male sex [24, 27, 48, 50] Socio-economic: Low income [43], Unemployment [44], Labor migration [44]	Socio-demographic: Being female [19, 60, 63, 68],Being male [24, 27, 48, 50],Being housewife [19], Higher family size [27], Poor literacy [27],Urban residence [24, 60],Long distance to nearest HF [24, 25, 44], Older age [24, 60], General caste [48]
Behavioral: Evil/bad luck perception [29], Knowledge of coughing > 3 wks as PTB symptom [58], Poor knowledge of PTB symptoms [25, 37, 48, 49, 57, 59, 61], Perceived social stigma [31, 51], Perceived inability to pay for care [23], Perception that PTB is common [21, 36], Belief of PTB is associated with HIV [59, 61, 64], Perceiving symptoms as non-serious [22, 43], Belief of PTB is curable [21, 64]	Clinical: Good functional status [35], No cough [56], Unusual symptoms other than common ones [53], Normal chest X-ray [56], Presence of fever [54], Fibrotic changes on chest x-ray ® [52], Smear negativity [28, 37, 53, 54, 58]	Behavioral: Perceived stigma [25, 27], Sanitation as perceived cause [19],1st visit to informal provider (traditional, religious [24, 25], Self-medication [44], Smoking [45]
Initial Care seeking: 1st visit at informal provider (traditional, religious) [25, 29, 31, 35, 37, 58], Self-medication [31, 32, 44, 51, 52, 62, 63], Alcoholism [44], smoking /tobacco use [47, 63]	Initial Care seeking: 1st visit to private facilities (clinics, drug vendors) [29–31, 35, 44, 50, 58], 1st visit to informal provider (traditional, religious) [23, 24], 1st visit to lower level HF [30, 32, 46, 49], Contact with more than two health providers [35]	Initial Care seeking: Prior antibiotics medication, 1st visit to private facility [44, 50, 60], Multi-facility visit [25]
Clinical: Smear positivity [29, 47], HIV positivity [44], Being new case [58], Chronic/persistent cough [44, 56, 63], Pulmonary co morbidity [37, 63], Mild severity of illness [35], MTB lineage 7 [66], Hemoptysis® [55, 62, 63], Chest pain® [61], Multiple symptoms® [63]		Clinical: Chronic cough [19, 44, 63], Only chest pain [19], Immunosuppressive therapy (62)

Key: ®: representsthe association is negative (preventive)
HF Health facility, *MTB Mycobacterium tuberculosis*

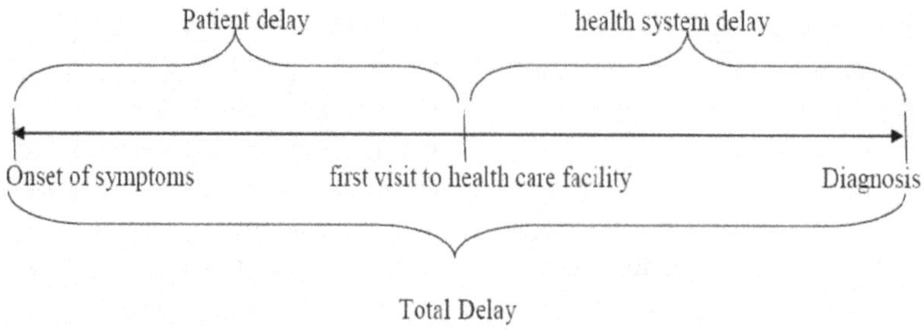

Fig. 1 Illustration of patient, health system and total delay

Patient delay

The time interval between the onsets of patient recognized PTB symptom(s) recognize and the patient's first consultation to a healthcare provider.

Health system delay

The time interval between the patient's first consultation with a health care provider and the date of diagnosis.

Diagnosis/Total delay

The time interval between the onset of PTB symptom(s) and the date of diagnosis. Alternatively, the sum of patient delay and health system delay (Fig. 1).

Data analysis

Systematic review

The data organized on excel spreadsheet were exported to SPSS version 21 for analysis. The median delay (in days) was summarized using median, box plots, inter quartile ranges (25th and 75th percentile), and 95% confidence interval and ranges. Since the distribution of median delays was skewed, the pooled median delay was taken rather than the mean to compare delays between Sub-Saharan Africa and other LMICs. The median differences were estimated using the non-parametric Mann-Whitney test which was used to test the statistical difference of pooled median delays between Sub-Saharan Africa and other LMICs. In addition, the 95% confidence interval was calculated using bootstrap method.

Meta-analysis

The data for each of the six predictor variables were entered into the Comprehensive Meta-analysis software version 2. The effect size measurement computed were odds ratio (pooled and individual) and prevalence of patient delay at 30 days cutoff point. Forest plots were drawn to visualize effect size (odds ratio with 95%CI). Both fixed and random effect models were used for pooled analysis based on the heterogeneity level of studies included. Heterogeneity was evaluated using Cochrane Q and I^2 tests as well as Q/df (degree of freedom) ratio. Cochrane Q test ($p = 0.1$), Q/df = 1and $I^2 = 50\%$ were considered as cutoff points to mark heterogeneity and to select the effect model for combined analysis.

As initial test of pooled analysis, we used fixed effect model to combine individual effect sizes. If there was no heterogeneity observed during initial test using fixed effect model (i.e. $P > 0.1$ and $I^2 \leq 50\%$ and $Q/df \leq 1$ **or** $p \leq 0.1$ but $I^2 \leq 50\%$), we used fixed model as final model to estimate combined effect sizes. However, if there was significant heterogeneity observed (i.e. $p \leq 0.1$ and $I^2 > 50\%$, **or** $p > 0.1$ but $Q/df > 1$), we used random effect model. The sources of heterogeneity were assessed by subgroup analysis based on clinical heterogeneity of the studies mainly using smear status of participants. Funnel plot and Egger's regression test were used for checking graphic and statistical publication biases, respectively. Sensitivity test was done to check the effect of each study on combined effect size.

Results

Description of selected studies

A total of 40 eligible studies were retrieved for systematic review; 19 (47.5%) from sub-Saharan Africa, 20 (50%) from other LMICs, and 1 (2.5%) study involved three countries (Bangladesh, India and Malawi). Among these, 14 studies were found to be eligible for meta-analysis, two with 15 days and 12 with 30 days cutoff points to categorize patient delay (Fig. 2). The numbers of studies which measured patient, health system and total median delays were 35, 27 and 30 respectively (Tables 3 and 4). All but one study used cross-sectional study design with either one time or prospective participant recruitment strategy.

There was certain level of variation on categorization of delays across reviewed studies. Majority of the studies categorized time in diagnosis into 'delayed' and 'not delayed' using cutoff point. However, there was no uniform cutoff point across all studies. Some studies used the median of their finding, and others used 2 weeks (15 days), 3 weeks (21 days), 1 month (30 days). With no justification, one study used 6 and 12 weeks as cutoff

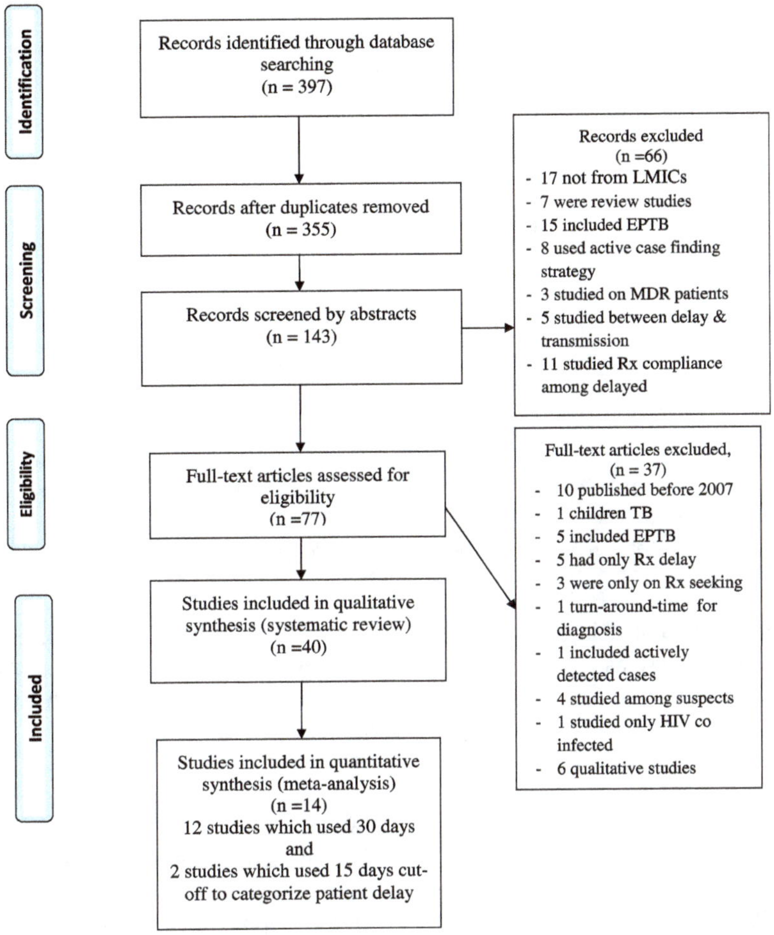

Fig. 2 PRISMA flow diagram for article selection and screening

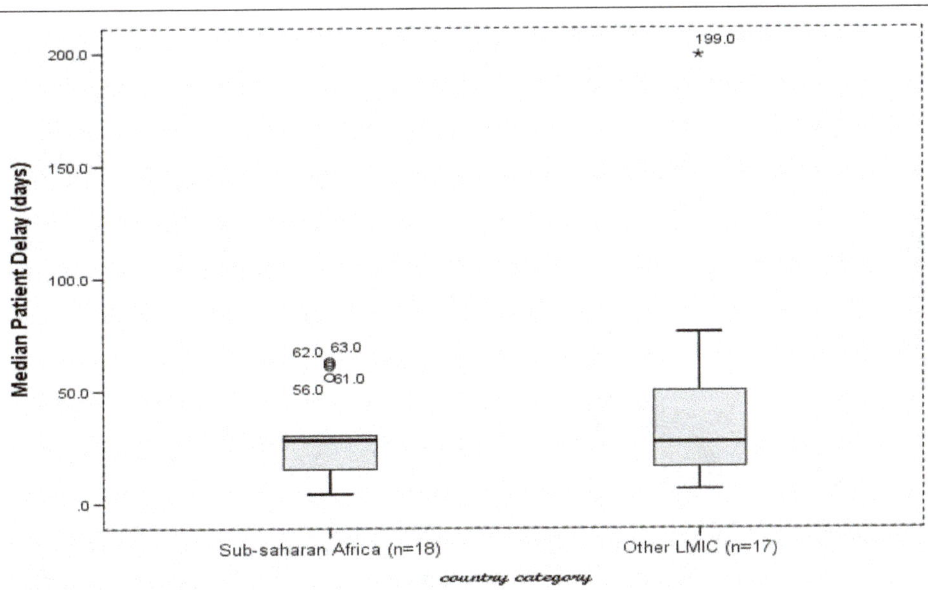

Fig. 3 median patient delay in Sub-Saharan Africa and other Low- and Middle-Income countries, 2007 to 2015

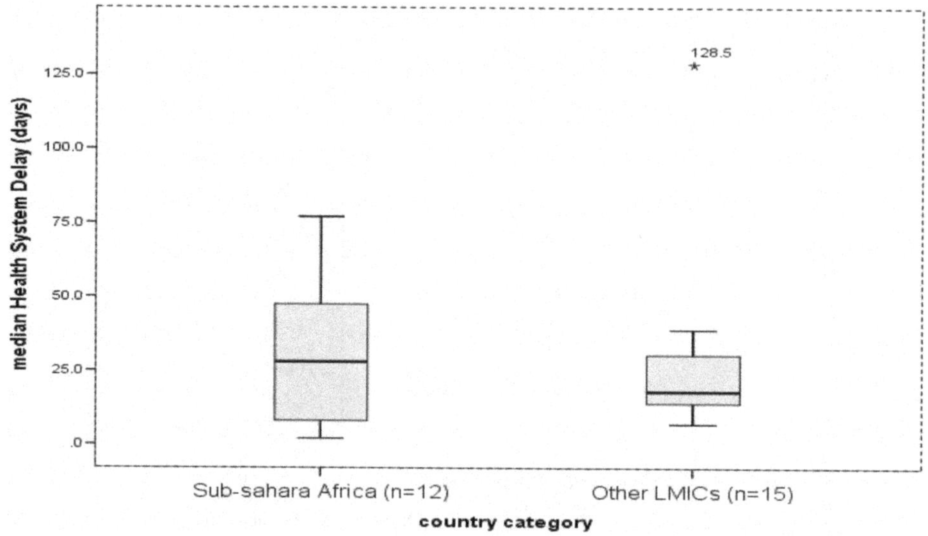

Fig. 4 median health system delay in Sub-Saharan Africa and other Low- and Middle-Income countries, 2007 to 2015

point to determine patient and total delays, respectively [30]. A few studies considered delay as continuous variable, and computed linear regression, ANOVA and Mann-Whitney test.

Diagnosis delay overview

The overall median delay in LMICs ranged from 4 to 199 days (25th & 75th percentile = 15 & 50) for patient delay, 2 to 128.5 days (25th & 75th percentile = 12 & 34) for health system delay, and 30 to 366.5 days (25th& 75th percentile = 44 & 78.8) for total delay. All of the highest median patient (199), health system (128.5) and total (366.5) delays were reported from Afghanistan [31]. The mean patient delay (35.5 days, 95%CI = 24.4–55.4) was similar to mean health system delay (28.7 days, 95%CI = 19.7–45.8), $p > 0.05$.

Patient delay

The median patient delay in Sub-Saharan Africa varied from 4 days in Sudan to 63 days in Ethiopia, and median of the reported median delays was 28 days (95%CI = 18.9–41.7). In other LMICs, it varied from 6 in India to 199 days in Afghanistan, and median of the reported median delays was 27 days (95%CI = 16.5–55.4). There

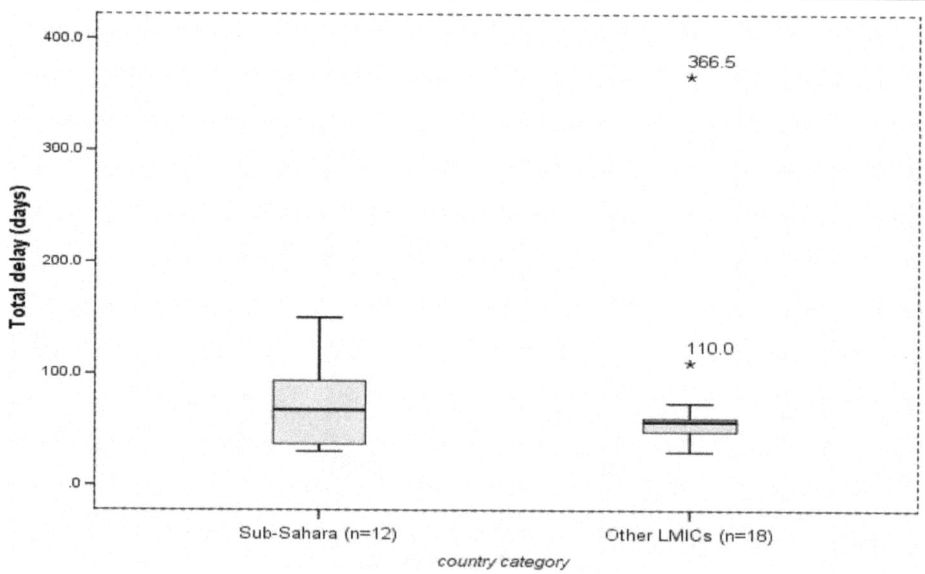

Fig. 5 median total delay in Sub-Saharan Africa and other Low- and Middle-Income countries, 2007 to 2015

Study name	Event Rate	Lower Limit	Upper Limit	Z-Value	P-Value
Yimer	0.29	0.238	0.36	-6.10	0.00
Mesfin	0.53	0.501	0.56	2.03	0.04
Mfinanga	0.35	0.314	0.39	-7.09	0.00
Ngadaya	0.38	0.320	0.45	-3.31	0.01
Maciel	0.50	0.444	0.55	0.00	1.00
Asefa	0.50	0.446	0.55	0.00	1.00
Deponti	0.50	0.425	0.58	0.08	0.94
Maamari	0.41	0.378	0.44	-4.81	0.00
Takarinda	0.48	0.433	0.53	-0.66	0.50
Biya	0.41	0.345	0.49	-2.04	0.04
Cambanis	0.25	0.201	0.31	-7.38	0.00
	0.419	**0.366**	**0.474**	**-2.864**	**0.004**

Statistics for each study

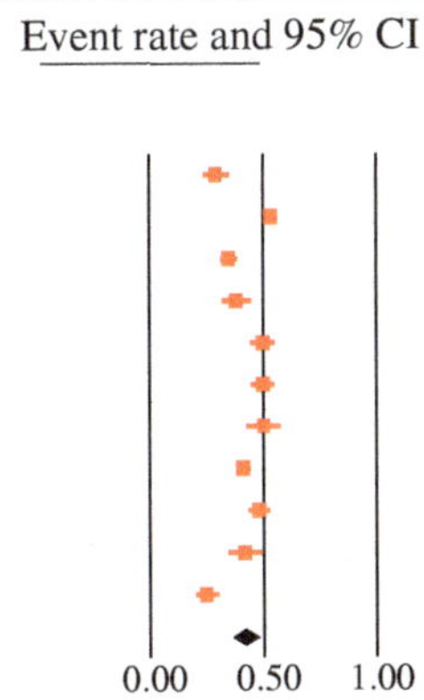

Fig. 6 Forest plot showing the pooled proportion of patient delayed above 30 days to seek formal medical care

was no statistically significant difference observed between the two groups, $p = 0.49$ (Fig. 3).

Our review identified a wide range of factors affecting patient delay that were related to individual, health system and clinical characteristics. Some of the individual factorswere poor literacy, first care seeking from informal providers, self-medication, sex (mostly female), wrong perceptions and rural residence among others. The clinical factors were being a new case, mild severity of illness, chronic/persistent cough and pulmonary co--morbidity. On the contrary, the presences of hemoptysis, chest pain and multiple symptoms reduced patient delay (Table 5).

Health system delay

The median health system delay in Sub-Saharan countries ranged from the lowest of 2 days in Zimbabwe to 77 days in Uganda and the median of reported median delays was 28 days (95%CI: 14–35.9). In other LMICs, it varied from 7 days in Vietnam and Uzbekistan to 128.5 days in Afghanistan, and the median of reported median delays was 18 days (95%CI: 14–30). However, no median difference between the two groups was observed, $p = 0.35$ (Fig. 4).

Individual factors related to health systems delay were poor literacy, sex (mainly being female), being unemployed and labor migrant while good functional status, absence of cough, presence of unusual symptoms, normal chest X-ray, and smear negativity results were among the clinical factors. First care seeking at private or lower-level health facility was also identified as determinant of health system delay (Table 5).

Total delay

The median total delay in Sub-Saharan countries ranged from the lowest of 30 days in Zimbabwe to 150 days in Mozambique, and the median of reported median total delays was 67 days (95%CI: 37–90). In other LMICs, it varied from the lowest median delay of 30 days in Vietnam to 366.5 days in Afghanistan, and the median of reported median total delays was 57 days (95%CI: 49–66.8). There was no median difference between the two groups, $p = 0.31$. Outlier median total delays of 110 and 366.5 were reported from Brazil and Afghanistan, respectively (Fig. 5).

Statistics for each study

Study name	Odds Ratio	Lower Limit	Upper Limit	Z-Value	P-Value
Yimer	0.88	0.50	1.57	-0.42	0.67
Mesfin	1.25	0.96	1.62	1.68	0.09
Mfinanga	1.51	1.07	2.13	2.34	0.02
Ngadaya	0.60	0.32	1.10	-1.65	0.10
Maciel	1.08	0.52	2.23	0.21	0.84
Asefa	1.00	0.65	1.54	0.00	1.00
Deponti	0.98	0.46	2.11	-0.05	0.96
Takarinda	0.88	0.59	1.31	-0.63	0.53
Biya	1.45	0.76	2.77	1.14	0.25
Maamari	0.94	0.70	1.27	-0.38	0.70
	1.08	0.95	1.23	1.18	0.24

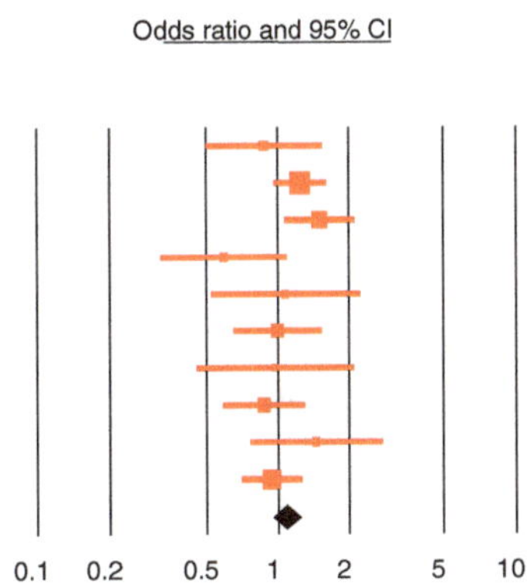

Fig. 7 Forest plot showing the association between sex and patient delay at 30 days cutoff

Study name	Statistics for each study				
	Odds Ratio	Lower Limit	Upper Limit	Z-Value	P-Value
Hussen 2012	2.306	0.693	7.675	1.362	0.173
Ngangro2012	1.131	0.687	1.860	0.484	0.628
	1.255	0.792	1.988	0.968	0.333

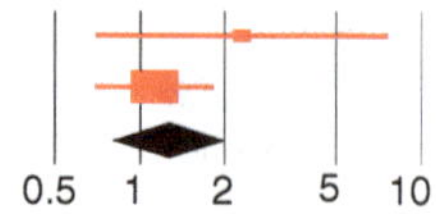

Fig. 8 Forest plot showing the association between sex and patient delay at 15 days cutoff

The determinants of total delay were a mix of factors affecting patient or health system delay (Table 5).

Summary of findings from meta-analysis

The combined analysis of 12 studies indicated that 42% (95%CI = 37–47%) of PTB patients delayed a month or more without seeking formal medical care (Q = 123, $p <$ 0.1, df = 10, I^2 = 91%). Significant heterogeneity existed following subgroup analysis by smear type (any type and smear positive) (Fig. 6).

Pooled effect sizes were estimated to determine the independent effect of sex, residence, educational status, first care seeking from informal provider and HIV status on patient delay, and 11, 4, 9, 4 and 3 studies (with 30 days cutoff point) were analyzed, respectively. In addition, 2 studies (with 15 days cutoff) were also pooled.

The majority of studies identified females were more likely to delay but the quantitative summary indicated no statistically significant difference in patient delay between female and male PTB patients at 30 days [pooled OR = 1.08, 95%CI = 0.95–1.23, $p = 0.24$] (Fig. 7) and 15 days cutoff points [pooled OR = 1.26, 95%CI = 0.79–1.99] (Fig. 8). No heterogeneity was observed at both cutoff points (Fig. 9). Similarly, there was no statistically significant difference in patient delay between rural and urban PTB patients at 30 days cutoff [pooled OR = 1.06, 95%CI = 0.66–1.71, $p = 0.81$] (Fig. 10) but observed at 15 days cutoff [pooled OR = 2.4, 95%CI = 1.4–4.1, $p =$ 0.002] (Fig. 11).

Literacy had significant association [pooled OR =1.5, 95%CI = 1.1–1.9, $p = 0.01$], and the odds of patient delay was greater among illiterate PTB patients as compared to those who had formal educition. Significant heterogeneity was observed [Q = 14.3, p = 0.01, df = 5, I^2 = 65%] (Fig. 12). First care seeking from informal providers had statistically significant association with patient delay at 30 days cutoff [pooled OR = 3, 95%CI = 2.3–3.9, $p <$ 0.05]; PTB patients who sought first care at informal providers were 3 times more to delay by a month or more to seek care compared to their counterparts. No heterogeneity was observed [Q = 1.7, $p = 0.64$, df = 3, I^2 = 0%] and Egger's regression test, $p = 0.23$ (Fig. 13). The patient delay had no statistically significant association with HIV [pooled OR = 0.98, 95%CI = 0.79–1.21, $p =$ 0.84] (Fig. 14).

Discussion

Our systematic review and meta-analysis indicated that the extent of delay in diagnosis of PTB remains a serious

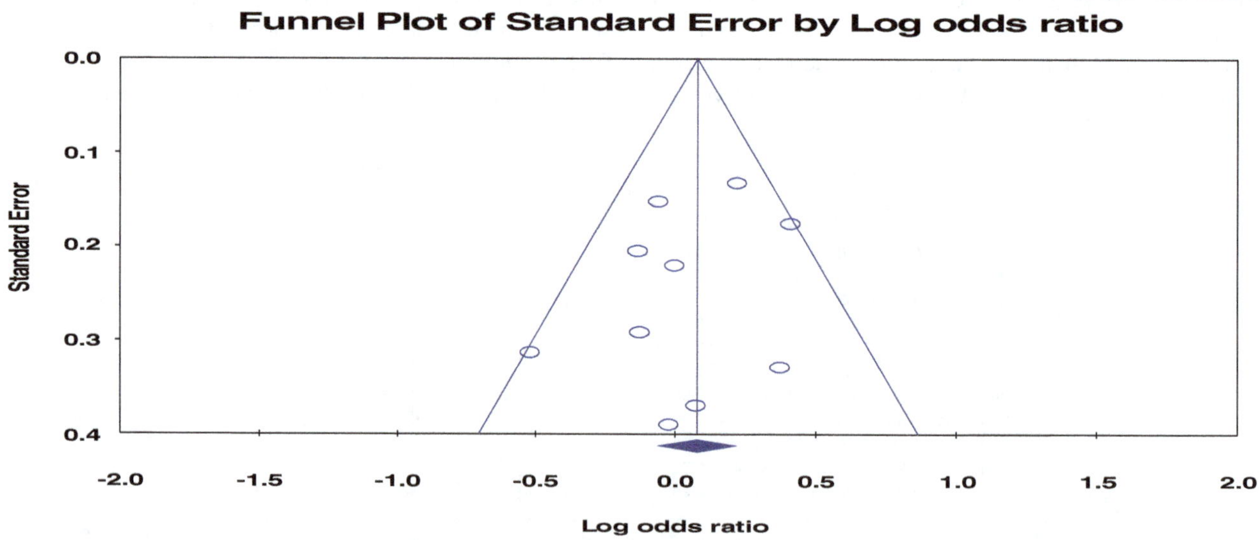

Fig. 9 funnel plot of the standard error of pooled proportion of patient delaye above 30 days

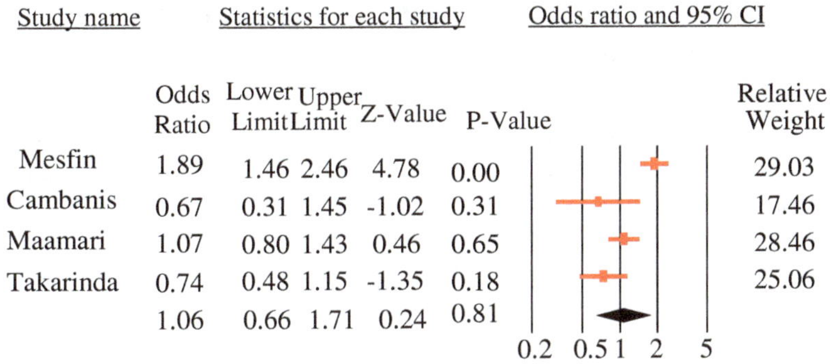

Fig. 10 Forest plot showing the association between residence and patient delay at 30 days cutoffs

challenge for TB control programs in low- and middle-income countries. Half of the studies in this review reported a median diagnosis delay higher than 2 months, both patient and health system delays made comparable contributions.

This review shows the extent of delays in diagnosis of PTB continued to be as bad as it was a decade ago [6]. Our review showed no significant difference in patient, health system and total delays of PTB cases between Sub-Saharan Africa and other LMICs. Delays have been a common problem to all LMICs which harbor a large share of global TB burden. The minimum median total delay in diagnosis was 30 days in this review [30, 32] which has been indicated as a turning point at which a significant increase in risk for TB transmission occurs [33]. WHO recommends diagnosis within 2 to 3 weeks of symptom initiation [20] though the acceptable time delay is not known. Considering the WHO cutoff point recommendations, this review has, therefore, indicated unacceptable level of delay occurring in LMICs, and actual delays may even be worse than reported here as patients are likely to recall the date when the illness gets severe but not exact date of illness onset.

In this review, the qualitative and quantitative summary of studies indicated the observed patient, and health system delays in LMICs were attributed by a set of individual and health system related factors. The individual factors are related to characteristics of the patients and skill of healthcare providers that influence the health seeking behavior of patients, and suspicion and detection of the disease by healthcare providers. These include demographic, socio-economic, knowledge, beliefs, perceived barriers, behaviors, clinical features and provider skills (*the details stated below*). The health system factors comprise factors which drive within the health system, and hinder access to health facilities and limit availability of diagnosis services. These include limited access of health facilities near to villages, lack of TB diagnosis services in easily accessible health facilities such as private facilities, drug vendors and lower level facilities (e.g. health posts), high cost of some diagnostics (pathology and X-ray), and existence of informal healers (traditional and religious) providing unlimited therapeutic services.

Even though higher number of studies (five) reported that female patients were more likely to wait longer periods without medical consultation, the pooled analysis indicated that sex was not the independent determinant of patient delay ($p = 0.24$). This may be due to gender based social influence in health decision making that might vary across cultures and countries. Similarly, our pooled analysis showed residence was not the independent determinant of patient delay, but three studies in Ethiopia [29, 34, 35] reported rural residence and three other studies from Iran, Nigeria and Sudan [24, 36, 37] reported urban residence as independent determinants

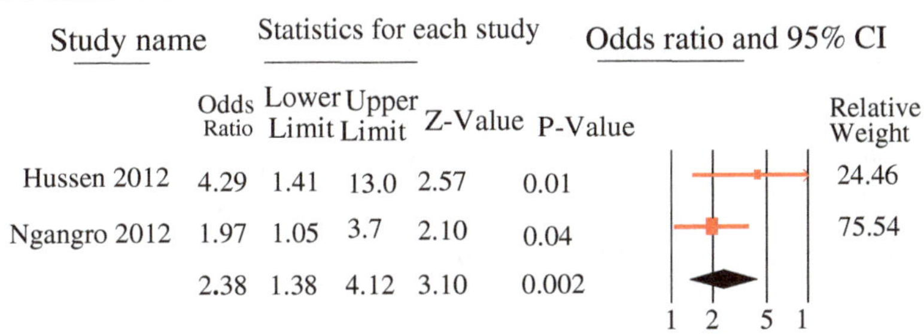

Fig. 11 Forest plot showing the association between residence and patient delay at 15 days cutoffs

Study name	Odds Ratio	Lower Limit	Upper Limit	Z-Value	P-Value	Relative Weight
Yimer	1.63	0.92	2.88	1.68	0.09	13.49
Mesfin	1.94	1.49	2.53	4.94	0.00	22.65
Mfinanga	1.67	1.14	2.45	2.65	0.01	18.81
Ngadaya	0.80	0.45	1.41	-0.77	0.44	13.54
Maamari	1.07	0.79	1.45	0.45	0.65	21.37
Maciel	2.08	1.00	4.31	1.97	0.05	10.14
	1.45	1.08	1.94	2.50	0.01	

Statistics for each study

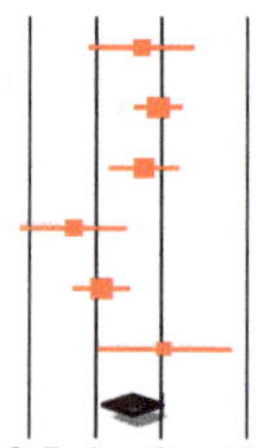

Fig. 12 Forest plot showing the association between educational status and patient delay at 30 days cutoff

of patient delay. This may be owing to the health system of the respective countries. For instance, most patients in rural areas of Ethiopia have primary access to the health post (first level of the health system) where there are no TB diagnostic services [38] and patients might have to walk for some hours to access hospitals or health centers. This is supported by considerable number of studies in our review that indicated patients who travel long distance to access healthcare services experienced longer patient delays in both settings.

Our pooled analysis showed that illiterate patients were more likely to delay in seeking care compared to those patients who had formal education (pooled OR = 1.5; 95% CI = 1.1–1.9). Illiteracy may limit patients' access to written health education and communication materials that are commonly utilized to increase public awareness about the disease [5]. Our review also found poor knowledge of PTB sign and symptoms, cause and treatment lengthened patient delay in LMICs. Patients who believed the cause of TB is evil/bad luck, perceived the symptoms are common and not dangerous, feared social stigmatization/embarrassment, and associated PTB with HIV sought medical consultation after long suffer from the disease. This is because such limited knowledge and perceived barriers direct patients to hide their illness, self-medicate and practice traditional healing [39]. In addition, poor understanding of the disease in the community results in being discriminated by peers, friends, neighbors and so on [40].

Our meta-analysis identified first care seeking from informal providers as a key determinant of patient delay (pooled OR = 3; 95%CI = 2.3–3.9). Similarly, another review identified patients consulting traditional healers first have experienced patient delay usually in rural residents of Sub-Saharan Africa [11]. This is because patients who have poor knowledge of PTB cause and/or believe PTB is acquired from evil curse deemed trust on treatment by traditional healers or religious leaders to be freed from evil spirits [41]. This implies traditional/religious healers are still preferred destinations for substantial number TB patients. Therefore, engaging them could help to identify presumptive cases early, establish referral link to TB care centers, avoid traditional therapy, and to target community misperceptions and wrong beliefs that hassled healthcare seeking.

Patients who had chronic cough, pulmonary comorbidity and mild severity of illness delayed seeking care. This may be because patients with such type of symptoms may suspect other common respiratory syndromes that are not considered serious. However, the presence of hemoptysis, chest pain and multiple symptoms reduced the possibility of patient delay. Beyond delaying care seeking, clinical presentations affected the time of diagnosis once patients consulted health care providers. Patients presented with good functional status, no cough and had unusual symptoms obtained delayed diagnosis from the health system. These appearances may hinder PTB suspicion by heath care providers or they may fail to suspect

Study name	Odds Ratio	Lower Limit	Upper Limit	Z-Value	P-Value
Mesfin	3.235	2.354	4.447	7.234	0.000
Ngadaya	3.095	1.282	7.472	2.513	0.012
Cambanis	3.040	1.422	6.500	2.868	0.004
Takarinda	1.921	0.937	3.935	1.784	0.074
	2.988	2.305	3.874	8.267	0.000

Statistics for each study

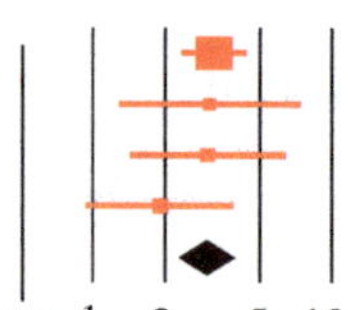

Fig. 13 forest plot showing the association between 1st care seeking from informal provider and patient delay of PTB patients (30 days cutoff)

Study name	Odds Ratio	Lower Lim	Upper Limit	Z-Value	P-Value	Relative Weight
Yimer 2015	0.80	0.39	1.62	-0.63	0.53	8.95
Mesfin 2009	0.92	0.71	1.19	-0.64	0 .52	65.96
Takarinda 2015	1.24	0.82	1.90	1.01	0.31	25.09
	0.98	**0.79**	**1.21**	**-0.20**	**0.84**	

Statistics for each study; Odds ratio and 95% CI

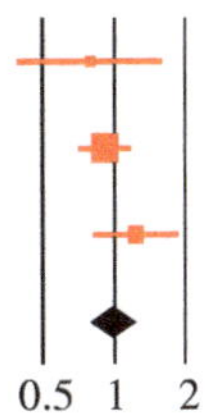

Fig. 14 Forest plot showing the association between HIV status and patient delay at 30 days cutoff

PTB as of poor skill in identifying rare symptoms. Normal chest X-ray and smear negative results at initial diagnosis have also delayed PTB diagnosis. This may be related to the poor skill of healthcare providers in detecting the disease or poor sensitivity of diagnostic methods to detect cases at early stage [42].

Our review indicated that considerable number PTB patients in LMICs sought initial care from private clinics, drug vendors and lower level public health facilities where TB diagnosis services are unavailable [30]. So, if these health providers are engaged in TB services, they will contribute greatly in identification of presumptive cases and refer to nearby higher health facilities in their setting. Patients who sought care from multiple providers are likely to experience health system delay [35]. In addition, unemployment, labor migration and low income were also reported as factors of health system delay. This might be due to the high costs for pathological and x-ray diagnosis which are not free of charge globally unlike the rest of TB services [43].

Despite these findings and scientific arguments, it appears to have some methodological limitations that arose from either individual studies or the review process. Only English articles were reviewed. There could be many articles written in other languages that might be different with respect to size and quality. All included studies except one were cross-sectional. Therefore, methodological bias and confounding which are common in cross-sectional studies might have been introduced. Furthermore, there was lack of detailed information and inconsistent reporting among retrieved studies. Some studies computed separate median patient delay (stratified analysis), few reported *p*-value only [44], no clear cutoff point to categorize delay, and the variability of predictor variables across the studies. This limited the number of studies and predictor variables considered in the meta-analysis that could affect the power of the pooled analysis.

Conclusion

This systematic review and meta-analysis confirms delays in diagnosis of PTB have remained higher similar to the preceding periods. Both patient and health system delays have contributed for observed delay all over the high burden low- and middle- income countries. This implies that the existing strategies and efforts under implementation did not appear to improve the desired early PTB case presentation, detection and prompt treatment initiation in low- and middle- income countries.

Multiple patient, provider and health system related factors seemed to contribute for the observed high diagnosis delays. The pooled analysis confirmed poor literacy and preference to seek care from informal healers significantly associated with patient delay. Substantial numbers of PTB patients still sought initial TB care from private healthcare facilities, traditional/religious healers and low level/community health workers. Hence, systematic engagement of these parties would potentially improve case finding strategies. If they are engaged in presumptive case identification and active referral network with TB care facilities established, early care seeking and detection can substantially be improved. Continuous community awareness activities should also be strengthened.

Abbreviations

CI: Confidence interval; HIV: Human immuno-deficiency virus; IQR: Inter-Quartile Range; LMICS: Low- and Middle-Income Countries; NTP: National tuberculosis control programs; OR: Odds Ratio; PRISMA: Preferred reporting items for systematic reviews and meta-analyses; PTB: Pulmonary Tuberculosis; TB: Tuberculosis; WHO: World Health Organization

Acknowledgements

We are very grateful to the authors of the articles included in this review. Our heartfelt gratitude extends to Haramaya University for facilitating the review process. We are very thankful to PhD fellows and faculty at the School of Public Health, Haramaya University, for their constructive comments. Our especial gratitude goes to Manendante Mulugeta (PhD in TEFL) for his language edition.

Authors' contributions

FG initiated the conception of this review, conducted literature search, assessed the studies, carried out the systematic review and meta-analysis, and wrote the first draft of the manuscript. MD enriched the conception, revised and approved the final manuscript. NA directed the design, assisted and supervised the review starting from the scratch and commented on the earlier drafts of the manuscripts. BM directed the design, supervised the review and commented on the earlier drafts of the manuscripts. AW commented on the final draft and revised the manuscript. All the authors read and approved the final version of the manuscript to be sent for publication. The sequence of authorship depends on their level of contribution to this paper.

Consent for publication

Not applicable.

Competing interests

The authors declare that they have no competing interests.

Author details

[1]Department of Public Health, College of Medicine and Health Sciences, Jigjiga University, PO Box = 1020, Jigjiga, Ethiopia. [2]Addis Continental Institute of Public Health, Addis Ababa, Ethiopia. [3]School of Public Health, College of Health and Medical Sciences, Haramaya University, Harar, Ethiopia. [4]School of Public Health, College of Health Sciences, Addis Ababa University, Addis Ababa, Ethiopia.

References

1. WHO. Global tuberculosis report 2017. Geneva: World Health Organization; 2017. Available at http://apps.who.int/iris.
2. WHO. The global plan to stop TB 2011-2015: Transforming the fight towards elimination of tuberculosis. World Health Organization; 2010.
3. WHO. Systematic screening for active tuberculosis: principles and recommendations. Geneva: World Health Organization; 2013.
4. WHO. Treatment of tuberculosis: guidelines. Geneva: World Health Organization; 2010.
5. Li Y, Ehiri J, Tang S, Li D, Bian Y, Lin H, et al. Factors associated with patient, and diagnostic delays in Chinese TB patients: a systematic review and meta-analysis. BMC Med. 2013;11(1):156.
6. Sreeramareddy CT, Panduru KV, Menten J, Van den Ende J. Time delays in diagnosis of pulmonary tuberculosis: a systematic review of literature. BMC Infect Dis. 2009;9:91.
7. Storla DG, Yimer S, Bjune GA. A systematic review of delay in the diagnosis and treatment of tuberculosis. BMC Public Health. 2008;8:15.
8. Shah NS, Yuen CM, Heo M, Tolman AW, Becerra MC. Yield of contact investigations in households of patients with drug-resistant tuberculosis: systematic review and meta-analysis. Clin Infect Dis. 2014;58(3):381–91.
9. Jia ZCS, Ma Y, Zhang Y, Bai L, Xu W, He X, Zhang P, Zhao J, Christiani DC. Tuberculosis burden in China: a high prevalence of pulmonary tuberculosis in household contacts with and without symptoms. BMC Infect Dis. 2014;14: 64.
10. Cheng S, Chen W, Yang Y, Chu P, Liu X, Zhao M, et al. Effect of diagnostic and treatment delay on the risk of tuberculosis transmission in Shenzhen, China: an observational cohort study, 1993-2010. PLoS One. 2013;8(6): e67516.
11. Finnie RK, Khoza LB, van den Borne B, Mabunda T, Abotchie P, Mullen PD. Factors associated with patient and health care system delay in diagnosis and treatment for TB in sub-Saharan African countries with high burdens of TB and HIV. Tropical Med Int Health. 2011;16(4):394–411.
12. FMOH. Guidelines for clinical and Programatic Manageent of TB, leprosy and TB/HIV in Ethiopia. In: TB L, TB/HIV. 5th ed. Addis Ababa: Federal Ministry Of Health of Ethiopia; 2012.
13. Fox GJ, Barry SE, Britton WJ, Marks GB. Contact investigation for tuberculosis: a systematic review and meta-analysis. Eur Respir J. 2013;41(1):140–56.
14. Uplekar M, Figueroa-Munoz J, Floyd K, Getahun H, Jaramillo E. The stop TB strategy: building on and enhancing DOTS to meet the TB-related millennium development goals. Geneva: World Health Organization; 2006. WHO/HTM/TB/2006.368.
15. LA Moher D, Tetzlaff J, Altman DG. Preferred reporting items for systematic reviews and meta-analyses: the PRISMA statement. PLoS Med. 2009;6(6): e1000097.
16. Matthews JR, Matthews RW. Successful scientific writing: a step-by-step guide for the biological and medical sciences. New York: Cambridge University Press; 2014. Available at www.cambridge.org/9780521699273.
17. National Collaborating Center for Environmental Health. A Primer for Evaluating the Quality of Studies on Environmental Health: Critical Appraisal of Cross-Sectional Studies. Ottowa: National Collaborating Centre for Environmental Health; 2011.
18. National Heart, Lung, and Blood Institute. "Quality assessment tool for observational cohort and cross-sectional studies". Bethesda: National Institutes of Health, Department of Health and Human Services; 2014.
19. Gosoniu GD, Ganapathy S, Kemp J, Auer C, Somma D, Karim F, Weiss MG. Gender and socio-cultural determinants of delay to diagnosis of TB in Bangladesh, India and Malawi. Int J Tuberc Lung Dis. 2008;12(7):848–55.
20. WHO. Early detection of tuberculosis: an overview of approaches, guidelines and tools. Geneva: World Health Organizatiom; 2011. WHO/HTM/STB/PSI/ 2011.21.
21. Ford CM, Bayer AM, Gilman RH, Onifade D, Acosta C, Cabrera L, et al. Factors associated with delayed tuberculosis test-seeking behavior in the Peruvian Amazon. Am J Trop Med Hyg. 2009;81(6):1097–102.
22. Ekinci GH, Karakaya E, Ongel EA, Haciomeroglu O, Yilmaz A. Patient and doctor delays in smear-negative and smear-positive pulmonary tuberculosis patients attending a referral hospital in Istanbul, Turkey. The Scientific World Journal. 2014; Article ID 158186.
23. Tamhane A, Ambe G, Vermund SH, Kohler CL, Karande A, Sathiakumar N. Pulmonary tuberculosis in Mumbai, India: factors responsible for patient and treatment delays. Int J Prev Med. 2012;3(8):569–80.
24. Ukwaja KN, Alobu I, Nweke CO, Onyenwe EC. Healthcare-seeking behavior, treatment delays and its determinants among pulmonary tuberculosis patients in rural Nigeria: a cross-sectional study. BMC Health Serv Res. 2013; 13:25.
25. Maamari F. Case-finding tuberculosis patients: diagnostic and treatment delays and their determinants. East Mediterr Health J. 2008;14(3)
26. Yimer SA, Norheim G, Namouchi A, Zegeye ED, Kinander W, Tønjum T, et al. Mycobacterium tuberculosis lineage 7 strains are associated with prolonged patient delay in seeking treatment for pulmonary tuberculosis in Amhara region, Ethiopia. J Clin Microbiol. 2015;53(4):1301–9.
27. Asefa A, Teshome W. Total delay in treatment among smear positive pulmonary tuberculosis patients in five primary health Centers, southern Ethiopia: a cross sectional study. PLoS One. 2014;9(7):e102884.
28. Gebeyehu E, Azage M, Abeje G. Factors associated with Patient's delay in tuberculosis treatment in Bahir Dar City Administration, Northwest Ethiopia. BioMed Res Int. 2014;2014:701429.
29. Mesfin MM, Newell JN, Walley JD, Gessessew A, Madeley RJ. Delayed consultation among pulmonary tuberculosis patients: a cross sectional study of 10 DOTS districts of Ethiopia. BMC Public Health. 2009;9:53.
30. Huong NT, Vree M, Duong BD, Khanh VT, Loan VT, Borgdorff MW, et al. Delays in the diagnosis and treatment of tuberculosis patients in Vietnam: a cross-sectional study. BMC Public Health. 2007;7(1):110.
31. Sabawoon W, Sato H, Kobayashi Y. Delay in the treatment of pulmonary tuberculosis: a report from Afghanistan. Environ Health Prev Med. 2012; 17(1):53–61.
32. Takarinda KC, Harries AD, Nyathi B, Ngwenya M, Mutasa-Apollo T, Sandy C. Tuberculosis treatment delays and associated factors within the Zimbabwe national tuberculosis programme. BMC Public Health. 2015;15(1):29.
33. Lin X, Chongsuvivatwong V, Lin L, Geater A, Lijuan R. Dose–response relationship between treatment delay of smear-positive tuberculosis patients and intra-household transmission: a cross-sectional study. Trans R Soc Trop Med Hyg. 2008;102(8):797–804.
34. Gebeyehu E, Azage M, Abeje G. Factors associated with Patient's delay in tuberculosis treatment in Bahir Dar City Administration, Northwest Ethiopia. Biomed Res Int. 2014;2014
35. Hussen A, Biadgilign S, Tessema F, Mohammed S, Deribe K, Deribew A. Treatment delay among pulmonary tuberculosis patients in pastoralist communities in bale zone, Southeast Ethiopia. BMC Res Notes. 2012;5:320.

36. Mohamed E, Abdalla S, Khamis A, Abdelbadea A, Abdelgadir M. Factors associated with patient delay in accessing pulmonary tuberculosis care. Sudan: Gezira State; 2009. p. 2013.
37. Saifodine A, Gudo PS, Sidat M, Black J. Patient and health system delay among patients with pulmonary tuberculosis in Beira city, Mozambique. BMC Public Health. 2013;13(1):559.
38. Yimer SA, Bjune GA, Holm-Hansen C. Time to first consultation, diagnosis and treatment of TB among patients attending a referral hospital in northwest, Ethiopia. BMC Infectious Diseases. 2014;14:19.
39. Kuznetsov VN, Grjibovski AM, Mariandyshev AO, Johansson E, Bjune GA. Two vicious circles contributing to a diagnostic delay for tuberculosis patients in Arkhangelsk. Emerg Health Threats J. 2014;7 10.3402/ehtj.v3407.24909.
40. Valerie A. Paz-Soldan REA, Jones CD, Powell AR and Richard A. Oberhelman: patient reported delays in seeking treatment for tuberculosis among adult and pediatricTB patients andTB patients co-infected with HIV in lima, Peru: a qualitative study. FrontiersinPublicHealth | InfectiousDiseases. 2014; 2|Article281.
41. Verhagen LM, Kapinga R, van Rosmalen-Nooijens KAWL. Factors underlying diagnostic delay in tuberculosis patients in a rural area in Tanzania: a qualitative approach. Infection. 2010;38(6):433–46.
42. Chen CC, Chiang CY, Pan SC, Wang JY, Lin HH. Health system delay among patients with tuberculosis in Taiwan: 2003–2010. BMC Infect Dis. 2015;15: 491.
43. Pradhan A, Kielmann K, Gupte H, Bamne A, Porter JD, Rangan S. What'outliers' tell us about missed opportunities for tuberculosis control: a cross-sectional study of patients in Mumbai, India. BMC Public Health. 2010;10(1):263.
44. Belkina TV, Khojiev DS, Tillyashaykhov MN, Tigay ZN, Kudenov MU, Tebbens JD, et al. Delay in the diagnosis and treatment of pulmonary tuberculosis in Uzbekistan: a cross-sectional study. BMC Infect Dis. 2014;14(1):624.
45. Mohammad S, Alavi PB, Albagi A: Factors associated with delay in diagnosis and treatment of pulmonary tuberculosis. undishapur J Microbiol 2015; 8(3): e19238. DOI: 19210.15812/jjm.19238.
46. Ayé R, Wyss K, Abdualimova H, Saidaliev S. Patient's site of first access to health system influences length of delay for tuberculosis treatment in Tajikistan. BMC Health Serv Res. 2010;10(1):10.
47. Basnet R, Hinderaker SG, Enarson D, Malla P, Mørkve O. Delay in the diagnosis of tuberculosis in Nepal. BMC Public Health. 2009;9:236.
48. Behera BK, Jain RB, Gupta KB, Goel MK. Extent of delay in diagnosis in new smear positive patients of pulmonary tuberculosis attending tertiary care hospital. Int J Prev Med. 2013;4(12):1480–5.
49. Biya O, Gidado S, Abraham A, Waziri N, Nguku P, Nsubuga P, et al. Knowledge, care-seeking behavior, and factors associated with patient delay among newly-diagnosed pulmonary tuberculosis patients, Federal Capital Territory, Nigeria, 2010. Pan African Med J. 2014;18(Suppl 1)
50. Buregyeya E, Criel B, Nuwaha F, Colebunders R. Delays in diagnosis and treatment of pulmonary tuberculosis in Wakiso and Mukono districts, Uganda. BMC Public Health. 2014;14(1):586.
51. Cambanis A, Ramsay A, Yassin MA, Cuevas LE. Duration and associated factors of patient delay during tuberculosis screening in rural Cameroon. Tropical Med Int Health. 2007;12(11):1309–14.
52. Deponti GN, Silva DR, Coelho AC, Muller AM, Paulo de Tarso RD. delayed diagnosis and associated factors among new pulmonary tuberculosis patients diagnosed at the emergency department of a tertiary care hospital in Porto Alegre, South Brazil: a prospective patient recruitment study. BMC Infect Dis. 2013;13(1):538.
53. Jurcev-Savicevic A, Mulic R, Kozul K, Ban B, Valic J, Bacun-Ivcek L, et al. Health system delay in pulmonary tuberculosis treatment in a country with an intermediate burden of tuberculosis: a cross-sectional study. BMC Public Health. 2013;13(1):250.
54. Kansiime C, Kiwuwa SM, Levi M, Asiimwe BB, Katamba A. Health service delay among pulmonary tuberculosis patients presenting to a National Referral Hospital, Kampala, Uganda: a cross sectional study. Pan African Med J. 2013;15:84.
55. Li X, Jiang S, Li X, Mei J, Zhong Q, Xu W, et al. Predictors on delay of initial health-seeking in new pulmonary tuberculosis cases among migrants population in East China. PLoS One. 2012;7(2):e31995.
56. Maciel E, Golub J, Peres R, Hadad D, Fávero J, Molino L, et al. Delay in diagnosis of pulmonary tuberculosis at a primary health clinic in Vitoria, Brazil. Int J Tuberc Lung Dis. 2010;14(11):1403–10.
57. Maior ML, Guerra RL, Cailleaux-Cezar M, Golub JE, Conde MB. Time from symptom onset to the initiation of treatment of pulmonary tuberculosis in a city with a high incidence of the disease. J Bras Pneumol. 2012;38(2):202–9.
58. Makwakwa L, Sheu ML, Chiang CY, Lin SL, Chang PW. Patient and health system delays in the diagnosis and treatment of new and retreatment pulmonary tuberculosis cases in Malawi. BMC Infect Dis. 2014;14(1):132.
59. Mfinanga SG, Mutayoba BK, Kahwa A, Kimaro G, Mtandu R, Ngadaya E, et al. The magnitude and factors associated with delays in management of smear positive tuberculosis in Dar es salaam, Tanzania. BMC Health Serv Res. 2008; 8:158.
60. Nasehi M, Hassanzadeh J, Rezaianzadeh A, Zeigami B, Tabatabaee H, Ghaderi E. Diagnosis delay in smear positive tuberculosis patients. J Res Med Sci. 2012;17(11):1001–4.
61. Ngadaya E, Mfinanga G, Wandwalo E, Morkve O. Delay in tuberculosis case detection in Pwani region, Tanzania. A cross sectional study. BMC Health Serv Res. 2009;9:196.
62. Ngangro NN, Ngarhounoum D, Ngangro MN, Rangar N, Siriwardana MG, des Fontaines VH, et al. Pulmonary tuberculosis diagnostic delays in Chad: a multicenter, hospital-based survey in Ndjamena and Moundou. BMC Public Health. 2012;12(1):513.
63. Rabin A, Kuchukhidze G, Sanikidze E, Kempker R, Blumberg H. Prescribed and self-medication use increase delays in diagnosis of tuberculosis in the country of Georgia. Int J Tuberc Lung Dis. 2013;17(2):214.
64. Sendagire I, Van der Loeff MS, Mubiru M, Konde-Lule J, Cobelens F. Long delays and missed opportunities in diagnosing smear-positive pulmonary tuberculosis in Kampala, Uganda: a cross-sectional study. PLoS One. 2010; 5(12):e14459.
65. Woith WM, Rappleyea ML. Emotional representation of tuberculosis with stigma, treatment delay, and medication adherence in Russia. J Health Psychol. 2014;1359105314538349.
66. Yimer S, Bjune G, Alene G. Diagnostic and treatment delay among pulmonary tuberculosis patients in Ethiopia: a cross sectional study. BMC Infect Dis. 2005;5:112.
67. Li Y, Ehiri J, Tang S, Li D, Bian Y, Lin H, et al. Factors associated with patient, and diagnostic delays in Chinese TB patients: a systematic review and meta-analysis. BMC Med. 2013;11:156. http://www.biomedcentral.com/1741-7015/1711/1156.
68. Alavi SM, Bakhtiyariniya P, Albagi A. Factors associated with delay in diagnosis and treatment of pulmonary tuberculosis. Jundishapur J Microbiol. 2015;8(3).

Miliary tuberculosis with co-existing pulmonary cryptococcosis in non-HIV patient without underlying diseases

Toyomitsu Sawai[1*], Takumi Nakao[1], Satoru Koga[1], Shotaro Ide[1], Sumako Yoshioka[1], Nobuko Matsuo[1] and Hiroshi Mukae[2]

Abstract

Background: Tuberculosis and cryptococcosis co-infection usually occurs in immunosuppressed patients with impaired cell-mediated immunity. However, there are few reports about such co-infection in non-HIV patients without underlying diseases. Here, we report a case of miliary tuberculosis with co-existing pulmonary cryptococcosis in non-HIV patient without underlying diseases.

Case presentation: An 84-year-old Asian female presented to our hospital with complaints of a 1-week history of abdominal pain and appetite loss. Chest computed tomography (CT) showed diffuse micronodules in random patterns in both lung fields. Liver, skin and bone marrow biopsies showed epithelioid cell granuloma. Polymerase chain reaction of gastric aspirate was positive for *Mycobacterium tuberculosis*. According to these findings, miliary tuberculosis was suspected and antimycobacterial therapy was initiated. After a 6-month treatment course, chest radiograph showed new multiple nodules in the right middle lung field. Chest CT showed that a right S6 small nodule was increased and new multiple nodules appeared in the right lower lobe. Flexible fiberoptic bronchoscopy was subsequently perfomed. Cytology of the bronchial lavage showed a small number of Periodic acid-Schiff-positive bodies, suggesting *Cryptococcus* species. Moreover, serum cryptococcal antigen testing was positive. According to these findings, pulmonary cryptococcosis was diagnosed, although the culture was negative. Oral fluconazole therapy was subsequently initiated. After a 6-month treatment course, chest radiograph showed gradual improvement.

Conclusion: Although tuberculosis and cryptococcosis co-infection is relatively rare in immunocompromised hosts, such as those with acquired immunodeficiency syndrome, clinicians should be aware that these infections can co-exist even in non-HIV patients without underlying diseases.

Keywords: Miliary tuberculosis, Pulmonary cryptococcosis, Co-infection, Non-HIV patient without underlying diseases

* Correspondence: toyosawai@yahoo.co.jp
[1]Department of Respiratory Medicine, Nagasaki Harbor Medical Center, 6-39 Shinchi-machi, Nagasaki 850-8555, Japan
Full list of author information is available at the end of the article

Background

There are an increasing number of cases of either tuberculosis or cryptococcosis due to impaired cellular immunity in immunocompromised patients such as those with acquired immunodeficiency syndrome (AIDS) and diabetes mellitus or receiving corticosteroids or immunosuppressive agents [1]. However, tuberculosis and cryptococcosis co-infection is seldom reported even in immunocompromised patients. Particularly, co-infection of these diseases is extremely rare in immunocompetent patients. Here, we present a case of miliary tuberculosis with co-existing pulmonary cryptococcosis in non-HIV patient without underlying diseases.

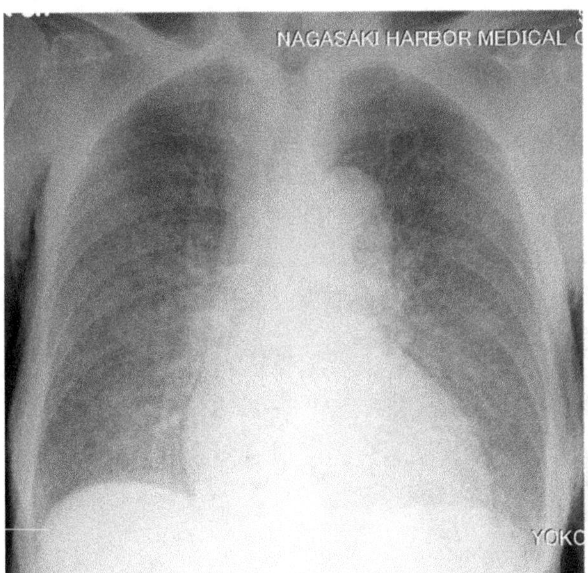

Fig. 1 Chest radiography on admission showed diffuse micronodules in both lung field

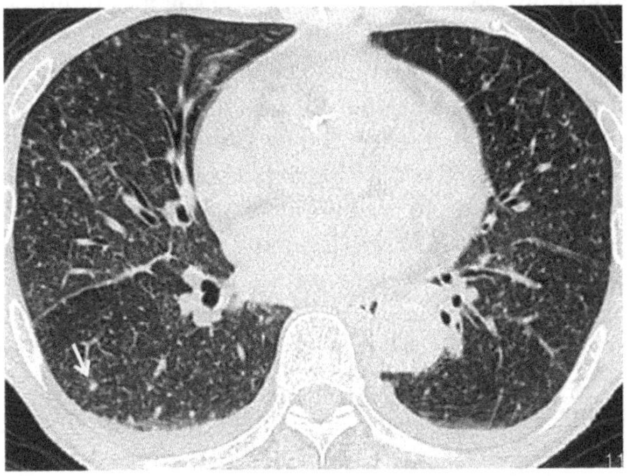

Fig. 2 Chest CT on admission showed diffuse micronodules at random pattern in both lung field and a small nodule in the right S6 (white arrow)

Case presentation

An 84-year-old woman presented to our hospital with complaints of a 1-week history of abdominal pain and appetite loss. The patient had no history of cough, sputum, fever, chills, weight loss, or night sweats. She had no history of tobacco smoking, tuberculosis or exposure to individuals with tuberculosis. She did not have a history of malignancy, diabetes mellitus, cytotoxic therapy or corticosteroid use. Her family history was unremarkable. Physical examination revealed a heart rate of 90 beats/min, blood pressure of 157/76 mmHg, respiratory rate of 24 breaths/min, temperature of 37.8 °C and oxygen saturation of 98% on room air. Respiratory, cardiac and abdominal examination were unremarkable. Chest radiograph showed multiple small nodules in both lung fields and chest computed tomography (CT) showed diffuse micronodules in random patterns in both lung lobes, cardiomegaly and bilateral pleural effusion (Figs. 1 and 2). White blood cell count, C-reactive protein and procalcitonin levels were 2800 /μl, 7.50 mg/dl (normal range 0.00–0.10 mg/dl) and 0.373 ng/ml (normal range 0.000–0.046 ng/ml), respectively. Serum carcinoembryonic antigen, carbohydrate antigen 19–9 and soluble IL-2 receptor were elevated at 9.4 ng/ml (normal range 0.0–5.0 ng/ml), 188.4 U/ml (normal range 0.0–37.0 U/ml) and 6163 U/ml (normal range 0–500 U/ml), respectively. Angiotensin-converting enzyme, mycoplasma antibody and blood sugar were within normal ranges. Serum QuantiFERON testing was positive. CD4/8 ratio, CD4 count and CD8 count were 1.73 (normal range 0.6–2.9), 422 /μl (normal range 344–1289) and 244 /μl (normal range 110–1066), respectively. IgG, IgA and IgM were 998 mg/dl (normal range 870–1700), 128 mg/dl (normal range 110–410), 59 mg/dl (normal range 46–260), respectively. Testing for human immunodeficiency virus infection was negative. Expectorated sputum smears were negative for bacteria and acid-fast bacilli. Urinary antigen testing (Binax NOW; Binax, Inc., Portland, ME) for *Streptococcus pneumoniae* and *Legionella pneumophila* was negative. According to these results, we initially suspected intraabdominal malignancy including malignant lymphoma. However, abdominal CT and magnetic resonance imaging showed no abnormalities. Therefore, we suspected miliary tuberculosis or pulmonary sarcoidosis. Liver, skin and bone marrow biopsies were subsequently performed and showed epithelioid cell granuloma without caseous necrosis. Gastric aspirate smear was positive for acid-fast bacilli and polymerase chain reaction (Loopamp; Eiken Chemical Co., Ltd. Tokyo, Japan) was positive for *Mycobacterium tuberculosis*. Although these microbiological findings might indicate the presence of non-viable *M. tuberculosis*, miliary tuberculosis was suspected and antimycobacterial therapy [oral isoniazid (INH) 200 mg/day, rifampicin (RFP) 300 mg/day and ethambutol (EB) 500 mg/day] was initiated on hospital day 12. Gastric aspirate culture was positive for *M. tuberculosis* after 1 week of culture. After a 2-month treatment course, chest radiograph showed gradual improvement, oral EB was discontinued and the patient was discharged. Although INH and RFP therapy was continued, chest radiograph showed new multiple nodules in the right middle lung field after a 6-month treatment course. Chest CT showed that a right S6 small nodule, presumed to be miliary tuberculosis, had increased and new multiple nodules appeared in the right lower lobe (Fig. 3). The patient's white blood cell count and C-reactive protein at this time were 2400 /μl and 0.09 mg/dl, respectively. Flexible fiberoptic bronchoscopy was subsequently perfomed. Microbiological testing of bronchial lavage fluids did not reveal any bacteria, mycobacteria or fungi. However, cytology showed a small number of Periodic acid-Schiff-positive bodies, suggesting *Cryptococcus* species (Fig. 4). Moreover, serum cryptococcal antigen testing (Serodirect "EIKEN" Cryptococcus; Eiken Chemical Co., Ltd. Tokyo, Japan) was positive (×128). According to these findings, pulmonary cryptococcosis was diagnosed, although the culture was negative. Oral fluconazole (FLCZ; 300 mg/day) was subsequently initiated. After a 6-month treatment course, chest radiograph showed gradual improvement and oral FLCZ was discontinued. The patient received a total of 12 months of antimycobacterial therapy. On follow-up, she has remained asymptomatic with suspect to pulmonary disease, with no recurrence.

Discussion and conclusions

Both tuberculosis and cryptococcosis have a wide range of clinical presentations, varying from pulmonary infection to the systemic infection. These diseases are more common in patients with impaired cell-mediated immunity such as those with AIDS, hemodialysis, hematologic malignancies, cancer and diabetes mellitus or receiving corticosteroids or immunosuppressive agents [1, 2]. Especially, this co-infection is almost always indicative of compromised cell-mediated immunity. Thus, its occurrence is extremely rare in immunocompetent patients. The first report of concomitant tuberculosis and cryptococcosis in immunocompetent patients was reported in 1966 [3]. Since that initial report, several cases of concurrent infection of tuberculosis and cryptococcosis in immunocompetent patients have been reported [3–12] (Table 1). Most reported cases with tuberculosis and cryptococcosis co-infection involved the lung and central nervous system, respectively. Aydemir H et al. reported a case of *C. neoformans* meningitis in an HIV-negative patient suspected of having miliary tuberculosis [13]. However, the authors did not definitively diagnose the patients with miliary tuberculosis. To our knowledge, a case of miliary tuberculosis with co-existing pulmonary cryptococcosis, even in immunocompromised patients, has not been reported previously. Additionally, despite an extensive evaluation, we found no evidence of immunodeficiency in our patient. In conclusion, the described patient was diagnosed with military tuberculosis with a co-existing pulmonary cryptococcal infection in non-HIV patient without underlying diseases.

In this case, CT images on the day of admission showed diffuse micronodules in random patterns in both lung fields and a small nodule in the right S6. Although both miliary tuberculosis and disseminated cryptococcosis present diffuse micronodules in random patterns in chest CT images, diffuse micronodules decreased following antimycobacterial treatment. Accordingly, these images were compatible with a diagnosis of miliary tuberculosis. However, the small nodule in the right S6 increased in size despite antimycobacterial therapy but reduced in size after antifungal treatment. Therefore, the small nodule was considered to be a primary focus of pulmonary cryptococcosis. The radiological findings of pulmonary cryptococcosis are well known. The common CT findings are nodular lesions, alveolar infiltrates, ground glass attenuation, cavitation, linear opacities, septal thickening, pleural effusion and lymphadenopathy [14]. In our case, the diagnosis of cryptococcosis was delayed because we believe that the small nodule was suggestive of miliary tuberculosis or post-inflammatory

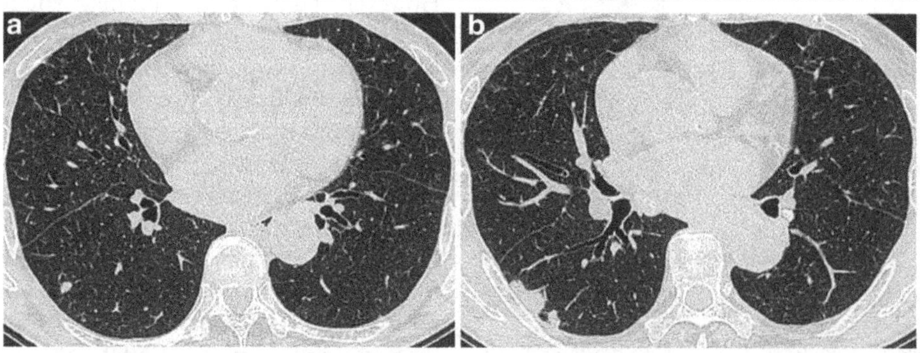

Fig. 3 Chest CT showed that a right S6 small nodule was increased (**a**) and new multiple nodules appeared in the right lower lobe (**b**)

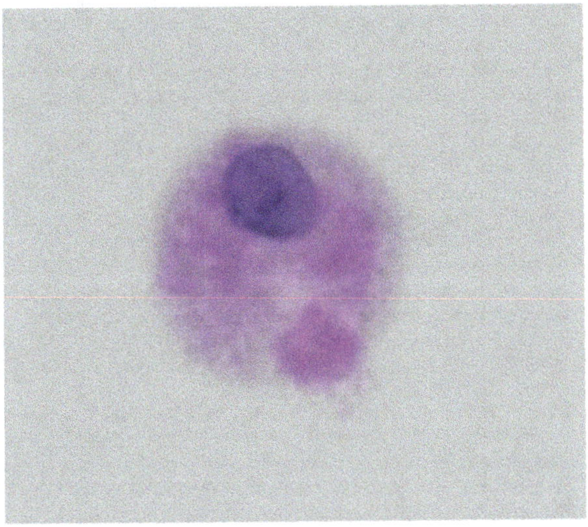

Fig. 4 Cytology of the bronchial lavage showed small amount of body suspicious for *Cryptococcus* species (Periodic acid-Schiff stain, ×400)

change. When pulmonary cryptococcosis appears as a small nodule combined with miliary tuberculosis, it might be very difficult to distinguish between these two diseases. We usually consider abnormal shadows to have the same etiology. However, pulmonary tuberculosis and pulmonary cryptococcosis are known to exhibit non-specific CT findings, such as alveolar infiltrates, nodules, micronodules, lymph node swelling and pleural effusion, and there are no characteristic findings [15]. Therefore, helpful diagnostic tools such as QuantiFERON test and serum cryptococcal antigen test should be considered. However, Dotsu et al. reported that sensitivity of the serum cryptococcal antigen test was decreased when the nodule size measured <15 mm [16]. Although we did not examine serum cryptococcal antigen on admission, its result would likely have been negative due to the small nodule size in this case.

Although impaired cellular-mediated immunity is a known risk factor for both mycobacterial and cryptococcal infections, the results of CD4 and CD8 counts and immunoglobulins in the present case were normal. Previous studies have demonstrated that tuberculosis causes alternations in cellular immunity and is recognized as a predisposing factor for developing cryptococcosis [17, 18]. However, high melanin-producing strains of *C. neoformans* inhibit T cell-mediated immunity such as the production of tumor necrosis factor-alpha and lymphoproliferation, thereby predisposing patients to tuberculosis reactivation or infection [19]. Thus, there is some evidence that both infections have immunomodulatory effects on host defenses. However, it is difficult to determine whether tuberculosis preceded cryptococcosis or vice versa in this case.

Because miliary tuberculosis with co-existing pulmonary cryptococcosis is not common, its presence may easily be overlooked, especially, if the nodule is very small. The present case emphasizes the fact that radiological findings of the two infections may be confusing when both co-exist in the lungs. Clinicians should take into consideration that these infections can co-exist even in immunocompetent patients.

In conclusion, we described a case of miliary tuberculosis with co-existing pulmonary cryptococcosis in non-HIV patient without underlying diseases. Although rare, clinicians should be aware of the possibility that these infections can co-exist even in immunocompetent patients.

Table 1 Reported case of co-infection tuberculosis and cryptococcosis in non-HIV patient without underlying diseases

Case/Ref	Age/sex	Region	Pathological lesions (tuberculosis/cryptococcosis)	Treatment (tuberculosis/cryptococcosis)	Outcome
1/3)	61/M	United States	Lung/CSF	INH, SM/AMPH-B	Recovered
2/4)	69/M	United States	Lung/Lung	INH, RFP/KCZ	Recovered
3/5)	51/M	Spain	CSF/CSF	INH, RFP, EB, PZA/AMPH-B, 5-FC	Recovered
4/6)	34/F	Saudi Arabia	Lymph node/Vertebra	INH, RFP, EB, PZA/FLCZ	Recovered
5/7)	25/F	Italy	CSF/CSF	INH, RFP, EB, PZA, SM/FLCZ, L-AMB	Recovered
6/8)	18/F	Canada	Lung/CSF, Lymph node	INH, RFP, EB, PZA/AMPH-B, 5-FC, FLCZ	Recovered
7/9)	65/M	India	Lung/Lung	NA/AMPH-B, ITCZ	Recovered
8/10)	58/F	Taiwan	Lymph node/Lung	NA/FLCZ	Recovered
9/11)	70/M	Iran	Lung/CSF, Lung	INH, RFP, EB, PZA/AMPH-B	Died
10/12)	61/M	Rwanda	Lung, Bone marrow, Liver/CSF	INH, RFP, EB/AMPH-B, FLCZ	Recovered
11/present case	84/F	Japan	Lung, Bone marrow, Liver, Skin/Lung	INH, RFP, EB/FLCZ	Recovered

NA Not available, *CSF* Cerebrospinal fluid, *INH* Isoniazid, *SM* Streptomycin, *AMPH-B* Amphotericin B, *RFP* Rifampicin, *KCZ* Ketoconazole, *EB* Ethambutol, *PZA* Pyrazinamide, *5-FC* 5-fluorocytosine, *FLCZ* Fluconazole, *L-AMB* Liposomal amphotericin B, *ITCZ* Itraconazole, *HIV* Human immunodeficiency virus

Abbreviations
EB: Ethambutol; FLCZ: Fluconazole; INH: Isoniazid; RFP: Rifampicin

Acknowledgements
Not applicable.

Funding
Not applicable.

Authors' contributions
TS managed the patient and reviewed the literature. TN, SK and SI contributed to the collection of patient data. SY and NM analyzed the radiologic findings. TS was the main writer of the manuscript. HM moderated the manuscript. Final approval: TS, TN, SK, SI, SY, NM and HM. All authors read and approved the final manuscript.

Consent for publication
Written informed consent was obtained from the patient's daughter for publication of this case report and any accompanying images.

Competing interests
All authors declare that they have no competing interests.

Author details
[1]Department of Respiratory Medicine, Nagasaki Harbor Medical Center, 6-39 Shinchi-machi, Nagasaki 850-8555, Japan. [2]Second Department of Internal Medicine, Nagasaki University Hospital, 1-7-1 Sakamoto-machi, Nagasaki, Japan.

References

1. Godbole G, Gant V. Respiratory tract infections in the immunocompromised. Curr Opin Pulm Med. 2013;19:244–50.
2. Kakeya H, Izumikawa K, Yamada K, Obata Y, Nishino T, Takazono T, Kosai K, Kurihara S, Nakamura S, Imamura Y, Miyazaki T, Tsukamoto M, Yanagihara K, Tashiro T, Kohno S. Three cases of concurrent infection with *Mycobacterium tuberculosis* and *Cryptococcus neoformans*. Intern Med. 2014;53:1685–92.
3. Chomicki J. Coexistence of pulmonary tuberculosis with pulmonary and meningeal cryptococcosis: report of a case. Dis Chest. 1966;50:214–6.
4. Kahn FW, England DM, Jones JM. Solitary pulmonary nodule due to *Cryptococcus neoformans* and *Mycobacterium tuberculosis*. Am J Med. 1985;78:677–81.
5. Gomez-Aranda F, Lopez-Dominguez JM, Munoz Malaga A, Blanco Ollero A. Meningitis simultaneously due to *Cryptococcus neoformans* and *Mycobacterium tuberculosis*. Clin Infect Dis. 1993;16:588–9.
6. Al-Tawfiq JA, Ghandour J. *Cryptococcus neoformans* abscess and osteomyelitis in an immunocompetent patient with tuberculous lymphadenitis. Infection. 2007;35:377–82.
7. Manfredi R, Calza L. Severe brain co-infection with *Cryptococcus neoformans* and *Mycobacterium tuberculosis* in a young, otherwise healthy student recently immigrated from China. Intern. J Infect Dis. 2008;12:438–41.
8. Van Tongeren L, Shaipanich T, Fleetham JA. Coinfection with *Cryptococcus gattii* and *Mycobacterium tuberculosis* in an otherwise healthy 18-year-old woman. Can Respir J. 2011;18:e62–3.
9. Thomas R, Christopher DJ, Balamugesh T, James P, Thomas M. Endobronchial pulmonary cryptococcosis and tuberculosis in an immunocompetent host. Singap Med J. 2012;53:e32–4.
10. Huang CL, Chen CT, SW W, Lin TY. Simultaneous coinfection with *Cryptococcus neoformans* and *Mycobacterium tuberculosis* in an adult. Q J Med. 2014;107:223–4.
11. Nabaei G, Afhami S. Disseminated cryptococcosis and active pulmonary tuberculosis co-infection in an otherwise healthy adult. Iran J Neurol. 2015;14:174–6.
12. Musabende M, Mukabatsinda C, Riviello ED, Ogbuagu O. Concurrent cryptococcal meningitis and disseminated tuberculosis occurring in an immunocompetent male. BMJ Case Reports. 2016;10:1136.
13. Aydemir H, Piskin N, Oztoprak N, Celebi G, Tekin IO, Akduman D. *Cryptococcus neoformans* meningitis in a HIV negative miliary tuberculosis-suspected patient. Mikrobiyol Bul. 2008;42:519–24.
14. Lindell RM, Hartman TE, Nadrous HF, Ryu JH. Pulmonary cryptococcosis: CT findings in immunocompetent patients. Radiology. 2005;236:326–31.
15. Diamond RD. Cryptococcus Neoformans. In: Mandell GL, Bennett JE, Dolin R, editors. Bennett's principles and practice of infectious diseases. 5th edn. London: Churchill Livingstone; 2000. p. 2707–18.
16. Dohtsu Y, Ishimatsu Y, Takatani H, Minami K, Inoue K, Kohara N, Yanagihara K, Higashiyama Y, Miyazaki Y, Hirakata Y, Kohno S. Clinical studies of sixteen cases with pulmonary cryptococcosis mainly with respect to serum level of cryptococcal antigen. Kansenshogaku zasshi. 2005;79:656–63.
17. Nagrajan S, Gugnani HC, Kowshik T. Case report. Meningitis due to *Cryptococcus neoformans* Var. Neoformans serotype AD association with pulmonary tuberculosis. Mycoses. 2000;43:679.
18. Bottasso O, Bay ML, Besedovsky H, del Rey A. Immunoendocrine alterations during human tuberculosis as an integrated view of disease pathology. Neuroimmunomodulation. 2009;16:68–77.
19. Huffnagle GB, Chen GH, Curtis JL, McDonald RA, Strieter RM, Toews GB. Down-regulation of the afferent phase of T cell-mediated pulmonary inflammation and immunity by a high melanin-producing strain of *Cryptococcus neoformans*. J Immunol. 1995;155:3507–16.

20

Tuberculosis treatment outcome and predictors in northern Ethiopian prisons

Kelemework Adane[1,2*], Mark Spigt[2,3] and Geert-Jan Dinant[2]

Abstract

Background: The prison situations are notorious for causing interruptions of tuberculosis (TB) treatment and occurrence of unfavorable outcomes. In Ethiopian prisons, though TB treatment programs exist, treatment outcome results and factors contributing to unsuccessful outcome are not well documented. In this study, we assessed the treatment outcome of TB cases and identified risk factors for unsuccessful outcome in northern Ethiopian prisons.

Methods: A retrospective record review was conducted for all prisoners diagnosed with TB between September 2011 and August 2015. Outcome variables were defined following WHO guidelines.

Results: Out of the 496 patients, 11.5% were cured, 68% completed treatment, 2.5% were lost to follow-up, 1.6% were with a treatment failure, 1.4% died, and 15% were transferred out. All transferred out or released prisoners were not appropriately linked to health facilities and might be lost to treatment follow-up. The overall treatment success rate (TSR) of the 5 years was 94% among the patients who were not transferred out. The odds of unsuccessful outcome were 4.68 times greater among re-treatment cases compared to the newly treated cases. The year of treatment was also associated with variations in TSR; those treated during the earlier year were more likely to have unsuccessful outcome. Sputum non-conversion at the second-month check-up was strongly associated with unsuccessful outcome among the smear-positive cases.

Conclusions: The mean TSR of the prisoners in the study prisons was quite satisfactory when gauged against the target level set by the End TB Strategy. However, the lack of appropriate linkage and tracking systems for those prisoners transferred or released before their treatment completion would have a negative implication for the national TB control program as such patients might interrupt their treatment and develop drug-resistant TB. Being in a re-treatment regimen and sputum non-conversion at the second-month check-up were significantly associated with unsuccessful treatment outcome among the all forms of and smear-positive TB cases, respectively.

Keywords: Tuberculosis, Treatment outcome, Prisons, Ethiopia

* Correspondence: ingoldmlt@gmail.com
[1]Department of Medical Microbiology and Immunology, College of Health Sciences, Mekelle University, PO Box 1871, Mekelle, Ethiopia
[2]Department of Family Medicine, Maastricht University/CAPHRI School for Public Health and Primary Care, PO Box 616, Maastricht, the Netherlands
Full list of author information is available at the end of the article

Background

Globally, the burden of tuberculosis (TB) is higher in vulnerable populations such as prisoners and is reported to be up to 100 times higher than in the general population [1]. In Sub-Saharan African prisons, TB remains as one of the fastest growing epidemics [2, 3]. The high prevalence of human immunodeficiency virus (HIV) infection and the lack of well-organized TB diagnostic and treatment systems [2, 4] contribute to the disproportionate burden of TB in the Sub-Saharan African prisons.

Inadequate TB treatment will lead to the emergence of drug-resistant strains [5]. The prison situations are notorious for causing interruptions of TB treatment and occurrence of unfavorable outcomes [6]. In some prisons, up to 24% of the TB cases have been shown to harbor multidrug-resistant TB (MDR-TB) which makes TB control efforts very complicated [7]. In Russian and Brazilian prisons, 12% [8] and 8% [9] of the TB cases have been reported to default their treatment, respectively. In a Ugandan prison, 43% of the prisoners with TB had defaulted their treatment [10]. The TB treatment category, HIV co-infection, smoking, alcoholism, and a lack of family support have been indicated as factors affecting TB treatment success in prisons [8, 9, 11].

In Ethiopian prisons, TB treatment programs exist and are integrated within the national TB control program where the prison health staff provides treatment based on the national guidelines [12]. However, treatment outcome results and the potential factors for unsuccessful outcome are not well documented. According to a report in 2013 from the prison of North Gondar, the treatment success rate (TSR) of the prisoners ranged from 42 to 80% within the 10 years period [13]. However, this study was not comprehensive in that it did not assess the potential factors that might be affecting the treatment success. Evaluating the treatment outcome results and identifying the risk factors for the unsuccessful outcome will help to identify the gaps between the national TB treatment policy and practice in prisons and initiate evidence-based interventions. This study was designed to assess the treatment outcome of TB cases and identify risk factors for unsuccessful outcome in northern Ethiopian prisons.

Methods

Study setting and diagnostic criteria

This study was carried out in prisons of the Tigray Regional State, northern Ethiopia. Out of the nine prisons in Tigray, four prisons, located in the cities Alamata, Humera, Mekelle and Shire, were randomly selected and included in the study. Information regarding the TB diagnostic and treatment services in these settings have been described elsewhere [14]. In general, conditions of the four prisons were comparable where the prisons had only poorly equipped clinics staffed with diploma holding nurses. There were also no sputum microscopy, GeneXpert or drug susceptibility testing (DST) services in the clinics of the prisons and the TB diagnosis relied merely on a referral of prisoners to health facilities outside prisons [14]. The diagnosis was carried out at the referral sites using the direct smear microscopy and/or chest X-ray, and pathological investigation following the national guidelines [15]. Accordingly, a presumptive TB case with at least two initial sputum smear examinations positive for AFB (acid-fast bacilli) by direct smear microscopy or one sputum examination positive for AFB and having radiographic abnormalities consistent with active pulmonary TB is considered as a smear-positive TB (PTB+) case. A patient having symptoms suggestive of TB with at least three initial smear examinations negative for AFB on the direct microscopy and with radiological abnormalities consistent with pulmonary TB is defined as a smear-negative TB (PTB−) case. On the other hand, if a patient has TB involving organs other than lungs as proven by histopathological evidence from a biopsy or based on strong clinical evidence consistent with active extra-pulmonary TB (EPTB) he/she is categorized as having EPTB.

Prisoners diagnosed with TB were linked to the directly observed treatment short-course (DOTS) clinics of the nearby health facilities where they were registered and started the treatment according to the national guidelines [15]. Afterwards, the prison health personnel collected drugs weekly from such facilities and continued the treatment within prisons. The treatment is given based the patients' treatment category. Newly diagnosed TB cases are provided with the 6 months treatment regimen where they take a combination of four drugs (rifampicin, isoniazid, pyrazinamide, and ethambutol) during the first 2 months of the intensive phase and continue with two of the drugs (rifampicin and isoniazid) for the remaining 4 months. On the other hand, the previously treated cases are treated for 8 months. This regimen consists of 8 weeks treatment with streptomycin, rifampicin, isoniazid, pyrazinamide, and ethambutol followed by 4 weeks treatment with rifampicin, isoniazid, pyrazinamide, and ethambutol during the intensive phase, followed by 5 months with rifampicin, isoniazid, and ethambutol. Bacteriological follow-up examinations (sputum smear checkups) are done at the end of the second, fifth, and sixth month of therapy for all new sputum-positive patients and at the end of the intensive phase of treatment (the third month), and at the end of the fifth and eighth months of treatment for the previously treated sputum smear-positive patients. The treatment follow-up data was regularly reported back to the health facilities for registration as the study prisons lacked standardized logbooks to register.

Study design and data collection

This was a retrospective analysis in which the profile and treatment outcomes of all prisoners diagnosed with TB between September 2010 and August 2015 was retrieved from the TB treatment follow-up clinics of the four selected prisons. Patients' information such as age, sex, the type of TB case, the treatment category, the date of treatment initiation and completion, weight at the time of treatment initiation, HIV status, and other related data were recorded by the prison nurses using a standardized recording format.

Outcome definition

The referral sites and/or the DOTS centers use the standard national TB case definitions and treatment outcomes adopted by WHO [16]. The categories of outcome include: cured (a TB patient who was smear- or culture-positive at the beginning of the treatment but who became smear- or culture negative in the last month of treatment and on at least one previous occasion), treatment completed (finished the treatment with resolution of symptoms but without smear or culture result), treatment failure (remained or became smear-positive at the end of 5 months or later), lost to follow-up (missed treatment for at least eight consecutive weeks), transferred out (transferred to another site during the treatment), died (patients who died from any cause during the course of treatment). We further grouped the outcomes into successful treatment (sum of cured and treatment completed) and unsuccessful treatment which is the sum of treatment failure, loss to follow-up, and death as per the WHO standard definition [17].

Data analysis

Data were entered using Epi Data entry version 3.1 software and analyzed using SPSS version 21. We compared prisoners with unsuccessful treatment outcome with those having successful outcome. Even though it was already one of the elements of the unsuccessful outcome, death was specifically considered as an additional outcome variable because we were interested to see its relationship with body weight at treatment initiation. Bivariate and multivariate logistic regression analyses were performed to examine the association of independent variables with our outcome variables. Covariates with p-values of ≤0.25 and collinearity matrix index of ≤0.7 in the bivariate analysis were considered for inclusion in the multivariate model. A p-value of ≤0.05 was considered to define a statistical significance.

Results

Socio-demographic and clinical characteristics

The baseline characteristics of TB patients ($n = 496$) are shown in Table 1. The majority (97%) was male, and the mean age was 30 years (range 15–18 years). Extra-pulmonary TB patients accounted for 43% of the TB cases; 30% of total cases had PTB–. Out of the 123 (25%) PTB+ cases, repeated smear was done for 119 (97%) at the end of the 2nd month of treatment and nine were still smear-positive. Eleven percent of the TB cases were HIV-infected; the co-infection rate being slightly higher among EPTB cases (13%). However, the difference was not statistically significant.

Table 1 Socio-demographic and clinical characteristics of the 496 patients with tuberculosis in northern Ethiopian prisons, 2011–2015

Characteristic	*n* (%)
Sex	
Male	480 (97)
Female	16 (3)
Age, years	
15–24	201 (40)
25–34	173 (35)
≥35	122 (25)
Weight at treatment initiation (Kg)	
<50	221 (45)
≥50	275 (55)
Form of TB	
PTB+	123 (25)
PTB–	150 (30)
EPTB	211 (43)
EPTB & PTB	12 (2)
Treatment category	
New case	481 (97)
Retreatment case	15 (3)
HIV status	
Negative	424 (85)
Positive	54 (11)
Unknown	18 (4)
Antiretroviral treatment (ART)[a]	
On ART at time/within in 3 months of TB treatment	46 (85)
Not on ART	3 (6)
Unknown	5 (9)
Use of co-trimoxazole prophylaxis[a]	
On co-trimoxazole at time/within 3 months of TB treatment	40 (74)
Not on co-trimoxazole	14 (26)
Site	
Alamata	73 (14)
Humera	163 (33)
Mekelle	183 (37)
Shire	77 (16)

[a]The denominator is HIV co-infected patients ($n = 54$); *HIV* human immunodeficiency virus, *TB* tuberculosis, *PTB+* smear-positive pulmonary tuberculosis, *PTB–* smear-negative pulmonary tuberculosis, *EPTP* extra-pulmonary tuberculosis

Trend of the TB types

The 5-year trend of all the TB types is shown in Fig. 1. The number of PTB− cases showed variation across years steadily increasing in the recent year; more than half of the TB cases (51.8%) were PTB− between the September 2014 and August 2015. On the other hand, the number of EPTB cases roughly decreased over the 5 years.

Treatment outcome and trends

The mean treatment success rate (TSR) of the 5 years was 94% (395/422) among the patients who were not transferred out. As shown in Fig. 2, the TSR steadily increased from 87% during September 2010–August 2011 to 97% in September 2013–August 2014. Overall, 57 (11.5%) were cured, 338 (68%) had completed treatment, 12 (2.5%) were lost to treatment follow-up, 8 (1.6%) were with treatment failure, 7 (1.4%) died, and 74 (15%) were transferred out with outcome unknown. All the prisoners transferred to other prisons or released during the course of their TB treatment were not appropriately linked to health facilities.

Treatment success rate and associated factors

The treatment success rate and associated predictors are shown in Table 2. After excluding the transferred out prisoners and dichotomizing the outcome variable, further analysis was done for the 422 cases. In the multivariable analysis, the odds of having unsuccessful outcome was significantly higher among the retreatment cases compared to the newly treated ones (AOR = 4.68; 95% CI = 1.02–21.4). Prisoners that were treated during September 2010–August 2011 were also more likely to have unsuccessful outcome, compared to those treated during September 2011–August 2012 (AOR = 0.28; 95% CI = 0.08–0.92), September 2012–August 2013 (AOR = 0.24; 95% CI = 0.06–0.98), and September 2013–August 2014 (AOR = 0.17; 95% CI = 0.05–0.67). Sputum non-conversion at the second-month check-up was strongly associated with unsuccessful outcome among the smear-positive cases. There was no association between unsuccessful outcome and HIV status, the weight at treatment initiation, the study site, and the form of the TB case. When we perform the analysis considering death as an outcome variable, the odds of dying among patients with a weight at initiation of <50 Kg was 8.4 times higher (OR = 8.39; 95% CI = 1.01–70.34) compared to the other group.

Discussion

In this study, the overall treatment success was found to be 94% for the prisoners that complete their treatment while in prison. However, all the prisoners transferred to other prisons or released during their treatment were not appropriately linked to health facilities and might be lost to treatment follow-up. TB treatment category, the year of treatment, and sputum non-conversion at the second-month check-up (for smear-positive cases) were statistically associated with unsuccessful treatment outcome.

The observed treatment success rate (94%) is slightly higher than the findings from similar studies in the general population of Tigray (89.2%) [18], northeast Ethiopia (90.1%) [19] and is in the range of the target level set by End TB Strategy (a TSR of ≥90%) [20]. It also remains remarkably higher than reports from Southern (85.2%) [21], Western (70.8%) [22] and Northwest (85.6%) [23] Ethiopia. More specifically, the loss to follow-up

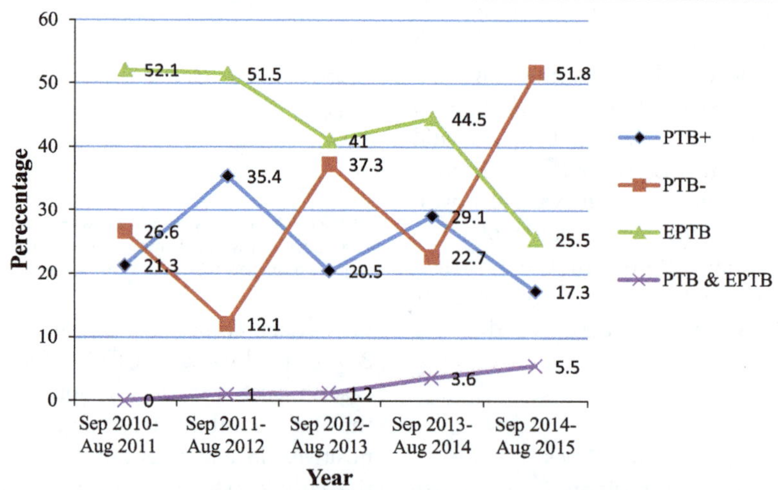

Fig. 1 Trends of all forms of registered TB cases ($n = 496$) in the DOTs center of four northern Ethiopian prisons, 2010–2015. Aug: August, Sep: September; PTB+: smear-positive pulmonary tuberculosis; PTB−: smear-negative pulmonary tuberculosis; EPTP: extra-pulmonary tuberculosis

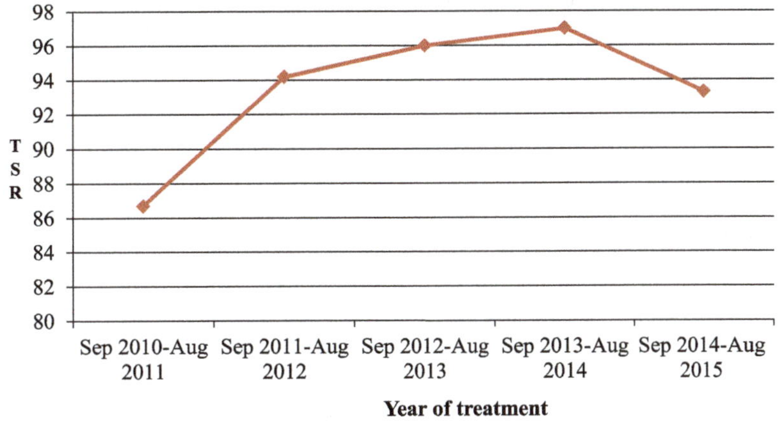

Fig. 2 Trends of treatment success rate for all forms of the TB cases ($n = 496$) from four northern Ethiopian prisons, 2010 to 2015. Aug: August; Sep: September; TSR: Treatment Success Rate; TB: Tuberculosis

(2.5%) and death rates (1.4%) in our study are lower than the loss to follow-up and death rates recorded in the previous studies [18, 21, 22] which ranged from 3.2 to 35.5% and 3.3 to 58.8%, respectively. In all the above-mentioned studies, the TSR was calculated in a similar way with our study where the transferred out patients were not considered. The discrepancy with findings could partly be attributed to differences in settings that might account for the variation in the DOTs performance. In prisons, it easier to administer DOTs and monitor the progress as the patients are accessible to the prison health personnel [24]. In addition, we observed that the prison health personnel provided the TB drugs under strict supervision not only during the first 2 months but also during the 4 months of the continuation phase, which might result in an increased likelihood of better treatment outcome in prisons.

When compared with prison specific studies, the overall TSR in this study (94%) is higher than the findings from the prison in Gondar which ranged from 42 to 80% across the 10 years [13]. The time difference could not exclusively be the reason for this discrepancy because the TSRs in this study were still smaller than the TSR in our study during the years that overlapped with our study period. Other factors such as differences in the healthcare delivery service between the prisons of the two regions and the commitment of the prison health personnel in delivering the DOTS service might be possible reasons. Higher rates of loss to follow-up were reported elsewhere in prisons in Uganda (43.0%) [10], and Brazil (13.0%) [9]. Similarly, the 1.4% death rate observed in this study is lower than those recorded in Ugandan (5.0%) [10], South African (1.8%) [11] and Brazilian (2.0%) prisons [9]. One possible explanation for this variation could be the difference in the burden of HIV co-infection, which has been shown to be associated with unsuccessful treatment outcome [19, 25]. For example, 54% of the study participants in the South African prison [11] were co-infected with HIV [11] whereas only 11% of the TB cases had HIV co-infection in our study.

Our study demonstrates that the DOTS program is effectively functioning for prisoners that complete their TB treatment while in the study prisons. However, the absence of appropriate linkage for those prisoners transferred to other prisons or released during their treatment raises a public health concern. It is more likely for such patients to end up with a loss to follow-up or treatment failure if not death. Those patients who survived would be at high risk to develop of drug-resistant TB [10]. This also implies that the community would be at risk of being infected with a resistant strain from these patients. For the national TB program to be successful, governmental and non-governmental organizations (NGOs) should take the initiative in establishing improved linkage between the prison and public health facilities. For example, a mobile-based communication system involving the prison health personnel, the health professionals at a public health facility, and the released prisoners could be a good approach in tracking released prisoners and reducing loss to treatment follow-up [26].

In this study, as it could be expected, previously treated cases were more likely to have unsuccessful treatment outcome compared to new cases which is consistent with several previous reports [11, 18]. One of the reasons could be the high level of treatment failure and hence possible development of drug-resistant strains in retreatment cases [27]. In addition, patient-related behavior might also have contributed to the unsuccessful outcome; a study indicated patients that were already lost to follow-up previously could be reluctant and tend to interrupt their treatment again [28]. Due attention should be given to such patients to make sure that they are taking the full

Table 2 Factors related to unsuccessful treatment outcome among northern Ethiopian prisoners with tuberculosis in the bivariate and multivariate logistic regression analysis (n = 422). AOR: adjusted odds ratio; COR: crude odds ratio; CI: confidence interval; ref = reference

Characteristic	Treatment outcome		COR (95% CI)	P-value	AOR (95% CI)	P-value
	Unsuccessful n (%)	Successful n (%)				
Sex						
Female	2 (14.3)	12 (85.7)	2.56 (0.54-12.04)	0.26	-	
Male	25 (6.2)	383 (93.8)	ref			
Age, years						
15-24	8 (4.6)	164 (95.4)	0.62 (0.23-1.71)	0.36	-	
25-34	11 (7.9)	129 (92.1)	0.86 (0.86-1.09)			
≥ 35	8 (7.3)	102 (92.7)	ref			
Weight at initiation (Kg)						
< 50	15 (8.4)	164 (91.6)	1.76 (0.83-3.86)		1.72 (0.75-3.98)	0.2
≥ 50	12 (4.9)	231 (95.1)	ref			
Form of TB[a]						
PTB+	8 (7.6)	97 (92.3)	1.22 (0.48-3.14)	0.48	-	
PTB -	8 (6.1)	124 (93.9)	0.96 (0.37-2.45)	0.38		
EPTP	11 (6.3)	163 (93.7)	ref			
Non-conversion at the 2nd month[b]						
Yes	2 (12.5)	4 (87.5)	9.1 (1.33-62.16)	0.02	-	
No	5 (5.2)	91 (94.8)				
Type of TB case						
Retreatment case	3 (25.0)	9 (75.0)	5.36 (1.36-21.11)	0.01	4.68 (1.02-21.4)	0.04
New case	24 (5.8)	386 (94.2)	ref			
HIV status[C]						
Positive	4 (8.5)	43 (91.5)	1.36 (0.45-4.14)	0.58	-	
Negative	23 (6.4)	338 (93.6)	ref			
Year						
Sep 2010-Aug 2011	10 (13.3)	65 (86.7)	ref			
Sep 2011-Aug 2012	5 (5.8)	81 (93.2)	0.41 (0.13-1.23)	0.11	0.28 (0.08-0.92)	0.04
Sep 2012-Aug 2013	3 (4.2)	69 (95.8)	0.28 (0.07-1.07)	0.06	0.24 (0.06-0.98)	0.047
Sep 2013-Aug 2014	3 (3.0)	97 (97.0)	0.21(0.05-0.76)	0.018	0.17 (0.05-0.67)	0.01
Sep 2014-Aug 2015	6 (6.7)	83 (93.3)	0.48 (0.16-1.36)	0.16	0.45 (0.14-1.43)	0.18
Site						
Mekelle	12 (8.6)	127 (91.4)	ref			
Alamata	1 (1.4)	72 (98.6)	0.15 (0.02-1.15)	0.07	0.14 (0.02-1.18)	0.07
Shire	5 (6.8)	68 (93.2)	0.78 (0.26-2.30)	0.65	0.53 (0.16-169)	0.28
Humera	9 (6.6)	128 (93.4)	0.74 (0.3-1.83)	0.52	0.64 (0.23-1.72)	0.38

[a]Patients with both PTB & EPTB were not included; [b]Analysis limited to the smear-positive cases; [c]Analysis limited to patients with known HIV status; *HIV* human immunodeficiency virus; *Kg* kilogram; *PTB+* smear-positive pulmonary tuberculosis; *PTB-* smear-negative pulmonary tuberculosis; *EPTB* extra-pulmonary tuberculosis

course of treatment and immediate referral should be done for MDR screening if they already had a treatment failure. Year of treatment was also associated with variations in treatment outcome; in general, those treated during the earlier year (September 2010–Augst 2011) were more likely to have unsuccessful outcome compared to the latest years, indicating improvements in the DOTS performance over years. This could be due to the increasing efforts of the national TB control program in introducing and implementing the TB/HIV collaborative activities in healthcare settings and prisons in recent years [29].

Unlike several previous reports [11, 19, 25], in this study, HIV co-infection was not associated with unsuccessful outcome. The difference in the sample size and burden of the co-infection rate might be possible reasons for this. In addition, the prison health personnel reported that they routinely supervise the TB treatment progress of prisoners including those co-infected with HIV which might have contributed to the improved outcome in both groups. Though it was not associated with unsuccessful outcome, body weight at initiation of anti-TB treatment (<50 Kgs) was found to be a significant predictor of death of the patients, which is in agreement with previous reports [30, 31]. The relationship between TB and malnutrition is bidirectional. Severe TB disease renders patients to be malnourished and malnourished individuals are at a high risk to develop severe TB diseases and end up with unfavorable treatment outcomes [32]. Hence, the death of patients might be attributed to the severity of the TB disease itself or due to the malnutrition and associated consequences. Closer nutritional monitoring and earlier initiation of nutrition support are important to rescue severely malnourished TB patients [32]. In smear-positive cases, sputum non-conversion at the second-month check-up was a predictor of unsuccessful outcome. This might be partly related to the drug resistance development. In 2015, the incidence of multidrug-resistant/rifampicin-resistant (MDR/RR-TB) in Ethiopia was estimated to be 2.7% among the new and 14% among retreatment TB cases [20]. In the Tigray region of Ethiopia, 55% of the presumptive MDR cases have been shown to harbor MDR strains [33]. We suggest that such prisoners should be immediately referred for DST.

Furthermore, an overview of the TB profile data showed that the majority of the patients in our study were EPTB and PTB– cases, which is consistent with the previous reports from the general population in Ethiopia [34, 35]. The exact causes for the high proportion of EPTB in Ethiopia remain unknown, however, the high potential for a wrong diagnosis (due to the poor diagnostic facility), and poor immunologic and nutritional status have been shown to be associated with high rates of EPTB and PTB– cases [36, 37]. This might suggest the need to incorporate a more accurate diagnostic test, such as the GeneXpert MTB/RIF assay, in Ethiopian prisons.

This study has some limitations mainly inherited from the retrospective design. As we relied on historical records, we were not able to add some important variables such as alcoholism, smoking, substance abuse, nutritional status, and lack of family support, which are known to be related to the variations in the TB treatment outcome [38]. Tracking the prisoners transferred between prisons was also not possible, as the information was not clearly indicated in the treatment recording protocol.

Conclusions

The mean treatment success rate of the prisoners in the study prisons was quite satisfactory when gauged against the target level set by the End TB Strategy. However, the lack of appropriate linkage and tracking systems for those prisoners transferred or released before their treatment completion would have a negative implication for the national TB control program as such patients might interrupt their treatment and develop drug-resistant TB. Being in a re-treatment regimen and sputum non-conversion at the second-month check-up were significantly associated with unsuccessful outcome among all forms of and smear-positive TB cases, respectively. The concerned authorities should take an urgent action to help establish improved linkages between the prison and public health facilities to prevent possible loss to follow-up of released prisoners and due attention should be given to the previously treated cases.

Abbreviations

AFB: Acid-fast bacilli; DOTS: Directly observed treatment short-course; DST: Drug susceptibility testing; EPTB: Extra-pulmonary tuberculosis; HIV: Human immunodeficiency virus; MDR-TB: Multidrug-resistant tuberculosis; PTB–: Smear-negative pulmonary tuberculosis; PTB+: Smear-positive pulmonary tuberculosis; TB: Tuberculosis; TSR: Treatment success rate; WHO: World Health Organization

Acknowledgements

The authors would like to thank staffs of the Prison Administration Office of Tigray and the Amhara Regional States, especially Commander Tsegay Uqubay and Commander Workneh Gashe for their invaluable support during the data collection.

Funding

This study was financially supported by Maastricht University through Nuffic scholarship (NFP-PHD 14/139) and Mekelle University. The funder had no role in study design, data collection and analysis, decision to publish, or preparation of the manuscript.

Authors' contributions

KA, MS, and GJD were all involved in the study conception and design. KA was involved in the data analysis and drafting of the manuscript. KA, MS, and GJD were all involved in the write-up and refinement of the manuscript. All authors have read and approved the final version of the manuscript.

Consent for publication

Not applicable

Competing interests

The authors declare that there is no any competing interest.

Author details
[1]Department of Medical Microbiology and Immunology, College of Health Sciences, Mekelle University, PO Box 1871, Mekelle, Ethiopia. [2]Department of Family Medicine, Maastricht University/CAPHRI School for Public Health and Primary Care, PO Box 616, Maastricht, the Netherlands. [3]General Practice Research Unit, Department of Community Medicine, UiT the Arctic University of Norway, PO Box 6050, Tromsø, Norway.

References

1. World Health Organization. Tuberculosis in prisons. Geneva: World Health Organization; 2011.
2. O'Grady J, Mwaba P, Bates M, Kapata N, Zumla A. Tuberculosis in prisons in sub-Saharan Africa: a potential time bomb. S Afr Med J. 2011;101(2):107.
3. O'Grady J, Hoelscher M, Atun R, et al. Tuberculosis in prisons in sub-Saharan Africa–the need for improved health services, surveillance and control. Tuberculosis. 2011;91(2):173–8.
4. Johnstone-Robertson S, Lawn SD, Welte A, Bekker L-G, Wood R. Tuberculosis in a south African prison: a transmission modelling analysis. S Afr Med J. 2011;101(11):809–13.
5. Kliiman K, Altraja A. Predictors of poor treatment outcome in multi-and extensively drug-resistant pulmonary TB. Eur Respir J. 2009;33(5):1085–94.
6. Reyes H. Pitfalls of TB management in prisons, revisited. Int J Prison Health. 2007;3(1):43–67.
7. World Health Organization. Tuberculosis in prisons: address TB/HIV, MDR/XDR-TB and other challenges; 2012.
8. Shin SS, Pasechnikov AD, Gelmanova IY, et al. Treatment outcomes in an integrated civilian and prison MDR-TB treatment program in Russia. Int J Tuberc Lung Dis. 2006;10(4):402–8.
9. Ribeiro Macedo L, Reis-Santos B, Riley L, Maciel E. Treatment outcomes of tuberculosis patients in Brazilian prisons: a polytomous regression analysis. Int J Tuberc Lung Dis. 2013;17(11):1427–34.
10. Schwitters A, Kaggwa M, Omiel P, Nagadya G, Kisa N, Dalal S. Tuberculosis incidence and treatment completion among Ugandan prison inmates. Int J Tuberc Lung Dis. 2014;18(7):781–6.
11. Mnisi T, Tumbo J, Govender I. Factors associated with pulmonary tuberculosis outcomes among inmates in Potchefstroom Prison in north west province: original research. S Afr J Infect Dis. 2013;28(2):96–101.
12. Federal Ministry of Health. Tuberculosis, Leprosy and TB/HIV prevention and control programme manual. Addis Ababa: Federal Ministry of Health; 2008.
13. Moges B, Amare B, Asfaw F, Mulu A, Tessema B, Kassu A. High prevalence and poor treatment outcome of tuberculosis in North Gondar Zone Prison, Northwest Ethiopia. Int J Med Med Sci. 2013;5(9):425–9.
14. Adane K, Spigt M, Ferede S, Asmelash T, Abebe M, Dinant G-J. Half of pulmonary tuberculosis cases were left undiagnosed in prisons of the Tigray region of Ethiopia: implications for tuberculosis control. PLoS One. 2016; 11(2):e0149453.
15. Federal Democratic Republic of Ethiopia. Guidelines for the clinical and programmatic management of TB, TB/HIV and leprosy in Ethiopia. Addis Ababa: Federal Ministry of Health; 2013.
16. World Health Organization. Definitions and reporting framework for tuberculosis – 2013 revision, Multi-country global workshop on TB prevalence surveys and TB surveillance, 29 April–3 May 2013. Accra: World Health Organization; 2013.
17. World Health Organization. TB case definitions revision; 2011.
18. Berhe G, Enquselassie F, Aseffa A. Treatment outcome of smear-positive pulmonary tuberculosis patients in Tigray region, northern Ethiopia. BMC Public Health. 2012;12(1):537.
19. Tesfahuneygn G, Medhin G, Legesse M. Adherence to anti-tuberculosis treatment and treatment outcomes among tuberculosis patients in Alamata District, northeast Ethiopia. BMC Res Notes. 2015;8(1):503.
20. World Health Organization Geneva. Global tuberculosis report. Geneva: World Health Organization; 2016.
21. Gebrezgabiher G, Romha G, Ejeta E, Asebe G, Zemene E, Ameni G. Treatment outcome of tuberculosis patients under directly observed treatment short course and factors affecting outcome in southern Ethiopia: a five-year retrospective study. PLoS One. 2016;11(2):e0150560.
22. Ejeta E, Chala M, Arega G, et al. Outcome of tuberculosis patients under directly observed short course treatment in western Ethiopia. J Infect Dev Ctries. 2015;9(07):752–9.
23. Tessema B, Muche A, Bekele A, Reissig D, Emmrich F, Sack U. Treatment outcome of tuberculosis patients at Gondar University Teaching Hospital, Northwest Ethiopia. A five-year retrospective study. BMC Public Health. 2009;9(1):371.
24. Dara M, Acosta CD, Melchers NW, et al. Tuberculosis control in prisons: current situation and research gaps. Int J Infect Dis. 2015;32:111–7.
25. Kayigamba FR, Bakker MI, Mugisha V, et al. Adherence to tuberculosis treatment, sputum smear conversion and mortality: a retrospective cohort study in 48 Rwandan clinics. PLoS One. 2013;8(9):e73501.
26. West D. How mobile devices are transforming healthcare. Issues Technol Innov. 2012;18:1–14.
27. Espinal MA, Kim SJ, Suarez PG, et al. Standard short-course chemotherapy for drug-resistant tuberculosis: treatment outcomes in 6 countries. JAMA. 2000;283(19):2537–45.
28. Muñoz-Sellart M, Cuevas L, Tumato M, Merid Y, Yassin M. Factors associated with poor tuberculosis treatment outcome in the southern region of Ethiopia. Int J Tuberc Lung Dis. 2010;14(8):973–9.
29. Reves R, Angelo S. As Ethiopia moves toward tuberculosis elimination, success requires higher investment. Washington DC: Center for Strategic and International Studies; 2016.
30. Getahun B, Ameni G, Biadgilign S, Medhin G. Mortality and associated risk factors in a cohort of tuberculosis patients treated under DOTS programme in Addis Ababa, Ethiopia. BMC Infect Dis. 2011;11(1):127.
31. Vasantha M, Gopi P, Subramani R. Survival of tuberculosis patients treated under DOTS in a rural tuberculosis unit (TU), south India. Indian J Tuberc. 2008;55(2):64.
32. World Health Organization. Guideline: nutritional care and support for patients with tuberculosis. Geneva: World Health Organization; 2013.
33. Tesfay K, Tesfay S, Nigus E, Gebreyesus A, Gebreegziabiher D, Adane K. More than half of presumptive multidrug-resistant cases referred to a tuberculosis referral laboratory in the Tigray region of Ethiopia are multidrug resistant. Int J Mycobacteriol. 2016;5(3):324–7.
34. Mekonnen D, Derbie A, Mekonnen H, Zenebe Y. Profile and treatment outcomes of patients with tuberculosis in northeastern Ethiopia: a cross sectional study. Afr Health Sci. 2016;16(3):663–70.
35. Beza MG, Wubie MT, Teferi MD, Getahun YS, Bogale SM, Tefera SB. A five years tuberculosis treatment outcome at kolla diba health center, dembia district, northwest Ethiopia: a retrospective cross-sectional analysis. J Infect Dis Ther. 2013;1(1):1–6.
36. Cegielski J, McMurray D. The relationship between malnutrition and tuberculosis: evidence from studies in humans and experimental animals. Int J Tuberc Lung Dis. 2004;8(3):286–98.
37. Iwnetu R, Van Den Hombergh J, Woldeamanuel Y, et al. Is tuberculous lymphadenitis over-diagnosed in Ethiopia? Comparative performance of diagnostic tests for mycobacterial lymphadenitis in a high-burden country. Scand J Infect Dis. 2009;41(6–7):462–8.
38. Abera SF, Adane K. One-fourth of the prisoners are underweight in northern Ethiopia: a cross-sectional study. BMC Public Health. 2017;17(1):449.

21

Potential effect of household environment on prevalence of tuberculosis in India

S. K. Singh[1], Gyan Chandra Kashyap[1*] and Parul Puri[2]

Abstract

Background: Tuberculosis (TB) has been a major health problem globally since ages, and even today, it is a major cause of morbidity in millions of people each year. In 2015 alone, TB accounted for about 1.4 million deaths globally, with India carrying the biggest burden of the disease. The physical environment of the household, an individual living in, has a significant influence on the incidence of TB. Thus, an understanding of the socio-economic, demographic and environmental factors that individuals are exposed to is of importance. The objective of present study is to examine the association of household environment with the prevalence of Tuberculosis in India.

Methods: The study utilizes data from the fourth round of National Family Health Survey (NFHS-4), 2015-16, which was collected from self-reported information pertaining to Tuberculosis in the household questionnaire. The specific question was, "Does any usual resident of your household suffer from tuberculosis?" the response to which helped in the detection of Tuberculosis. Binary Logistic regression was performed from which appropriate inferences are drawn on the association of household environment with Tuberculosis.

Results: Prevalence of TB was found to be the highest among elderly people (0.9%), no education (0.4%) and people belonging to the poorest wealth quintile (0.53%). Family members who were regularly (daily) exposed to smoke (second-hand smoke) inside the house were more prone to getting tuberculosis (OR = 1.49; CI = 1.39-1.61) as compared with households where people do not smoke inside the house. Further, households having a finished wall (OR = 0.7; CI = 0.6-0.8) are less likely to get TB than the households with mud walls. Households that shared their toilets with other households are more likely to get hold of Tuberculosis (OR = 1.2; CI = 1.1-1.4).

Conclusions: Results strongly suggest that a contaminated household environment increases the risk of tuberculosis in India. There are multiple risk factors that are strongly associated with Tuberculosis: smoke inside house, type of cooking fuel, separate kitchen, floor, roofing and wall material, number of persons sleeping in a room, sharing toilet and potable water with other households; and individual characteristics such as age, sex, educational attainment, marital status, place of residence and wealth index.

Keywords: Household, Environment, Prevalence of Tuberculosis, India

* Correspondence: statskashyap@gmail.com
[1]Department of Mathematical Demography & Statistics, International Institute for Population Sciences, Govandi Station Road, Deonar Mumbai 400088, India
Full list of author information is available at the end of the article

Background

The Sustainable Development Goals (SDG, 2015) are aimed at building an inclusive, sustainable and resilient future by incorporating economic, social and environmental protection for people and planet in order to ensure good health and well-being for all [1]. "The future will either be green or not at all", said Australian environmentalist Robert James "Bob" Brown. A clean environment is mandatory for human health and well-being.

The best-known health impacts are related to environmental (air) pollution, poor water quality, and inadequate sanitation. Air pollution is an adulteration of the environment by any chemical, physical or biological agent that modifies the conventional characteristics of the atmosphere [2]. Owing to the increasing trends in the number of motor vehicles and industries, it is commonly believed that the problem is associated with developed urban areas. In reality, however, air pollution tends to be higher in developing regions. This is attributable to the combustion of biomass fuel indoors [3]. Indoor air pollution is not only dependent on the combustion of solid fuel, but it is also affected by overcrowded housing conditions and exposure to secondhand smoke inside the house.

Globally, around three billion people use solid fuel like wood, animal dung, crop waste and coal for cooking and keeping their houses warm. These fuels have low combustion efficiency and highly polluting emissions. Biomass smoke contains many harmful components, including suspended particulate matter, nitrogen oxides, carbon monoxide, etc. Regular exposure to these air pollutants can cause serious health problems [4–6]. Estimates suggest that over four million people die prematurely from illnesses attributable to the household air pollution resulting from cooking with solid fuels. In India, estimates from the National Family Health Survey (NFHS-4) suggest that about 55% of the household use solid fuel for cooking, among which about 99% use open fire/*chullah* for cooking. About 41% of household uses wood as their primary cooking fuel. Further, about half of all households do not have a separate kitchen [7].

Tuberculosis (TB) has been a major health problem globally since ages, and even today, it is a major cause of morbidity in millions of people each year. Tuberculosis (TB) is ranked among the top ten causes of deaths worldwide and as one of the leading causes of death from infectious disease. In 2015 alone, TB accounted for about 1.4 million deaths globally with India carrying the biggest burden of the disease [8]. The proportion of TB patients is higher in India because of poor socio-economic and environmental conditions. According to NFHS-4, the prevalence of TB is 316 per 100,000 persons in India [7].

The Indian government has envisaged a "TB-free India" by 2017, aimed at reducing the burden of TB in Indian sub-continent [9]. Studies show indoor air pollution as a significant risk factor for the occurrence of TB. However, the findings of most studies are based on small study populations [10, 11]. Existing literature suggests a number of factors associated with TB infection, including demographic, socio-economic and environmental factors, such as age, sex, level of education, marital status, place of residence, wealth, overcrowding, poor housing and household environment factors [3, 12–14].

The studies also highlight the higher prevalence of TB in men [14, 15], elderly, poor and malnourished [14], those belonging to urban areas, living in *kuchha* (usually made of mud) house and other environmental factors [10, 16]. About 26% of the cases of TB is attributed to Indoor Pollution [17]. However, the nature of the relationship between indoor air pollution and tuberculosis has not been in much focus. By considering the exposure to all environmental factors present in households, the present study tries to identify the potential household environmental factors which enhance the risk of prevalence of Tuberculosis in India.

Methods

The present study utilized data from the fourth round of the National Family Health Survey (NFHS-4). NFHS-4 provides district level estimates of important indicators on population, health and nutrition for India and each State / Union territory. It provides data on 601,509 households, 699,686 women, and 103,525 men. The study utilizes data, which was collected from self-reported information pertaining to Tuberculosis in the household questionnaire. The specific question was, "Does any usual resident of your household suffer from tuberculosis?" the response to which helped in the detection of Tuberculosis (Additional file 1). Auxiliary information retrieved from a national report from the third round of National Family Health Survey (NFHS-3, 2005-06) is used for analysis.

Sampling design and response rate

The NFHS-4 survey adopted a multistage stratified sampling design by considering the urban and rural areas as the natural strata. The 2011 census served as the sampling frame for the selection of Primary Sampling Units (PSUs). The PSUs in the survey were villages in rural areas. For urban areas, Census Enumeration Blocks (CEBs) were selected. Within each rural stratum, villages were selected from the sampling frame based on probability proportional to size (PPS). The final sample PSUs were selected through PPS sampling.

In urban areas, CEBs were also selected through PPS sampling. In every selected rural and urban PSU, selected PSUs with an estimated number of households were segmented. Two of the segments were randomly chosen for the survey using systematic sampling with probability proportional to segment size. Therefore, an NFHS-4 cluster is either a PSU or a segment of a PSU.

In the second stage, in every selected rural and urban cluster, households were randomly selected with systematic sampling. A total of 628,900 households were selected for the sample, of which 616,346 were occupied. Of the occupied households, 601,509 were successfully interviewed, a response rate of 98%. In the interviewed households, 723,875 eligible women age 15–49 years were identified for being interviewed individually of which 699,686 were interviewed, women, a response rate of 97%. Among males, there were 122,051 eligible men age 15–54 years in the households selected for the state module. Interviews were completed with 112,122 men, a response rate of 92%.

Variables used

Response variables

Self-reported presence of Tuberculosis (TB) is the outcome variable.

Predictor variables

Based on the factors discussed in past studies, literature, exposure variables include various socio-economic, demographic and environmental indicators like age (< 15 years, 15-59 years and 60 and above), sex (male/female), educational attainment (no education, up to primary, up to secondary and higher), marital status (never married, currently married and widowed/ divorced/ separated/ disserted), place of residence (rural/ urban), wealth Index (poorest, poorer, middle, richer, richest), frequency of smoke inside house (never, less than daily and daily), type of fuel used for cooking (non- solid and solid), presence of separate room for cooking (yes/no), material of floor, wall and roof (natural, rudimentary and finished), number of people sleeping in a room (< 3 persons, 3 to 4, 5 to 6, 7 & above), shared toilet (no/yes) and potable water(yes/no).

Statistical analysis

As the first step in the analysis, the study considered the prevalence of tuberculosis (TB) by background characteristics and then by household environment risk factors. This was followed by an estimation of the adjusted effects of the variables in the household environment, along with individual characteristics, on tuberculosis for the members in a household by using binary logistic regression model. The binary response (1 = presence of TB, 0 = absence of TB) for each respondent was related to a set of categorical predictors, X, by a *'logit'* link function:

$$\text{logit}\,[P(Y = 1)] = ß0 + ß^{*}X + \epsilon$$

The parameter ***ß0*** estimates the log odds of TB for the reference group, while ***ß*** estimates the maximum likelihood, the differential log odds of TB associated with the set of predictors X, as compared to the reference group and ϵ represents the residuals in the model.

All the estimates and standard errors were adjusted for the multistage sampling design and clustering at the primary sampling unit and were weighted at the state level to give results that are unbiased and representative of the population. The statistical analysis was done in MS-Excel and STATA 13 software (Stata Corp, College Station, Texas).

Results

Prevalence of tuberculosis by background characteristics

It is seen that the prevalence of Tuberculosis (TB) varies according to different background characteristics, such as age, sex, educational attainment, marital status, place of residence and wealth index (Table 1). The overall prevalence of TB in India was 0.32%. It was found to be the highest among elderly people (0.9%). The prevalence of TB was also found to be higher in males (0.4%) than females (0.2%). Education has a significant association with TB. The prevalence of TB varied with educational attainment — people without education had the highest prevalence of TB (0.4%), while it was lowest among the people had higher education (0.04%). Those living in rural areas showed a higher prevalence of TB (0.34%) than those in urban places. As expected, people belonging to the most deprived (poorest wealth quintile) had the highest prevalence of TB (0.53%).

The physical environment within the household is closely associated with TB. Environmental risk factors, such as smoke inside the house, type of fuel used for cooking, separate kitchen, the material used for floors, roof and walls, number of persons sleeping in a room, sharing of toilets with other households, and potable water are strongly associated with TB as shown in Table 2. The prevalence of TB was found to be higher in households where there was regularly (daily) exposure to smoke within the house (0.4%). It is also seen that there is a strong association of the fuel used for cooking with Tuberculosis. Prevalence of TB was found to be higher in households using solid fuel for cooking (0.37%), and those that did not have a separate area for cooking (0.39%).

Predictably, persons living in poor quality dwellings have a higher risk of Tuberculosis. The prevalence of TB was higher — respectively 0.42, 0.41, and 0.51% —in households with mud (or other naturally available material) floors, walls, and roofs. TB was considerably higher (0. 34%) in households that share toilets with other households, and those not using potable water (0.4%).

Table 1 Prevalence of Tuberculosis among household members by some selected background characteristics in India

Variables	Prevalence (%)	Number (N)
Age		
< 15 Years	0.06	847,380
15-59 years	0.33	1,737,560
60 & above	0.88	283,648
Sex		
Male	0.39	1,442,520
Female	0.22	1,426,523
Educational attainment		
No education	0.38	2,184,972
Up to primary	0.07	339,346
Up to secondary	0.08	325,790
Higher	0.04	18,688
Marital Status		
Never Married	0.16	596,279
Currently Married	0.45	1,373,339
Widowed/ Divorced/ Separated/ Disserted	0.68	167,581
Place of residence		
Urban	0.25	804,654
Rural	0.34	2,064,389
Wealth Index		
Poorest	0.53	609,790
Poorer	0.36	625,444
Middle	0.28	586,096
Richer	0.22	535,071
Richest	0.14	512,642
Overall	0.32	2,869,043

Table 2 Household environmental risk factors for Tuberculosis in India

Variables	Prevalence (%)	Number (N)
Smoke inside the house		
Never	0.26	1,462,050
Less than Daily	0.32	447,857
Daily	0.39	959,136
Fuel used for cooking		
Non-solid Fuel	0.21	1,023,975
Solid Fuel	0.37	1,601,004
Separate kitchen		
No	0.39	933,119
Yes	0.23	1,425,393
Material of floor		
Natural	0.42	1,139,694
Rudimentary	0.26	218,339
Finished	0.24	1,508,524
Material of wall		
Natural	0.41	568,060
Rudimentary	0.42	306,853
Finished	0.27	1,985,085
Material of roof		
Natural	0.51	206,653
Rudimentary	0.39	142,116
Finished	0.29	2,422,173
Number of persons sleeping per room		
< 3 persons	0.33	2,124,315
3 to 4	0.23	655,126
5 to 6	0.12	73,421
7 & above	0.18	15,766
Share toilet with other household		
No	0.23	1,508,130
Yes	0.34	246,380
Potability of water		
No	0.35	1,725,274
Yes	0.23	1,143,306
Overall	0.32	2,868,580

Comparison of state wise prevalence (number of persons suffering from TB per 100,000 usual residents of households) is shown in Fig. 1. Data from two rounds of National Family Health Survey (NFHS-3 and NFHS-4) was used. It is seen that there is a significant increase in the prevalence of TB in the states of Jammu & Kashmir, Nagaland, Karnataka, and Kerala. In the other states, a sharp decline is seen.

Table 3 presents the result of logistic regression, which helps in the understanding of the factors associated with the prevalence of TB in the Indian population. Two models were used to assess the factors: Model-1 is concerned with socio-economic variables (including age, sex, educational attainment, marital status, place of residence, wealth index), while Model-2 considers variables related to the household environment (smoke inside house, fuel used for cooking, separate kitchen, the material of floor, material of wall, the material of roof, a room used for sleeping, sharing of toilets with other households and use of potability of water) in addition to those considered in Model-1.

The adjusted effects, as estimated from Model-1, show that age, sex, educational attainment, marital status, place of residence, wealth index have a statistically significant association with Tuberculosis. Older people in the age group of 16–59 years (OR = 1.6; CI = 1.3-2.0) and those aged 60 years and above (OR = 3.1; CI = 2.4-3.8) are more prone to getting Tuberculosis as compared to individuals age less than 15 years. Females are less likely (OR = 0.51;

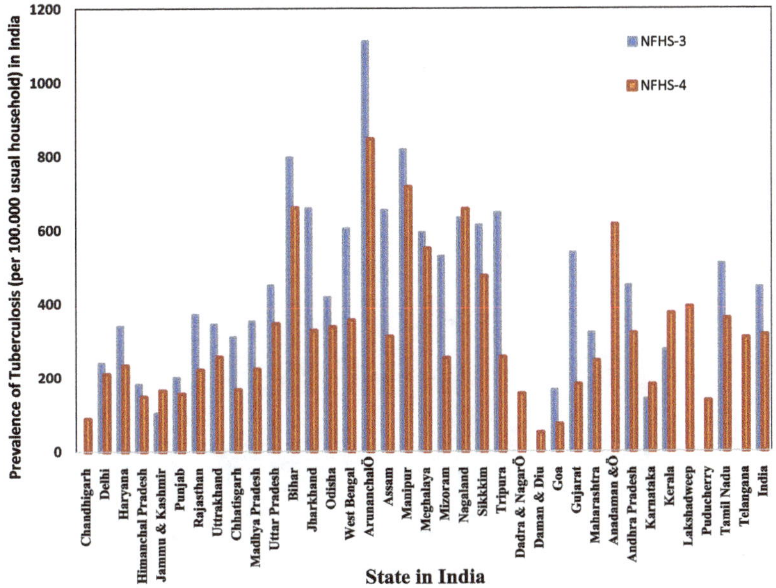

Fig. 1 Number of persons per 100,000 usual household residents suffering from any tuberculosis by state, India (2005-06, 2015-16)

CI = 0.5-0.6) to get Tuberculosis than males. It is also seen that educational attainment has a strong association with TB. Persons who had studied up to the secondary (OR = 0.5; CI = 0.4-0.6) level and higher (OR = 0.4; CI = 0.2-0.7) are seen to be at lower risk of getting tuberculosis as compared with those counterparts who had no education. Further, people living in urban areas are more prone to the infection then rural people. As anticipated, poor people are 78% more likely to get TB than the people belonging to the richest wealth quintile in India.

The variables associated with the household environment, which are considered in Model-2, also show statistically significant association with Tuberculosis. Persons who are regularly (daily) exposed to second-hand smoke inside their homes are more prone to getting tuberculosis (OR = 1.49; CI = 1.39-1.61) as compared those who are not. Households that use solid fuel for cooking and do not have a separate kitchen are more prone to infection with tuberculosis than those using non-solid fuel for cooking and having a separate room for cooking. The results are not statistically significant. Further, households having a finished wall (OR = 0.7; CI = 0.6-0.8) are less likely to get TB than those with mud walls. The predictor variables such as roof material and room for sleeping also have an association with TB; however, the results are not statistically significant. Households that shared their toilet with other households are more likely to get Tuberculosis (OR = 1.2; CI = 1.1-1.4) as compared to those that do not. Further, households that are not using potable water (or are not treating water to make it safer for consumption) are ten times more likely to get Tuberculosis than the households that use potable water.

Discussion

The World Health Organization has raised many important issues during discussions in various International fora. Among these, public health, environmental and social determinants of health are the most crucial. WHO (2017) has estimated that about 12.6 million deaths each year are attributable to morbid environments — almost one-fourth of total global deaths [18, 19]. Environmental risk factors, such as air, water and soil pollution, chemical exposures, climate change and ultraviolet radiation, contribute to more than 100 diseases and injuries. The objective of present study was to examine the association between household living environment and prevalence of Tuberculosis in India. The results demonstrate the effects of household environmental factors on Tuberculosis (TB), which suggests that the likelihood of the presence of self-reported TB is higher for elderly respondent i.e., those above 60 years of age. The elderly are 3.1 times more prone to tuberculosis. This finding is found to be consistent with the findings of other reported studies, suggesting that are difficulties in diagnosing the presence of TB in the elderly because only a small proportion of them suffer from respiratory disorders. Additionally, factors like tobacco use, low socio-economic status, previous disease, longer delays in seeking medical attention and very high rates of adverse reactions during treatment exacerbates the likelihood of TB in the Indian elderly [20]. Elderly suffer from multiple morbidities along with TB face a higher burden of TB, in terms of both health and monetary hardships. The 2010 report of Global Burden of Disease estimates that, globally, 57% of all tuberculosis deaths occur

Table 3 Adjusted effect of household environment and other selected variables on tuberculosis among member of household in India

Variables	Model-1		Model-2	
	Odds Ratio	95% C.I.	Odds Ratio	95% C.I.
Age				
< 15 Years®				
15-59 years	1.58*	1.27- 1.97	1.39	1.00-1.91
60 & above	3.06*	2.44-3.84	2.94*	2.11-4.09
Sex				
Male®				
Female	0.51*	0.48-0.53	0.58*	0.54-0.62
Educational attainment				
No education®				
Up to primary	1.05	0.68-1.63	1.25	0.66-2.38
Up to secondary	0.51*	0.44-0.60	0.61*	0.49-0.76
Higher	0.40*	0.24-0.68		
Marital Status				
Never Married®				
Currently Married	1.87*	1.74-2.02	1.58*	1.41-1.76
Widowed/ Divorced/ Separated/ Disserted	2.29*	2.07-2.53	1.80*	1.54-2.10
Place of residence				
Urban®				
Rural	0.82*	0.77-0.87	0.86*	0.79-0.93
Wealth Index				
Poorest®				
Poorer	0.70*	0.67-0.74	0.68*	0.59-0.78
Middle	0.54*	0.51-0.57	0.55*	0.47-0.64
Richer	0.40*	0.37-0.43	0.43*	0.36-0.52
Richest	0.22*	0.20-0.24	0.26*	0.21-0.32
Smoke inside the house				
Never®				
Less than Daily			1.38*	1.25-1.52
Daily			1.49*	1.39-1.61
Fuel used for cooking				
Non-solid Fuel®				
Solid Fuel			1.03	0.94-1.14
Separate kitchen				
No®				
Yes			0.95	0.88-1.03
Material of floor				
Natural®				
Rudimentary			1.27*	1.13-1.43
Finished			1.12*	1.01-1.25
Material of wall				
Natural®				
Rudimentary			1.07	0.95-1.20
Finished			0.74*	0.66-0.83

Table 3 Adjusted effect of household environment and other selected variables on tuberculosis among member of household in India *(Continued)*

Variables	Model-1		Model-2	
	Odds Ratio	95% C.I.	Odds Ratio	95% C.I.
Material of roof				
Natural®				
Rudimentary			0.82	0.66-1.02
Finished			0.90	0.79-1.04
Room used for sleeping				
< 3 person®				
3 to 4			0.95	0.88-1.03
5 to 6			0.87	0.70-1.09
7 & above			0.83	0.49-1.41
Share toilet with other household				
No®				
Yes			1.23*	1.13-1.36
Potability of water				
No®				
Yes			1.1*	1.03-1.18

Note: ® Reference category, *$P < 0.05$

among people aged 50 years or above, with more than half of these deaths in those aged more than 65 years of age. Estimates from studies suggest that around 51% of TB Disability-Adjusted Life Years (DALYs) are contributed by patients aged 50 years and older [21]. The major contributing factor is the increased level of susceptibility to infectious diseases and weakened immune system amongst the elderly [22–24]. Therefore, this group requires special attention which should include early screening and initiation of treatment, as well as proper nutritional supervision.

The results also show that the prevalence of TB was higher among males than females. Evidence from previous studies are also consistent with this finding. One of the major reasons could be that Indian men are more exposed to smoking and drinking [3]. Further, men are expected to be in greater contact with people who suffer from active Tuberculosis (TB) than women. While the World Health Organization (WHO) stated that the global male to female prevalence ratio of tuberculosis (TB) is in favour of males, which further widens with increasing age [25, 26]. However, today, TB is the leading cause of death for women globally [27]. The Sustainable Development Goals (SDGs) have stressed on gender equality and health, supported by specific targets to eliminate make available gender-specific data on TB incidence (target 3.3). TB has social stigmas attached to it which affects men and women differently. Studies in India suggest that women suffering from TB are ostracized and ill-treated. The consequences include social isolation, reduced chances of marriage, rejection, and harassment by in-laws and spouse. In the case of men, the likely consequences are social isolation, loss of income and economic hardships [9, 27, 28].

Place of residence also has a significant association with Tuberculosis. People living in urban areas are more prone infection than those in rural areas. Extant literature shows rural areas as pockets of TB which is further accelerated by dynamics of knowledge about the disease. These areas are marked by stigmatization, resulting in underutilization of treatment services, delay in diagnosis, and poor treatment fulfillment [29, 30]. Prevalence of TB is also seen to vary with educational attainment. People without education had the highest prevalence of TB. Educational attainment has a strong association with TB. Respondents who had studied up to the secondary level and higher are at a lower risk of getting Tuberculosis as compared to those who had no education.

The likelihood of TB was found to be higher (0.34%) among respondents whose households shared toilet facilities with others, and households with mud walls. TB was considerably higher in households where they usually share their toilet with other households. It was also higher (0.40%, and 1.2 times more likely) in households that did not use potable water. It was calculated that households that shared their toilet with other households are 1.2 times more likely to be infected with Tuberculosis as compared to the households that do not share.

Predictor variables such as the material used in roof and room used for sleeping also have an association with TB. Predictably, it was found that those living in the poor-quality housing (where the material of wall, roof, and the floor is made of mud or other natural material) are at higher risk of Tuberculosis. Prevalence of TB was higher — 0.42, 0.41 and 0.51% respectively in households where the floors, roofs, and walls were made of the mud or natural material. Households with finished walls are 0.7 times as less likely to be infected with TB than households with mud walls. Evidence from the Indian study which shows that ORs for poor-quality housing, toilet facilities and water supply were significant. In multivariate logistic regression analysis, the age, level of education, household crowding, type of housing and water supply in the household was found to be independently and significantly associated with a higher risk of TB [26].

Recent estimates in the World Bank's profile of India's poverty pointed out that one out of five Indian belong to the below poverty line (deprived section of society), or BPL group [31]. As expected, people belonging to the most deprived (the poorest wealth quintile) show the highest prevalence of TB (0.53%). As anticipated, poor people are 78% more likely to get TB than the people in India's richest wealth quintile. Owing to the living and working conditions, it is the impoverished class which is more vulnerable to the disease. Moreover, TB often results in a vicious circle of poverty and illness. Estimates suggest that on average, 20 – 30% of annual household income is lost due to TB [27, 32]. Studies also suggest that newly-diagnosed elderly TB patients are more likely to be lost to follow-up, die, or report drug side effects [33].

Earlier research suggests that the likelihood of TB is higher among respondents who were exposed daily to smoke in their homes. This study found that prevalence of TB was higher (0.40%) in households where there is daily exposure to smoke (0.4%). Households in which the family members are exposed to smoke (second-hand smoke) daily are 1.5 times more prone to getting tuberculosis as compared with households where people do not smoke inside the house. Smoke exposure may be caused by tobacco (from smoking or second-hand smoke), or from the burning of biomass. Similar inferences are also drawn from the present study [9]. Past studies strongly suggest that exposure to cooking smoke considerably increases the risk of tuberculosis in India [3, 10, 34, 35]. Often, women are more exposed to smoke inside household which puts them at greater risk of TB [36].

The risk of tuberculosis is influenced by factors, such as age, sex, nutrition levels (biological factors); tobacco smoking, alcoholism (behavioral factors); poverty, overcrowding and poor housing (socio-economic factors). The environment in which one lives has a major influence on the epidemiology of TB. Factors like exposure to smoke inside the house, exposure to second-hand smoke, number of people in each room (i.e., the crowing index), the material of construction of the house, sanitation facilities affect TB status [3, 37, 38]. There is a higher risk of TB if the households share their toilets and kitchens with people suffering from TB [3, 39]. The study also found the association of cooking fuel and Tuberculosis. Prevalence of TB was found to be higher in households that normally use solid fuel for cooking (0.37%), and those that did not have a separate kitchen for cooking (0.39%). Households using solid fuel for cooking and not having separate kitchen are more prone to TB infection in India than households using non-solid fuel for cooking and having a separate room for a kitchen space. There is also strong evidence that exposure to cooking smoke considerably increases the risk of tuberculosis in India. Because women are more exposed to kitchen smoke, they are more vulnerable to TB [3, 10, 34–36].

The use of a cross-sectional survey to collect data may have underestimated the true prevalence of Tuberculosis. The results of self-reported morbidities could be biased due to subjectivity in responses. Recall bias may also have affected the estimated prevalence of Tuberculosis.

Conclusion

However, the results of the analysis in this study provide compelling evidence that a contaminated household environment increases the risk of Tuberculosis in India. This is why a clean environment must be promoted to eliminate TB, still a significant cause of deaths in India. The study found environmental risk factors for TB, such as smoke inside the house, type of fuel used for cooking, separate kitchen space, floor, wall and roof materials, the number of persons sleeping in a room, sharing of toilets with other households, and non-use of potable water. Besides the environmental factors, individual characteristics like age, sex, educational attainment, marital status, place of residence and wealth index are also strongly associated with TB.

Abbreviations

CEBs: Census Enumeration Blocks; DALYs: Disability-Adjusted Life Years; NFHS: National Family and Health Survey; PSUs: Primary Sampling Units; SDGs: Sustainable Development Goals; TB: Tuberculosis; WHO: World Health Organization

Acknowledgements

Authors are thankful to all the project coordinators of National Family and Health Survey for their relentless efforts in producing such a vital information for community-based estimates of the prevalence of tuberculosis and its correlates.

Authors' contributions

SKS conceived the idea. GCK, SKS and PP designed the experiment and analyzed it, interpreted the results and drafted the manuscript. All the authors read and approved the final manuscript.

Competing interests

The authors declared that they have no competing interests.

Author details

[1]Department of Mathematical Demography & Statistics, International Institute for Population Sciences, Govandi Station Road, Deonar Mumbai 400088, India. [2]International Institute for Population Sciences, Govandi Station Road, Deonar Mumbai 400088, India.

References

1. United Nations sustainable development agenda: United Nations; 2016. Available from: http://www.un.org/sustainabledevelopment/development-agenda/.
2. WHO. Household air pollution and health: WHO; 2016. Available from: http://www.who.int/mediacentre/factsheets/fs292/en/.
3. Mishra VK, Retherford RD, Smith KR. Biomass cooking fuels and prevalence of tuberculosis in India. Available from: http://citeseerx.ist.psu.edu/viewdoc/download?doi=10.1.1.457.3473&rep=rep1&type=pdf.
4. Smith KR. Biofuels, air pollution, and health. Boston: Springer US; 1988. Available from: http://link.springer.com/10.1007/978-1-4613-0891-1.
5. Smith KR. Full-text. Annual review energy environment; 1993. p. 529–66.
6. Epidemiological, social and technical aspects of indoor air pollution from biomass fuel: Geneva; 1992. Available from: http://apps.who.int/iris/bitstream/10665/60069/1/WHO_PEP_92.3A.pdf.
7. IIPS. National family health survey - 4 - 2015-16: India fact sheet; 2015. p. 8.
8. Global Tuberculosis Report 2016. Available from: http://apps.who.int/medicinedocs/en/d/Js23098en/.
9. Singh J, Sankar MM, Kumar S, Gopinath K, Singh N, Mani K, et al. Incidence and prevalence of tuberculosis among household contacts of pulmonary tuberculosis patients in a Peri-urban population of South Delhi, India. PLoS One. 2013;8(7):1–11.
10. Jindal SK. Relationship of household air pollution from solid fuel combustion with tuberculosis? Indian J Med Res. 2014;140(2):167–70. Available from: http://www.pubmedcentral.nih.gov/articlerender.fcgi?artid=PMC4216490.
11. Slama K, Chiang C-Y, Enarson DA, Hassmiller K, Fanning A, Gupta P, et al. Tobacco and tuberculosis: a qualitative systematic review and meta-analysis. Int J Tuberc Lung Dis. 11(10):1049–61. Available from: http://citeseerx.ist.psu.edu/viewdoc/download?doi=10.1.1.381.7362&rep=rep1&type=pdf.
12. Kolappan C, Gopi PG, Subramani R, Narayanan PR. Selected biological and behavioural risk factors associated with pulmonary tuberculosis. Int J Tuberc Lung Dis. 11(9):999–1003. Available from: https://www.cap-tb.org/sites/default/files/documents/Gender.RiskFactors.Chennai.India.IJTLD.pdf.
13. Kim MJ, Kim HR, Hwang SS, Kim YW, Han SK, Shim YS, et al. Prevalence and its predictors of Extrapulmonary involvement in patients with pulmonary tuberculosis. J Korean Med Sci. 2009;24:237–41. Available from: https://www.ncbi.nlm.nih.gov/pmc/articles/PMC2672122/pdf/jkms-24-237.pdf.
14. Bhat J, Rao VG, Sharma RK, Muniyandi M, Yadav R, Bhondley MK. Investigation of the risk factors for pulmonary tuberculosis: a case- control study among Saharia tribe in Gwalior district, Madhya Pradesh, India. Available from: http://www.icmr.nic.in/ijmr/2017/july/0715.pdf.
15. Ananthakrishnan R, Kumar K, Ganesh M, Kumar AMV, Krishnan N, Swaminathan S, et al. The profile and treatment outcomes of the older (aged 60 years and above) tuberculosis patients in Tamilnadu, South India. PLoS One. 2013;8(7):6–11.
16. Prüss-Üstün A, Bonjour S, Corvalán C. The impact of the environment on health by country: a meta-synthesis. Environ Health. 2008;7(1):7. Available from: http://ehjournal.biomedcentral.com/articles/10.1186/1476-069X-7-7.
17. Narasimhan P, Wood J, MacIntyre CR, Mathai D. Risk factors for tuberculosis. Pulm Med. 2013;2013:1–11. Available from: http://www.ncbi.nlm.nih.gov/pubmed/23476764.
18. World Health Organization (WHO). Burden of NCDs and their risk factors in India (Excerpted from Global Status Report on NCDs -2014, vol. 2; 2014.
19. WHO. Global action plan for the prevention and control of noncommunicable diseases 2013-2020. World Health Organization. 2013. p. 102 Available from: http://apps.who.int/iris/bitstream/10665/94384/1/9789241506236_eng.pdf.
20. Challenges of dealing with TB in older people | HelpAge international. Available from: http://www.helpage.org/blogs/prakash-tyagi-869/challenges-of-dealing-with-tb-in-older-people-300/.
21. Negin J, Abimbola S, Marais BJ. Tuberculosis among older adults - time to take notice. Int J Infect Dis 2015;32:135–137. Available from: https://doi.org/10.1016/j.ijid.2014.11.018.
22. Byng-Maddick R, Noursadeghi M. Does tuberculosis threaten our ageing populations? BMC Infect Dis 2016;16(1):1–5. Available from: https://doi.org/10.1186/s12879-016-1451-0.
23. Stervbo U, Meier S, Mälzer JN, Baron U, Bozzetti C, Jürchott K, et al. Effects of aging on human leukocytes (part I): immunophenotyping of innate immune cells. Age (Omaha). 2015;37. Available from: https://www.ncbi.nlm.nih.gov/pubmed/26324155
24. Mahbub S, Brubaker AL, Kovacs EJ. Aging of the innate immune system: an update. Curr Immunol Rev. 2011;7(1):104–15. Available from: http://www.pubmedcentral.nih.gov/articlerender.fcgi?artid=3066013&tool=pmcentrez&rendertype=abstract
25. Boum Y, Atwine D, Orikiriza P, Assimwe J, Page AL, Mwanga-Amumpaire J, et al. Male gender is independently associated with pulmonary tuberculosis among sputum and non-sputum producers people with presumptive tuberculosis in southwestern Uganda. BMC Infect Dis. 2014;14(1):1–8.
26. Global Tuberculosis Report 2017. Geneva; 2017. Available from: http://www.who.int/tb/publications/global_report/Exec_Summary_13Nov2017.pdf?ua=1.
27. United Nations Development Programme. Discussion Paper: Gender and Tuberculosis. 2015;(December):14. Available from: https://www.undp.org/content/dam/undp/library/HIV-AIDS/Gender%20HIV%20and%20Health/Gender%20and%20TB%20UNDP%20Discussion%20Paper%20(1).pdf.
28. Raviglione MC, Uplekar MW. WHO's new stop TB strategy. Lancet. 2006; 367(9514):952–5.
29. Mushtaq MU, Majrooh MA, Ahmad W, Rizwan M, Luqman MQ, Aslam MJ, et al. Knowledge, attitudes and practices regarding tuberculosis in two districts of Punjab, Pakistan. Int J Tuberc Lung Dis. 2010;14(3):303–10.
30. World Health Organization. Stop TB Partnership. Available from: www.stoptb.org/.
31. Muniyandi M, Ramachandran R. Socioeconomic inequalities of tuberculosis in India. Expert Opin Pharmacother. 2008;9(10):1623–8. Available from: http://www.tandfonline.com/doi/full/10.1517/14656566.9.10.1623.
32. Singh SK, Tiwari KK. Clinicoradiological profile of lower Lung field tuberculosis cases among young adult and elderly people in a teaching Hospital of Madhya Pradesh, India. J Trop Med. 2015;2015(4).
33. Velayutham BR, Nair D, Chandrasekaran V, Raman B, Sekar G, Watson B, Charles N, Malaisamy M, Thomas A, Swaminathan S. Profile and response to anti-tuberculosis treatment among elderly tuberculosis patients treated under the TB Control programme in South India. PloS One. 2014;9(3): e88045.
34. Kan X, Chiang CY, Enarson DA, Chen W, Yang J, Chen G. Indoor solid fuel use and tuberculosis in China: a matched case-control study. BMC Public Health. 2011;11(1):498.
35. Behera D, Aggarwal G. Domestic cooking fuel exposure and tuberculosis in Indian women. Indian J Chest Dis Allied Sci. 2009;52:139–43.
36. Singh AL, Jamal S. Unhealthy cooking and prevalence of tuberculosis in Indian women: a case study. J Environ Protect. 2012;3(07):648-56.
37. Clark M, Riben P, Nowgesic E. The association of housing density, isolation and tuberculosis in Canadian first nations communities. Int J Epidemiol. 2002;31(5):940–5.
38. Chakraborty AK. Epidemiology of tuberculosis: current status in India. Indian J Med Res. 2004;120(4):248–76.
39. Guwatudde D, Nakakeeto M, Jones-Lopez EC, Maganda A, Chiunda A, Mugerwa RD, et al. Tuberculosis in household contacts of infectious cases in Kampala. Uganda Am J Epidemiol. 2003;158(9):887–98.

22

Delays to treatment initiation is associated with tuberculosis treatment outcomes among patients on directly observed treatment short course in Southwest Ethiopia

Abyot Asres[1,3*], Degu Jerene[2] and Wakgari Deressa[3]

Abstract

Background: Despite reported long delays to initiate anti-TB treatment and poor outcomes in different parts of Ethiopia and elsewhere, evidences on association between the delay and treatment outcomes are scanty.

Methods: A follow up study among 735 new TB cases registered at health facilities in districts of southwest Ethiopia was conducted from January 2015 to June 2016. Patients reported days elapsed between onset of illness and treatment commencement of 30 days cutoff was considered to ascertain exposure. Thus, those elapsed beyond 30 days to initiate anti-TB treatment since onset of illness were exposed and otherwise non-exposed. The cases were followed until earliest outcome was observed. Treatment outcomes was ascertained as per the World Health Organization standard definitions and dichotomized into 'successful' when cured or treatment completed and 'unsuccessful' when lost to follow-up or died or treatment failure. Bivariate and multiple log-binomial models were fitted to identify predictors of unsuccessful outcomes.

Results: The overall treatment success among the treatment cohort was 89.7% (88.4% vs. 94.2%, $p = 0.01$ respectively among those initiated treatment beyond and within of 30 days of onset of illness. Higher risk of unsuccessful outcome was predicted by treatment initiation beyond 30 days of onset [Adjusted Relative Risk (ARR) = 1.92, 95%CI:1.30, 2.81], HIV co-infection (ARR = 2.18, 95%CI:1.47, 3.25) and received treatment at hospital (ARR = 3.73, 95%CI:2.23, 6.25). On the other hand, lower risk of unsuccessful outcome was predicted by weight gain (ARR = 0.40, 95%CI:0.19, 0.83) and sputum smear negative conversion (ARR = 0.17,95% CI:0.09, 0.33) at the end of second month treatment.

Conclusion: Higher risk of unsuccessful outcome is associated with prolonged days elapsed between onset of illness and treatment commencement. Hence, promotion of early care seeking, improving diagnostic and case holding efficiencies of health facilities and TB/HIV collaborative interventions can reduce risk of unsuccessful outcome.

Keywords: TB, Delay, Follow-up, Log-binomial, Ethiopia

* Correspondence: abyotasres@gmail.com
[1]Department of Public Health, College of Health Sciences, Mizan Tepi University, Mizan Aman, Ethiopia
[3]Department of Preventive Medicine, School of Public Health, College of Health Sciences, Addis Ababa University, Addis Ababa, Ethiopia
Full list of author information is available at the end of the article

Background

Despite the fact that nearly all cases can be cured, tuberculosis (TB) remained to be among the major global public health problems. Globally, 10.4 million incident cases, of whom 6.1million notified and 1.4 million deaths were estimated to occur in 2015 [1]. Thus, the latest strategy, "End TB" has been designed in line with the sustainable development goals (SDG). The strategy aimed at reaching 90% case detection and treatment success by 2025 [2].

Tuberculosis has been recognized as a major public health problem in Ethiopia and efforts to control the disease has begun since early 1960s [3]. Nonetheless, TB has remained among the major public health problems in the country [4]. Accordingly, Ethiopia has been listed among the 14 TB, TB/HIV (Human Immunodeficiency Virus) and Multi-Drug Resistant TB (MDR TB) High Burden Countries (HBC) [1]. The first national TB prevalence survey conducted in 2011 revealed smear positive pulmonary TB(PTB) prevalence of 108/100,000; of which 55% were not detected before the survey [5] . In 2015, about 205,463 new cases [6] and 29,000 deaths were estimated to occur in the country [1] when only 125,801 (61%) were notified to National TB control Program (NTP) [6].

The ultimate goal of any TB control program is reduction of morbidity and mortality among patients and stop transmission through curing infectious cases [7]. Hence early detection and treatment of cases have been a pillar for the end TB strategy [2]. Nonetheless, studies from different parts of Ethiopia reported patients elapse too long time to initiate care seeking and treatment. TB patients elapse median of 30 [8, 9] in Northern Ethiopia and 63 days in Bale [10] to initiate care seeking and median of six in Addis Ababa [11] and 34 days in Bale [10] to commence treatment.

Delays to diagnosis and treatment of TB result in more serious illness, increased length of infectiousness and poor treatment outcomes including mortality and drug resistance [12–16]. It is also reported that the high mortality rate among people living with HIV is also partly explained by delays to TB treatment [16, 17]. In contrast, a study in Tel Aviv reported no association between treatment success and delay in treatment initiation [18].

Achieving high cure rates help to reduce transmission of TB and attract the great majority of existing cases to seek treatment [19]. As a result, treatment of TB is beyond treating an individual patient, rather it is considered as a public health intervention. Globally, 83% of cases successfully completed their treatment in 2015,and effective diagnosis and treatment of TB saved an estimated 49 million lives between 2000 through 2015 [1]. In Ethiopia, 89% (range: 69%–95%)of treatment cohort in different regions attained successful TB treatment [6]. However, cure rates of 81% (range: 38% to 92%) [4] across regions of the country have been reported.

Studies uncovered that patient demographics, clinical, bacteriologic and HIV co morbidity were associated with unsuccessful TB treatment outcomes [20–23]. Despite the prevailing long delays to initiate anti-TB treatment and poor outcomes in different parts of Ethiopia and elsewhere, evidences on effect of the delay on treatment outcomes are scanty. Hence, this study assessed effect of delayed treatment initiation on outcomes of TB. Evidences on the association between treatment delay and outcome is crucial to realize the targets of ending TB epidemic [2].

Methods

Study setting

The study was conducted in 14 health facilities (three hospitals and 11 health centers) in three zones of Southern Nation, Nationalities, and Peoples Region (SNNPR) of Ethiopia. The SNNPR is one of the nine Regional States in the country with an estimated 15.7million population in 2017 [24]. The three study Zones (Bench Maji, Kaffa and Sheka) are located at the southwestern part of Ethiopia bordering South Sudan and harbor an estimated 1.8million peoples [24]. The zones (an administrative unit that liaison *woredas* with the region) are organized into four town administrations and 26 *woredas*(administrative unit equivalent to districts). At the time of the study, three hospitals and 65 health centers were providing TB Directly Observed Treatment Short course (DOTS) services. However, all the hospitals and only 25 health centers were providing TB/HIV collaborative interventions [25].

Diagnosis and treatment of all forms of TB across Ethiopia has been based on national TB control guidelines that specify case definitions, diagnostic and treatment standards [26]. Thus all TB cases enrolled for this study were diagnosed using either sputum smear microcopy or clinical signs aided with x-ray. Those cases with sputum smear positive were labeled as smear positive pulmonary TB and negatives were smear negative pulmonary TB. Diagnosis of smear negative and extrapulmonary TB were made using diagnostic algorithm recommended by the national guideline [26]. Detail definitions for each cases presented in definition of terms section. Previously, TB diagnosis and treatment had been limited to public hospitals and health centers, but public private mix (PPM) DOTS and community DOTS to public health posts have been recently introduced. Thus, in 2011, 92% of public hospitals and 95% of health centers, 2100 health posts and 317 PPM–DOTS centers were providing DOTS based diagnosis and/or treatment of TB in the country [27].

Study design and sampling

A prospective cohort study among new TB cases was carried out from January 2015 through June 2016. The treatment cohorts were recruited from baseline survey designed to determine delays to initiate treatment. Since no standard cutoff point for delay to treatment, a clinical sound cutoff of 30 days was used to ascertain exposure. Thus TB cases who elapsed beyond 30 days to initiate treatment since onset of illness were labeled as exposed and those started treatment within 30 days of onset of illness were non exposed. Then the cases were followed until earliest treatment outcome. The sample size was computed using StatCalc program of EpiInfo at 95% significance level, 80% power, expected outcome (unsuccessful of 3% [15] among those delayed beyond 30 days) to detect a difference of 7% with those initiated treatment earlier and considering design effect of 1.5 and 10% lost to follow up a total of 640 cases were required., However, the sample size for assessing predictors of delaycomputed using the same procedure provided a total of 802 new cases . Hence, the same cases were followed for the outcome; the larger sample of 802 was taken the final sample size.

The sample was proportionally allocated to the zones, *woredas* and health facilities based on TB cases reported during the year preceding the study. Finally, consecutive consenting cases from were prospectively enrolled until the required sample was reached and followed until completion of the six-month treatment or earliest outcome. During the enrollment those new cases, older than 18 years of age, on intensive phase treatment were included and those transferred out and died before the interview were excluded from the study.

Data collection

A structured questionnaire adapted from tools used elsewhere [5, 28] and standard TB register book [26] was used to gather the data. Besides, data abstraction checklist was prepared to draw clinical, bacteriologic and treatment outcomes of the patients from TB register. The questionnaire was translated into national language (*Amharic*) spoken by almost all residents in the study area. Ten diploma graduate nurse data collectors and three public health specialist supervisors were recruited and trained for 3 days. The training included description of questionnaire, interviewing techniques and pretest among TB cases on DOTS at nearby health facilities not included in the study. Finally, eligible cases were traced from the unit TB register and interviewed for sociodemographic, health care seeking, and treatment practices.

Exposure ascertainment

The main exposure variable was delays to treatment measured by days elapsed between onsets of illness to initiation of anti-TB treatment (total delay). The total delay comprises both patient and provider delays. Patient delay was assessed by asking patients to recall and estimate date or number of days elapsed between onset of TB constitutional symptoms such as cough, fever, night sweats, chest pain, weight loss and loss of appetite until formal care seeking. Similarly, provider delay was estimated by asking date or number of days elapsed between first formal health care facility visits to anti-TB treatment initiation. Finally, total delay was computed as a sum of patient and provider delay or number of days elapsed between onsets of illness to initiation of anti-TB treatment. Since no standard cut off for delay, a clinically sound cut off of 30 days delay was taken to define exposure status. Therefore, cases who delayed beyond 30 days were categorized as exposed and those initiated within 30 days were grouped as non-exposed.

Outcome ascertainment

The main outcome variable was treatment outcome which was ascertained based on standard definitions [26, 29]. Accordingly, outcomes were categorized into successful when the TB patient completed treatment with or without evidence of cure and unsuccessful when died or lost to follow-up or treatment failure. So that, coding was made as unsuccessful outcomes = 1 and successful = 0.

Data processing

Data were entered in to Epi-Data V 3.5 and processed on SPSS version 21 and/or STATA version 13. The data were described using frequencies, proportions, mean, median, inter-quartile range and standard deviation as appropriate. Both the baseline and follow-up data were described and compared across the exposed and non-exposed groups. Categorical variables were compared using chi square test and numeric variables using independent and paired t tests as appropriate.

Information provision adequacy during treatment initiation was assessed based on 15 items constructed from TB treatment guidelines. The internal consistency of the items was checked by Cronbach's Alpha (α) =0.87). A score of one is given for proper information and zero otherwise. So that information adequacy index was computed and labeled adequate when above median and inadequate when below median scores.

Association between the exposure (exposed vs, non-exposed) and outcome (unsuccessful vs. successful) was determined by log-binomial regression. Accordingly, bivariate and multiple log-binomial regression models were fitted to estimate crude and adjusted relative risk (RR) of unsuccessful outcome. In all the statistical tests, significance was judged at p value < 0.05.

Ethical issues

The study was ethically approved by the Institutional Review Board (IRB) of college of Health Sciences at Addis Ababa University. Informed written consent was sought from patients before the two interviews, during the intensive phase and end of treatment.

Definition of terms

- New case those never been treated for TB or have taken anti-TB drugs for less than 1 month.
- Smear positive PTB is a patient with at least two sputum smear examinations positive for Acid Fast Bacilli (AFB) by direct microscopy.
- Smear negative pulmonary TB is a patient having symptoms suggestive of TB with at least three initial smear examinations negative for AFB by direct microscopy, and no response to a course of broad-spectrum antibiotics, and again three negative smear examinations by direct microscopy and radiological abnormalities consistent with pulmonary tuberculosis, and decision by a clinician to treat with a full course of anti- tuberculosis
- Extra pulmonary TB is TB in organs other than the lungs, proven by histo-pathological evidence from a biopsy, Or based on strong clinical evidence consistent with active EPTB and the decision by a physician to treat with a full course of anti-TB therapy.
- Cured: A bacteriologically confirmed pulmonary TB case at the beginning of treatment who was smear or culture-negative at last month of treatment and on at least one previous occasion.
- Treatment completed: A TB patient who completed treatment without evidence of failure BUT with no record to show that sputum smear or culture results in the last month of treatment and on at least one previous occasion were negative
- Treatment failure: TB patient whose sputum smear or culture is positive at month 5 or later during treatment.
- Died: TB patient who dies for any reason during the course of treatment.
- Lost to follow up: TB patient interrupted treatment for 2 or more consecutive months.
- Treatment outcome not evaluated TB patient for whom no treatment outcome is assigned including cases "transferred out" to another treatment unit.

Results

Profile of study participants

A total of 735 (91.6%) of TB cases required were enrolled from 11 health centers and 3 hospitals. The rest of cases 67(8.4%) were not retrieved due to refusals (9), inability to respond (3) and end of the survey time (55). Of the cases 574 (78.4%) and 161(21.9%) had initiated anti-TB treatment within and above 30 days of onset of illness, respectively. Of the cases enrolled, 699 (95.1%) had documented treatment outcome and analyzed (Fig. 1).

Baseline sociodemographic characteristics of study participants

The median age [inter-quartile range (IQR)] and of the cases was 27(20–37) years. Among the cases, 52.9% and 29.4% had completed elementary school and involved in subsistence farming respectively (Table 1).

Care seeking and treatment practices

Patients initially presented to healthcare facility after a median (IQR) 25(15–36) days (patient delay) since the onset of illness. Diagnosis of 623(84.7%) of the cases were made after an average (±SD) of 3.6(±2.4) visits to an average (±SD) of 2.2(±1.2) healthcare facilities at which time the patients had been treated with different medicines. The rest of the cases, 112(15.3%) were diagnosed at their first visit to the first health facilities. Thus diagnosis and initiation of anti-TB treatment took a median (IQR) of 22(9–48) days (provider delay) since the first visit to health care facilities. Generally, a median (IQR) 55(32–100) days (total delay) had been elapsed to initiate treatment since the onset of illness. Of the total cases, 373(50.7% were smear positive pulmonary in whom diagnosis was bacteriologicaly confirmed using sputum smear microscopy. All of the cases were offered HIV screening test, of whom 68 (9.3%) tested positive (95% CI: 7.2%–11.3%)). Of those TB/HIV co infected cases, 27(39.7%) and 32(47.1%) were respectively receiving antiretroviral therapy (ART) and Cotrimoxazole Prophylactic Therapy (CPT)(Table 2).

Follow-up and treatment outcomes

After initiation of treatment, patients had undergone weight and sputum smear monitoring as per the recommended schedules. Accordingly, 501(68.2%), 266(36.2%) and 239(32.5%) of the cases had documented weight at end of second, fifth and sixth months of treatment respectively. Thus, a statistically significant difference in mean weights were observed between baseline and end of second month ($t_{df=500} = 13.94$, $p < 0.001$), between sixth month and baseline weight ($t_{238} = 11.81$, $P < 0.001$). On the other hand, among those smear positive pulmonary TB cases (373(50.7%)) eligible for monitoring of sputum smear, 231(61.9%), 200(53.6%) and 178(47.5%) had documented sputum smear result at end of second, fifth and sixth months of treatment respectively. So, among those with documented follow-up sputum result, 225 (97.4%) from both groups converted to negatives at the end of second month treatment $p = 0.5$) (Table 3).

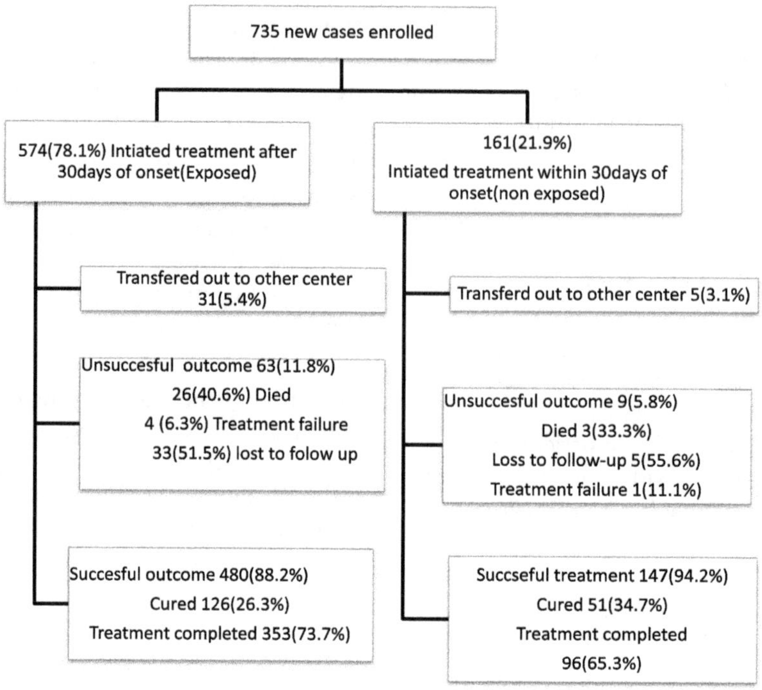

Fig. 1 Flow chart of exposure and outcome ascertainment of TB cases Southwest Ethiopia,January 2015 to June 2016

Table 1 Socidemographic characteristics and delays to treatment in southwest Ethiopia January to December 2015

Variable		Total delay(days)		*P* value	Total N(%)
		> 30 (Exposed) *N* = 574 n(%)	<=30 (Non exposed) *N* = 161 n(%)		
Gender	Male	345(60.1)	102(63.4)	0.6	447(60.8)
	Female	229(39.9)	59(36.6)		288(39.2)
Age group (years)	18–34	389(67.8)	114(70.8)	0.04	503(68.4)
	35–65	173(30.1)	43(26.7)		216(29.4)
	> 65	12(2.1)	4(2.5)		16(2.2)
Residence	Urban	280(48.9)	88(54.7)	0.7	368(50.1)
	Rural	294(51.1)	73(45.3)		367(49.9)
Marital status	Never married	208(36.2)	67(41.6)	0.3	275(37.4)
	Currently married	315(54.8)	89(55.3)		404(55.0)
	Divorced/widowed	51(9)	5(3.1)		56(7.6)
Educational status	Illiterate	168(29.3)	44(27.3)	0.2	212(28.8)
	Completed primary	309(53.8)	80(49.7)		389(52.9)
	Secondary & above	97(16.9)	37(23.0)		134(18.2)
Occupation	Employed	134(23.3)	38(23.6)	0.01	172(23.4)
	Farming	163(28.4)	53(32.9)		216(29.4)
	Unskilled work [a]	42(7.3)	9(5.6)		51(6.9)
	Dependents [b]	235(40.9)	61(37.9)		296(40.3)

[a]housemaid, daily laborer, [b]students, housewife

Table 2 Patient characteristics and time delays to treatment southwest Ethiopia January to December 2015

Variable		Total delay(days)			Total
		> 30 (Exposed) *N* = 574	<=30(non exposed) *N* = 161		
		n(%)	n(%)	*P* value	n(%)
Type of TB	Pulmonary positive	277(48.3)	96(59.6)	0.02	373(50.7)
	Pulmonary negative	167(29.1)	46(28.6)		213(29.0)
	Extra pulmonary	130(22.6)	19(11.8)		149(20.3)
HIV status	Positive	57(9.9)	11(6.8)	0.4	68(9.3)
	Negative	517(90.1)	150(93.2)		667(90.7)
Mode of TB diagnosis	Bacteriological	277(48.3)	96(59.6)	0.04	373(50.6)
	Clinical	297(51.7)	65(40.4)		363(49.4)
Treatment center	Hospital	206(35.9)	60(37.3)	0.02	266(36.2)
	Health center	368(64.1)	101(62.7)		469(63.8)
Action before HCF[a] visit	None	440(76.7)	146(90.7)	0.04	586(79.7)
	Took actions[b]	134(23.3)	15(9.3)		149(20.3)
Place TB diagnosis made	Public	493(85.9)	143(88.8)	0.09	636(86.5)
	Private	81(14.1)	18(11.2)		99(13.5)
Hospitalized for TB illness	Yes	15(2.6)	4(2.5)	0.5	19(2.6)
Knowledge about TB	Poor	159(27.7)	31(19.3)	0.8	190(25.8)
	Good	415(72.3)	130(80.7)		545(74.2)
Patient delay	Median(IQR)days	30(16–57)	14(10–17)	< 0.001	25(15–36)
Provider delay	Median (IQR)days	31(16–64)	7(3–10)	< 0.001	22(9–48)
Pre-diagnosis cost	Median(IQR) US$[c]	119.1(74.0–221.6)	48.2(36.3–66.8)	< 0.001	
Post-diagnosis cost	Median(IQR) US$[c]	93.7(56.9–141.3)	78.8(41.5–113.7)	< 0.001	
Treatment information adequate	Yes	279(48.6)	78(48.4)	0.04	357(48.6)
	No	295(51.4)	83(51.6)		378(51.4)
Initial weight	Mean(±SD) Kg	49.0(8.6)	47.7(8.5)	0.9	48.7(± 8.6)

[a]Healthcare Facility, [b]self treatment, traditional healer, holy water, [c](1US$ = 20.56Birr)

At the end of follow-up, 699(95.1%) TB patients had documented treatment outcome of whom 627(89.7%, 95%CI:87.2–91.7%) had successfully completed their treatment. However, among those smear positive TB cases, only 177(47.5%) were declared cured. The treatment success is significantly different among cases initiated treatment beyond and within 30 days of onset of illness (88.4% vs 94.2%, $P = 0.01$), respectively. Thus, significant difference in proportions of death (4.8% Vs 1. 9%), treatment failure (0.7% Vs 0.6%) and loss to follow-up (6.1% vs. 3.2%), respectively, among those initiated treatments beyond and within 30 days of onset $p = 0.04$. The treatment success across HIV positive and negatives respectively was 75.8% vs 91.1%, $p < 0.001$. Disaggregation of the treatment success among bacteriologicaly confirmed (smear positive pulmonary) and clinically diagnosed cases respectively revealed 90.1% vs 89.3%, $p = 0.7$. Furthermore, we found no statistically significant differences in treatment success among smear positive pulmonary (90.1%), smear negative pulmonary (88.0%) and extra pulmonary cases (91.1%) ($p = 0.6$).

Predictors of unsuccessful treatment outcomes

Treatment outcome of the study patients varied significantly across time elapsed for initiation of treatment. Patients delayed for > 30 days to initiate treatment had more than twice higher risk of having unsuccessful outcome Adjusted relative risk [(ARR) = 2.02, 95% confidence interval (CI); 1.03,3.95). Moreover, being older than 65 years, (ARR = 3.83,95% CI; 2.04,6.1), HIV co infection (ARR = 1.93,95% CI; 1.23,3.01) and treatment center being hospital (ARR = 3.78, 95% CI;2.25,6.36) independently predicted higher risk of unsuccessful outcomes. On the other hand, weight gain at the end of second month treatment (ARR = 0.45,95% CI;0.22,0.91) predicted lower risk of unsuccessful outcome. Those patients gained weight at the end of two-month treatment compared to the baseline had about 60% lower risk of having unsuccessful outcome (Table 4).

Subgroup analysis among smear positive pulmonary cases revealed delays to initiate treatment (ARR = 1. 56,95%CI;1.46,1.65), HIV co infection (ARR = 3.73,95%CI: 1.68,5.97), treatment center being hospital (ARR = 1.

Table 3 Follow-up characteristics and outcomes across delays to treatment southwest Ethiopia January 2015 to june 2016

Variable		Total delay(days)			
		> 30(exposed) *N* = 574	<=30 (non exposed) *N* = 161		Total
		n(%)	n(%)	*P* value	n(%)
Sputum smear end of 2[nd]month(*n* = 373)	Positive	3(1.1)	3(3.0)	0.5	6(1.6)
	Negative	158(57.9)	67(67.0)		225(60.3)
	Not available	112(41.0)	30(30.0)		142(38.1)
Sputum smear end of 5th month(*n* = 373)	Positive	4(1.5)	1(1.0)	0.4	5(1.3)
	Negative	137(50.1)	58(58.0)		195(52.3)
	Not available	132(48.4)	41(41.0)		173(46.4)
Sputum smear end of 6th month(*n* = 373)	Negative	127(46.5)	51(51.0)	0.3	178(47.7)
	Not available	146(53.5)	49(49)		195(52.3)
Sputum check up after diagnosis(*n* = 373)	None	112 (41.0)	30(30.0)	0.3	142(38.1)
	At least once	161(59.0)	70(70.0)		231(61.9)
Weight end of 2ndmonth	Mean(SD)	51.2(8.6)	50.2(8.6)	0.9	51.3(8.6)
Weight change end of 2nd month	Unchanged/lost	93(16.2)	30(18.6)	0.2	123(16.7)
	Gained	298(52.0)	80(49.7)		378(51.5)
	Unknown	183(31.8)	51(31.7)		234(31.8)
Weight end of 5[th]month	Mean(SD)	54.2(8.7)	51.8(9.5)	0.5	53.6(8.9)
Weight end of 6th month	Mean(SD)	54.2(10.3)	52.9(9.0)	0.1	53.9(9.9)
Treatment out come	Cured	126(21.9)	51(31.7)	0.04	177(24.2)
	Treatment complete	354(61.5)	96(59.6)		450(61.1)
	Loss to follow-up	33(5.7)	5(3.1)		38(5.2)
	Died	26(4.5)	3(1.9)		29(3.9)
	Treatment failure	4(0.7)	1(0.6)		5(0.7)
	Not evaluated[a]	31(5.4)	5(3.1)		36(4.9)
Treatment success (*n* = 699)	Unsuccessful	63(11.6)	9(5.8)	0.01	72(10.3)
	Successful	480(88.4)	147(94.2)		627(89.7)

[a]cases transferred out to other treatment centers

89,95%CI:1.04,3.45) and age older than 65 years (ARR = 6.49,95%CI:3.60,11.70) as independent predictors of unsuccessful outcomes. Similarly analysis among clinically diagnosed cases showed delayed treatment, HIV co-infection, treatment center being hospital and older than 65 years independently predicted higher risk of unsuccessful outcome. Weight gain at the end of second month (ARR = 0.16,95%CI: 0.05, 0.53) predicted higher risk of unsuccessful outcome among clinically diagnosed cases and having at least one sputum checkup after diagnosis (ARR = 0.17, 95%CI:0.09, 0.33) predicted higher risk of unsuccessful outcomes among smear positive cases. Analysis of treatment outcomes among HIV negatives showed initiated treatment after 30 days of onset (ARR = 2.52,95%CI:1. 55, 4.10), weight gain at the end of second month treatment (ARR = 0.27,95%CI:0.12, 0.64) and treatment center being hospital (ARR = 2.33,95%CI:1.33, 4.09) independently predicted unsuccessful treatment outcome (Additional file 1: Tables S1-S3).

Discussion

This follow-up study revealed patients elapse too long time (median of 55 days) to initiate anti-TB treatment since onset of the illness. Subsequently, we found statistically significant differences in treatment success (94.2% vs 88.4%) respectively among those who initiated treatment within and beyond 55 days of onset. Those patients initiated anti-TB treatment beyond 30 days of onset had higher risk of unsuccessful outcomes including death, lost to follow up and treatment failure. Patients initiated treatment within and beyond 30 days of onset had undergone significantly diverse healthcare seeking practices, patient and provider delays. However, both groups of patients had no significant differences in sputum smear conversion and weight changes at end of second month treatment. The longer delays to initiate treatment accompanied by higher risk of unsuccessful outcomes depict increased morbidity and mortality to patients and prolonged period of transmission to the community. The finding suggests need for prompt

Table 4 Predictors of TB treatment outcome in districts of southwest Ethiopia January 2015 to June 2016

Variable		Treatment success		Crude Relative Risk (CRR) (95%CI)	Adjusted relative risk (ARR) (95% CI)
		Unsuccessful n(%)	Successful n(%)		
Gender	Male	44(10.3)	382(89.7)	Ref.	Ref.
	Female	28(10.3)	245(89.7)	0.9(0.63,1.56)	0.87(0.61,1.25)
Age group(years)	18–34	48(10.0)	433(90.0)	Ref.	Ref.
	35–65	20(9.9)	183(90.1)	0.9(0.60,.62)	0.88(0.68,1.12)
	> 65	4(26.7)	11(73.3)	2.67(1.11,6.45)	3.82(2.4,6.10)*
Educational status	Illiterate	25(12.3)	178(87.7)	Ref.	Ref.
	Completed primary	37(9.9)	338(90.1)	0.8(0.50,1.29)	0.93(0.61,1.41)
	Secondary & above	10(8.3)	111(91.7	0.67(0.33,1.35)	1.00(0.64,1.56)
Treatment center	Hospital	31(12.6)	215(87.4)	1.39(0.9,2.16)	3.78(2.4,6.35)*
	Health center	41(9.1)	412(90.9)	Ref.	Ref.
Action before HCF [a]visit	None	57(10.3)	498(89.7)	Ref.	Ref.
	Took action	15(10.4)	129(89.6)	1.01(0.59,1.74)	0.81(0.50,1.30)
Mode of TB diagnosis	Bacteriological	35(9.9)	320(90.1)	Ref.	Ref.
	Clinical	37(10.7)	308(89.3)	1.09(0.7,1.7)	0.86(0.67,1.10)
HIV status	Positive	15(24.2)	47(75.8)	2.7(1.63,4.5)	1.93(1.23,3.01)*
	Negative	57(8.9)	580(91.1)	Ref.	Ref.
Weight change end of 2nd month	No change/lost	13(11.2)	103(88.8)	Ref.	Ref.
	Gained	15(4.1)	354(95.9)	0.36(0.18,0.74)	0.45(0.22,0.91)
	Unknown	44(20.6)	170(79.4)	1.83(1.03,3.26)	4.34(2.47.7.65)*
Total delay(days)	<=30	9(5.8)	147(94.2)	Ref.	Ref.
	> 30	63(11.6)	480(88.4)	2.01(1.02,3.95)	2.02(1.03,3.95)*
Treatment information provided	Inadequate	39(11.0)	314(89.0)	0.86(0.56,1.34)	1.06(0.70,1.63)
	Adequate	33(9.5)	313(90.5)	Ref.	Ref.

*statistically significant at $p < 0.05$ [a] Healthcare facility

detection and treatment of cases to ensure better outcomes among patients and reduce burden in community.

The higher risk of unsuccessful outcome among those patients delayed to initiate anti-TB treatment had been consistently reported in studies from Ethiopia [30] and elsewhere [15]. The increased risk of unsuccessful outcome among patients delayed treatment initiation could be explained by various factors. First, delayed initiation of treatment had been reported to be associated with severe clinical presentation [14, 31] which predict unsuccessful outcomes [32]. In this study, patients delayed to initiate treatment had relatively higher rate of hospitalization (3% vs 2.1%) that would be proxy measure of severe presentation. Second, a delay to treatment is associated with both prescribed and self-treatment those lead to poor treatment outcome [33–35]. In the current study, the majority (84.7%) of the cases had visited an average of 2.2 HCFs until diagnosis of TB at which time both self and prescribed medicines had been used. Third, delays to treatment often accompanied by higher direct and indirect costs that impoverish households [36, 37] and ultimately lead to poor treatment compliance and outcome [36]. In our study we observed significantly higher median pre diagnosis (US$119.1 vs 48.2, $p = 0.001$)and post diagnosis (US$93.7vs.98.8, $p < 0.001$) costs among those delayed to initiate treatment which could explain the increased risk of unsuccessful outcome.

Consistent with studies in Ethiopia [30, 38] and elsewhere [39–42], the current study revealed that HIV comorbidity increase risk of unsuccessful outcome. Hence, significantly lower (75.8% vs 91.1%, $p < 0.001$) treatment success with higher deaths (12.9% vs. 3.3%, $p = 0.002$) were observed among HIV co infected compared to negatives. The observed lower treatment success among HIV co infected is far below the targeted 90% success to be met by 2020 [2]. The increased risk of unsuccessful outcome among the HIV co infected could be due to significantly prolonged time to initiate care seeking (median of 29 vs.

24 days, $P = 0.04$) among HIV co infected patients. Thus HIV co morbidity had been reported to delay anti-TB treatment initiation [13, 43]that explain the high mortality among HIV co infected TB patients [16, 17]. In addition, HIV co infection independently increases risk of unsuccessful outcome due the complex and overlapping drug interactions and toxicities and TB-associated immune reconstitution inflammatory syndrome [44]. Furthermore the increased risk could also be explained by the low uptake of TB/HIV collaborative interventions (39.7% and 47.1% on ART and CPT, respectively) those proved to bring better outcome [45]and predict worse outcome in their absence [40].

We found patients took anti-TB treatment at hospital had higher risk of unsuccessful outcome compared to those treated at health center. This could be due to significantly higher proportion of delays to initiate anti-TB treatment (55.6% Vs46.3%, $p = 0.02$), HIV co infection (14.3% Vs 6.4%, $p < 0.001$) and hospitalization (5.3% Vs 1.1%, $p = 0.001$) among patients treated at hospitals. Studies reported HIV co infection [39, 40], hospitalization [32] and delays to treatment [15, 30] to predict higher risk of unsuccessful outcomes. Moreover, patients treated at hospitals were more of pulmonary negative (36.5% vs 24.7%, $p < 0.001$) and extra pulmonary (21.8% vs 19.4%, $p < 0.001$) those had been reported to predict unsuccessful outcome [46].

Regular monitoring of TB patients during treatment is among standard of TB care, which is used to assess response to therapy and facilitates treatment completion. Accordingly regular sputum and weight monitoring have been recommended TB patients on treatment [47]. Despite low sensitivity and modest specificity of sputum results at the end of intensive phase to predict failure and relapse [48], sputum conversion to negative among those positive at initiation of treatment had been taken as one of the indicator TB control program performance [47]. In the current study no significant differences was observed in sputum smear conversion at end of second month treatment in both patients initiated treatment within and beyond 30 days of onset. Consistent with studies in Ethiopia [46]and elsewhere [49] smear conversion to negative at the end of second month treatment had lower risk of unsuccessful outcome. In this study, 3/6(50%) of those treatment failure cases had positive smear at the end of second month treatment. The higher risk among those positives could be due to possible poor quality of initial therapy and co morbid conditions that interfere with adherence or response [47]. Similarly, weight gain at the end of second month treatment predicted lower risk of unsuccessful outcomes which is in line with reports from Vietnam [50].

This study has some limitations. First, exposure assessment relied upon patient recall of the onset of illness that might be subjected to recall bias and ultimate misclassification bias. But efforts had been made to minimize the bias through use of local and national event listing. The second limitation was inability to measure treatment adherence that could have effect on treatment outcome. Third, we did not test for drug susceptibility so that we could not associate delay with resistance. Lastly, we studied only new adult TB cases so that the findings will not apply to all TB cases. On the other hand, relatively large sample and geographic coverage, reduced selection bias through consecutive enrolment, being prospective design, direct estimation of risk and use of standard outcome ascertainment could be mentioned as strength of the study. Therefore, the study is valid and applies to new TB cases in similar settings.

Conclusion

TB patients in the study area elapse too long time to initiate anti-TB treatment. The delayed treatment initiation was associated with higher risk of unsuccessful outcome including death, treatment failure and lost to follow-up. Apart from the delayed treatment, HIV co infection, treatment center being hospital, weight change and sputum conversion at the end of second month treatment independently predicted unsuccessful outcomes. Therefore, promotion of early care seeking within community, improving diagnostic, and case holding efficiencies of HCF and TB/HIV collaborative interventions could enhance the TB treatment success. Time delays to TB diagnosis can be reduced by raising community level awareness on TB suggestive symptoms, involving traditional healer, religious and private healthcare institutions in TB case finding, equipping healthcare facilities with rapid diagnostic tests and building capacities of healthcare providers to suspect and diagnose TB.

Additional file

Additional file 1: Table S1. Predictors of unsuccessful outcomes among new smear positive pulmonary TB cases in districts southwest Ethiopia January 2015 to June 2016 ($n = 355$). Table S2 Predictors of unsuccessful outcomes among new clinically diagnosed TB cases in districts southwest Ethiopia January 2015 to June 2016 ($n = 344$). Table S3 Predictors of unsuccessful outcomes among not HIV coinfected TB cases in districts of southwest Ethiopia January 2015 to June 2016.

Abbreviations

ARR: Adjusted relative risk; ART: Antiretroviral therapy; CI: Confidence Interval; CPT: Cotrimoxazole prophylactic therapy; DOTS: Directly Observed Treatment Short course; HCF: Healthcare Facility; HIV: Human Immunodeficiency Virus; IQR: Inter-quartile Range; SD: Standard deviation; TB: Tuberculosis; US$: United States dollar

Acknowledgements

We are indebted to the data collectors, supervisors, study participants, and staffs of the study districts and health facilities for their cooperation and supports for realization of the study.

Funding
Financial and material support was obtained from Addis Ababa and Mizan-Tepi Universities based in Ethiopia. The funders did not have role in data collection, analysis, write up and publication of the manuscript.

Authors' contributions
AA conceived and designed the study, collected and analyzed data, prepared manuscript:
WD and DJ critically reviewed for intellectual content of the study protocol and manuscript as primary and co-supervisors respectively. All authors approved the final version of the manuscript for submission.

Competing interests
The authors declare that they have no competing interests.

Author details
[1]Department of Public Health, College of Health Sciences, Mizan Tepi University, Mizan Aman, Ethiopia. [2]Management Science for Health, Addis Ababa, Ethiopia. [3]Department of Preventive Medicine, School of Public Health, College of Health Sciences, Addis Ababa University, Addis Ababa, Ethiopia.

References
1. World Health Organization. Global Tuberculosis report. Switzerland: World Health Organization; 2016.
2. World Health Organization. The end TB strategy: global strategy and targets for tuberculosis prevention, care and control after 2015. Geneva: WHO; 2015.
3. Federal Minstry of Health of Ethiopia. Tuberculosis, leprosy and TB/HIV prevention and control Programme manual. 4th ed. Addis Ababa: Ministry of Health of Ethiopia; 2008.
4. Federal Democratic Republic of Ethiopia Minstry of Health. Health and health related indicators. Addis Ababa: Federal Democratic Republic of Ethiopia Minstry of Health; 2016.
5. Federal Minstry of Health of Ethiopia. First Ethiopian National Population Based Tuberculosis Prevalence Survey. Addis Ababa: Federal Ministry of Health Ethiopia; 2011.
6. Federal Republic of Ethiopia Ministry of Health. Annual performance report. Addis Ababa: Federal Repubilic of Ethiopia Minstry of Health; 2016.
7. Arandottir T. Tuberculosis and public health: policy and principles of tuberculosis control. Paris: International Union Against Tuberculosis and Lung Disease; 2009.
8. Mesfin M, Newel J, Walley J, Gessessew A, Madeley R. Delayed consultation among pulmonary tuberculosis patients: a cross sectional study of 10 DOTS districts of Ethiopia. BMC Public Health. 2009;9:53.
9. Yimer S, Bjune G, Alene G. Diagnostic and treatment delay among pulmonary tuberculosis patients in Ethiopia: a cross sectional study. BMC Infect Dis. 2005;5:112.
10. Hussen A, Biadgilign S, Tessema F, Mohammed S, Deribe K, Deribew A. Treatment delay among pulmonary tuberculosis patients in pastoralist communities in bale zone, Southeast Ethiopia. BMC Res Notes. 2012;5:320.
11. Demissie M, Lindtjorn B, Berhane Y. Patient and health service delay in the diagnosis of pulmonary tuberculosis in Ethiopia. BMC Public Health. 2002;2:23.
12. Ford C, Bayer A, Gilman R, Onifade D, Acosta C, Cabrera L, Vidal C, Evans C. Factors associated with delayed tuberculosis test-seeking behavior in the Peruvian Amazon. Am J Trop Med Hyg. 2009;81(6): 1097–102.
13. Finnie R, Khoza L, Van den Borne B, Mabunda T, Abotchie P, Mullen P. Factors associated with patient and health care system delay in diagnosis and treatment for TB in sub-Saharan African countries with high burdens of TB and HIV. Tropical Med Int Health. 2011;16(4):394–411.
14. Virenfeldt J, Rudolf F, Camara C, Furtado A, Gomes V, Aaby P, Petersen E, Wejse C. Treatment delay affects clinical severity of tuberculosis: a longitudinal cohort study. BMJ Open. 2014;4(6):e004818.
15. Jianzhao H, Van den Hof S, Lin X, Yubang Q, Jinglong H, Van der Werf M. Risk factors for non-cure among new sputum smear positive tuberculosis patients treated in tuberculosis dispensaries in Yunnan, China. BMC Health Serv Res. 2011;11:97.
16. Lusignani L, Quaglio G, Atzori A, Nsuka J, Grainger R, Da ConceiÃ§ao Palma M, Putoto G, Manenti F. Factors associated with patient and health care system delay in diagnosis for tuberculosis in the province of Luanda, Angola. BMC Infect Dis. 2013;13:168.
17. Kiwuwa M, Charles K, Harriet M. Patient and health service delay in pulmonary tuberculosis patients attending a referral hospital: a cross-sectional study. BMC Public Health. 2005;5:122.
18. Mor Z, Kolb H, Lidji M, Migliori G, Leventhal A. Tuberculosis diagnostic delay and therapy outcomes of non-national migrants in Tel Aviv, 1998-2008. Euro Surveill. 2013;18(12):43–50.
19. World Health Organization: An expanded DOTS framework for effective tuberculosis control. 2002.
20. Tessema B, Muche A, Bekele A, Reissig D, Emmrich F, Sack U. Treatment outcome of tuberculosis patients at Gondar University teaching hospital, Northwest Ethiopia. A five - year retrospective study. BMC Public Health. 2009;9:371.
21. Getahun B, Ameni G, Medhin G, Biadgilign S. Mortality and associated risk factors in a cohort of tuberculosis patients treated under DOTS programme in Addis Ababa, Ethiopia. BMC Infect Dis. 2011;11:127.
22. Berhe G, Enquselassie F, Aseffa A. Treatment outcome of smear-positive pulmonary tuberculosis patients in Tigray Region,Northern Ethiopia. BMC Public Health. 2012;12:537.
23. Shaweno D, Worku A. Tuberculosis treatment survival of HIV positive TB patients on directly observed treatment short-course in southern Ethiopia: a retrospective cohort study. BMC Research Notes. 2012;5:682.
24. Federal Democratic Republic of Ethiopia Central Statistical Agency. Population projection of Ethiopia for all regions at Wereda level from 2014–2017. Addis Ababa: Central Statistical Authority; 2013.
25. Southern Nation Nationalities Peoples Region Health Bureau. Annual performance report in. Hawassa: SNNPR HB; 2014.
26. Federal Minstry of Health of Ethiopia. Guidelines for clinical and programmatic management of TB, leprosy and TB/HIV in Ethiopia in. 5th ed. Addis Ababa: Ethiopian Federal Minstry of Health; 2012.
27. Federal Minstry of Health of Ethiopia. Annual performance report. In: Health sector development programme iv. Addis Ababa: Federal Minstry of Health. p. 2011.
28. Soliman S, Nasehi M, Nassir A, Agboatwala M, Abdilai A, Maamary F, Al-Absi N. Diagnostic and treatment delay in tuberculosis:an in-depth analysis of the health-seeking behaviour of patients and health system response in seven countries of the eastern Mediterranean region. Egypt: WHO; 2006.
29. World Health Organization. Definitions and reporting framework for tuberculosis – 2013 revision. Switzerland: WHO Library Cataloguing-in-Publication Data; 2013.
30. Gebreegziabher B, Bjune G, Yimer S. Total delay is associated with unfavorable treatment outcome among pulmonary tuberculosis patients in west Gojjam zone, Northwest Ethiopia: a prospective cohort study. PLoS One. 2016;11(7):e0159579.
31. Cheng S, Chen W, Yang Y, Chu P, Liu X, Zhao M, Tan W, Xu L, Wu Q, Guan H, et al. Effect of diagnostic and treatment delay on the risk of tuberculosis transmission in Shenzhen, China: an observational cohort study, 1993-2010. PLoS One. 2013;8(6):e67516.
32. Sacks L, Pendle S. Factors related to in-hospital deaths in patients with tuberculosis. Arch Intern Med. 1998;158(17):1916–22.
33. Wang J, Hsueh P, Jan I, Lee L, Liaw Y, Yang P, Luh K. Empirical treatment with a fluoroquinolone delays the treatment for tuberculosis and is associated with a poor prognosis in endemic areas. Thorax. 2006;61(10):903–8.
34. Chen TC, Lu PL, Lin CY, Lin WR, Chen YH. Fluoroquinolones are associated with delayed treatment and resistance in tuberculosis: a systematic review and meta-analysis. Int J Infect Dis. 2011;15(3):211–6.
35. Rabin A, Kuchukhidze G, Sanikidze E, Kempker R, Blumberg H. Prescribed and self-medication use increase delays in diagnosis of tuberculosis in the country of Georgia. Int J Tuberc Lung Dis. 2013;17(2):214–20.
36. Wingfield T, Tovar M, Huff D, Boccia D, Saunders M, Datta S, Montoya R, Ramos E, Lewis J, Gilman R, et al. Beyond pills and tests: addressing the social determinants of tuberculosis. Clin Med. 2016;16(Suppl 6):s79–91.

37. Mesfin M, Newell J, Madeley R, Mirzoev T, Tareke I, Kifle Y, Gessessew A, Walley J. Cost implications of delays to tuberculosis diagnosis among pulmonary tuberculosis patients in Ethiopia. BMC Public Health. 2010;10:173.
38. Asres A, Jerene D, Deressa W. Tuberculosis treatment outcomes of six and eight month treatment regimens in districts of southwestern Ethiopia: a comparative cross-sectional study. BMC Infect Dis. 2016;16(1):653.
39. Karo B, Krause G, Hollo V, Van der Werf M, Castell S, Hamouda O, Haas W. Impact of HIV infection on treatment outcome of tuberculosis in Europe. AIDS. 2016;30(7):1089–98.
40. Nglazi M, Bekker L-G, Wood R, Kaplan R. The impact of HIV status and antiretroviral treatment on TB treatment outcomes of new tuberculosis patients attending co-located TB and ART services in South Africa: a retrospective cohort study. BMC Infect Dis. 2015;15:536.
41. Heunis C, Kigozi G, Chikobvu P, Botha S, van Rensburg HD. Risk factors for mortality in TB patients: a 10-year electronic record review in a south African province. BMC Public Health. 2017;17(1):38.
42. Sanchez M, Bartholomay P, Arakaki-Sanchez D, Enarson D, Bissell K, Barreira D, Harries A, Kritski A. Outcomes of TB treatment by HIV status in National Recording Systems in Brazil, 2003–2008. PLoS One. 2012;7(3):e33129.
43. de Albuquerque M, Ximenes R, Lucena-Silva N, de Souza W, Dantas AT, Dantas O, Rodrigues L. Factors associated with treatment failure, dropout, and death in a cohort of tuberculosis patients in Recife, Pernambuco state, Brazil. Cad Saude Publica. 2007;23(7):1573–82.
44. Shankar E, Vignesh R, Ellegard R, Barathan M, Chong Y, Bador M, Rukumani D, Sabet N, Kamarulzaman A, Velu V, et al. HIV-mycobacterium tuberculosis co-infection: A 'danger-couple model' of disease pathogenesis. Pathog Dis. 2013; 70(2):110–8.
45. Kigozi G, Heunis C, Chikobvu P, Botha S, van Rensburg D. Factors influencing treatment default among tuberculosis patients in a high burden province of South Africa. Int J Infect Dis. 2017;54:95–102.
46. Munoz-Sellart M, Cuevas L, Tumato M, Merid Y, Yassin M. Factors associated with poor tuberculosis treatment outcome in the southern region of Ethiopia. Int J Tuberc Lung Dis. 2010;14(8):973–9.
47. World Health Organization. Treatment of tuberculosis: guidelines. Geneva: World Health Organization; 2010.
48. Horne D, Royce S, Gooze L, Narita M, Hopewell P, Nahid P, Steingart K. Sputum monitoring during tuberculosis treatment for predicting outcome: a systematic review and meta-analysis. Lancet Infect Dis. 2010;10(6):387–94.
49. Djouma FN, Noubom M, Ateudjieu J, Donfack H. Delay in sputum smear conversion and outcomes of smear-positive tuberculosis patients: a retrospective cohort study in Bafoussam, Cameroon. BMC Infect Dis. 2015;15:139.
50. Hoa N, Lauritsen J, Rieder H. Changes in body weight and tuberculosis treatment outcome in Viet Nam. Int J Tuberc Lung Dis. 2013;17(1):61–6.

Higher serum 25-hydroxyvitamin D concentrations are associated with active pulmonary tuberculosis in hospitalised HIV infected patients in a low income tropical setting

Cuthbert Musarurwa[1*], Lynn Sodai Zijenah[2], Doreen Zvipo Mhandire[1], Tsitsi Bandason[3], Kudakwashe Mhandire[1], Maria Mary Chipiti[2], Marshall Wesley Munjoma[4] and Witmore Bayayi Mujaji[1]

Abstract

Background: The inherent risk of developing tuberculosis (TB) in HIV- infected individuals is further enhanced by hypovitaminosis D. Interventions that offset HIV-associated immune deterioration potentially arrest disease progression and incidence of opportunistic infections including TB. Despite conflicting reports on association between vitamin D deficiency (VDD) and risk of TB, vitamin D (VD) supplementation remains a promising intervention.

Methods: We conducted a comparative cross-sectional study on 145 HIV^+/pulmonary TB^+ (PTB) and 139 HIV^+/PTB^- hospitalised patients to investigate association of vitamin D status and risk of PTB. Stratified random sampling was used to select archived serum specimens from participants enrolled in a randomised controlled trial (RCT) conducted to investigate the impact of using a point-of-care urine lipoarabinomannan strip test for TB diagnosis. PTB status was confirmed using sputum smear microscopy, culture or GeneXpert MTB/RIF. Serum 25-hydroxyvitamin D [25(OH) D] concentrations were assayed by competitive chemiluminescent immunoassay prior to commencement of anti-TB treatment. Effect of VD status on duration of hospital stay and patient outcomes on follow up at 8 weeks were also investigated. Median serum 25(OH) D concentrations were compared using Mann-Whitney test and covariates of serum VD status were assessed using logistic regression analysis.

Results: Overall VDD prevalence in the cohort was 40.9% (95% CI: 35.1–46.8). Median serum 25(OH)D concentrations were significantly higher in HIV^+/PTB^+ group (25.3 ng/ml, IQR:18.0–33.7) compared to the HIV^+/PTB^- group (20.4 ng/ml, IQR:14.6–26.9), $p = 0.0003$. Patients with serum 25(OH) D concentration ≥ 30 ng/ml were 1.9 times more likely to be PTB^+ compared to those with serum 25(OH) D concentrations < 30 ng/ml (odds ratio (OR) 1.91; 95% CI 1.1–3.2). PTB-related death was associated with higher odds of having 25(OH) D levels≥30 ng/ml. Age, gender, $CD4^+$ count, combination antiretroviral therapy (cART) status, efavirenz based cART regimen and length of hospital stay were not associated with vitamin D status.

Conclusions: The finding of an association between higher serum 25(OH) D concentrations and active PTB and TB-related mortality among hospitalised HIV-infected patients in the present study is at variance with the commonly reported association of hypovitaminosis and susceptibility to TB. Our findings though, are in concordance with a small pool of reports from other settings.

Keywords: Vitamin D deficiency, Pulmonary tuberculosis, HIV, Hospital stay, cART

* Correspondence: curtbertm@yahoo.com
[1]Department of Chemical Pathology, University of Zimbabwe, College of Health Sciences, P.O. Box A178, Avondale, Harare, Zimbabwe
Full list of author information is available at the end of the article

Background

Zimbabwe, ranked 13th of 22 high TB burden countries that account for 80% of global TB burden has an HIV co-infection rate of approximately 68% [1]. In a lifetime, 10% of immunocompetent individuals asymptomatically infected with *Mycobacterial tuberculosis* (MTB), progress to active TB compared to 10% per year of HIV-infected individuals [2].

In vitro studies suggest vitamin D supplementation minimises progression to active TB given the role of vitamin D in immune regulation [3, 4]. These studies reported further an association between hypovitaminosis D with decreased macrophage activation and suboptimal production of cathelicidin both of which blunt the host's ability to fight TB and other infections. One billion people worldwide are estimated to be vitamin D deficient [5]. HIV- infected individuals face a higher risk of hypovitaminosis D due to a unique risk profile associated with treatment or mere infection itself thus further enhancing susceptibility to TB [6]. HIV infection itself has been shown to increase metabolism of 25(OH) D into the active form, further driving vitamin D deficiency, due to gp120 induced CYP27B1 production [7].

Although some studies have associated VDD with poorer HIV infection outcomes and disease progression, in both cART-naive and treated patients [8, 9], the evidence for the association between VDD and increased TB risk is not sufficiently robust [10–12]. Clinical trials using 25(OH) D supplementation as adjunctive TB therapy reported no clinical benefits [13, 14] casting further doubt on the implied role of vitamin D on antimicrobial immunity. A study from The Gambia reported significantly higher median serum 25(OH) D concentrations in TB cases compared to tuberculin skin test positive controls and household contacts [10]. Another study conducted in Tanzania reported higher mean serum vitamin D levels in PTB patients compared to healthy controls but no significant difference between confirmed PTB$^+$ patients and PTB suspects who tested negative for PTB [15]. Both high and low serum vitamin D concentrations were associated with susceptibility to PTB in Greenlanders [16]. Furthermore, a meta-analysis concluded that the association between VDD and increased risk of TB was lacking in HIV-infected or -uninfected African populations [12].These conflicting findings may be attributed to underlying genetic differences, diet, exposure to sun or skin colour.

There is paucity of research on the relationship between vitamin D status and HIV-related outcomes, particularly in resource-limited settings where both HIV and TB are co-endemic. Interventions that offset immune deterioration associated with HIV infection can potentially arrest disease progression and incidence of opportunistic infections including TB. We examined the prevalence, covariates of VDD and risk of PTB among HIV- infected hospitalized patients with and without PTB.

Methods

Study setting and design

The study was conducted at Mabvuku Polyclinic and Parirenyatwa Group of Hospitals, Harare, Zimbabwe. Harare is located at an altitude of 1480 m, latitude 17° 55'S and longitude 31°7'E. The mean daily sunshine duration is about 8.2 h with the rainy season stretching from November to April. Study participants were enrolled from January 2013 to September 2014.

Two hundred and eighty four hospitalised, Black Zimbabwean patients comprising 145 HIV infected patients with active PTB (HIV$^+$/PTB$^+$) and 139 HIV infected patients without active PTB (HIV$^+$/PTB$^-$) were randomly selected from a cohort ($n = 920$) who participated in a randomised controlled trial (RCT) entitled 'A RCT to evaluate the impact of using a point-of-care urine lipoarabinomannan (LAM) strip test for TB diagnosis amongst hospitalized HIV-infected patients in resource-poor settings (RCT LAM)' whose details are described elsewhere [17, 18]. Briefly, to be eligible for inclusion into the RCT, potential participants were required to be HIV infected, presenting with any one of TB symptoms (fever, cough, drenching night sweats or self-reported weight loss) and sufficiently ill to warrant hospitalization. Patients demographic, clinical and laboratory data were abstracted from the RCT LAM database. Such data included length of hospital stay, and mortality outcomes 8-weeks post enrolment. Cause of death was recorded as tuberculosis, or not tuberculosis with the alternative cause of death specified. All data and specimens were anonymized before access was allowed to the current investigators.

Study patients

Consenting study patients aged ≥18 years were all dark skinned, unveiled, with faces and arms regularly exposed to the sun. All were indigenous Zimbabweans, HIV- infected and suspected of having TB. Participants from the RCT-LAM study were stratified by PTB status before stratified randomisation was used to select participants from the RCT-LAM study. Participants who had been immobilised by illness for more than 2 weeks were excluded as were those with liver or renal conditions. Individuals who had already commenced anti-TB treatment and those on vitamin supplements were also excluded. The estimated sample size was 138 participants for each of the PTB status strata.

Laboratory tests

Blood specimens were collected for enumeration of CD4 + T-lymphocytes, haemoglobin and plasma and serum processing within 6 h of venepuncture before participants commenced anti-TB treatment.

At enrolment, each patient submitted at least three sputum specimens utilised as follows (i) same day PTB testing (Xpert Mycobacterium tuberculosis/rifampicin (MTB/RIF) Version G4 and fluorescence smear microscopy) (ii) TB culture and (iii) archived for future studies. Sputum smear fluorescence microscopy, Xpert MTB/RIF assay and the Mycobacteria Growth Indicator Tube (MGIT BD Microbiology Systems, Cockeysville, MD, USA) culture to confirm PTB, were performed as previously described [17, 18].

25(OH) D assays

Serum specimens archived at -80 °C were retrieved and thawed only once before 25(OH) D assays were carried out. Serum 25(OH) D was measured as a marker of vitamin D status using a fully automated competitive chemiluminescent immunoassay analyser (Maglumi 2000 Snibe Co. Ltd. Shenzhen, 518,057 China) following manufacturer's instructions. Between-run precision coefficients of variation for the assay ranged from 6.04 to 6. 25% and within run precision coefficients of variation ranged from 3.01–3.45%.

Serum 25(OH) D concentrations reflect overall VD status because of a longer half-life of approximately 15 days compared to 15 h for the active form [19]. VDD was defined as serum 25(OH) D concentration < 20 ng/mL, vitamin D insufficiency as serum 25(OH) D concentration of 20–29 ng/mL, and sufficient vitamin D status as serum 25(OH) D ≥ 30 ng/ml [20]. Finally, 25(OH) D concentrations below 10 ng/ml were classified as severe VDD [21]. From these definitions, we further generated other dichotomies of vitamin D status as follows, optimal or suboptimal (≥ 30 ng/ml or < 30 ng/ml) and deficient or not deficient (< 20 ng/ml or ≥ 20 ng/ml).

Ethics statement

The study protocol was approved by the Medical Research Council of Zimbabwe (MRCZ/A/1906). All the patients in the parent study (RCT-LAM) consented to future use of their left-over archived specimens and data in future TB- and/or HIV-related studies.

Statistical analyses

Statistical analyses were conducted using STATA (version 13.0; Stata Corporation, College Station, Texas, USA). Counts and proportions (%) were used to summarise data. Medians and interquartile range (IQR) were used to summarise non-normally distributed variables and means ± standard deviations (SD) for normally distributed data. Differences in proportions were tested using the Chi-square test whilst differences between groups of continuous normally distributed data were tested using independent samples t-test and Mann-Whitney test for non-normal data. The prevalence of VDD was estimated in the whole sample and for the sub-groups (PTB^- and PTB^+) with 95% confidence intervals (95% CI). Logistic regression was used to identify factors associated with VDD with OR and 95% CI were reported for all such cases. For all statistical comparisons α was set at 0.05.

Results

Baseline clinico-demographic characteristics of the patients are presented in Table 1.

Of the 284 patients, 142(50%) were female with median age 38 (IQR32–46) years. There was however no significant difference in gender ($p = 0.893$), age ($p = 0.534$) and duration of cART ($p = 0.076$) between HIV^+/PTB^+ and HIV^+/PTB^- groups. Of 140 patients on cART, 109(77.9%) were on an efavirenz (EFV)-based cART regimen.

There was however, no significant difference in proportions of patients on EFV-based regimen between the two groups ($p = 0.061$). At 8-week follow-up, there was no significant difference in mortality rates ($p = 0.057$) between the two groups although the HIV^+/PTB^- patients stayed significantly longer in hospital compared to the HIV^+/PTB^+ ($p < 0.001$). Median CD4+ T- lymphocyte counts were significantly lower in HIV^+/PTB^+ patients ($p < 0.001$) as was mean haemoglobin concentration ($p = 0.03$).

The median serum 25(OH) D concentrations and vitamin D status for all participant groups are presented in Table 2.

Overall median serum 25 (OH) D concentration was 22. 1 ng/ml (IQR16.4–31.5). The HIV^+/PTB^+ group had significantly higher median serum 25(OH) D concentration 25.3 ng/ml (IQR18.0–33.7) compared to the HIV^+/PTB^- group 20.4 (IQR14.6–26.9) ($p < 0.0003$). However the medians of each group and overall median of the two groups were all within the vitamin D insufficient range.

Distribution of serum 25(OH) D concentrations by PTB status is further illustrated in Fig. 1.

An overall 40.9% (95% CI: 35.1–46.8) were vitamin D deficient, 31% (95% CI: 25.7–36.62) were vitamin D insufficient and 28.2% (95% CI: 23.0–33.8) had sufficient concentrations. Only 1.8% (95% CI: 0.6–4.1) had severe VDD and all were HIV^+/PTB^-. Prevalence of VDD at 33.8% (95% CI:26.2–42.1) was significantly lower in the HIV^+/PTB^+ compared to HIV^+/PTB^- group ($p = 0.014$). The HIV^+/PTB^- group had a significantly lower proportion of patients with optimal 25(OH) D concentration compared to HIV^+/PTB^+ group ($p = 0.016$).

Correlates of serum 25(OH) D levels

The Wilcoxon rank-sum test was used to compare median 25(OH) D concentrations by age, gender, CD4+ T-lymphocyte count, body mass index (BMI), efavirenz (EFV) based cART regimen and cART status. Univariate and multivariate logistic regression analysis were also conducted to ascertain the influence of the same variables on serum vitamin D status (Table 3). For logistic

Table 1 Participants clinico-demographic data

Variable	All $n = 284$	HIV^+/ PTB^+ $n = 145$	HIV^+/ PTB^- $n = 139$	p-value
Age median(IQR)	38 (32–46)	38 (32–44)	38 (32–47)	0.534
Female	142 (50)	72 (49.6)	70(50.4)	0.893
On cART	140(49.3)	62 (47.3)	78(56.1)	0.138
Duration of cART (months) Median(IQR)	21 (1–58)	10 (1–48)	32 (9–58)	0.076
Alive at Week-8 Follow-up	191(70.7)	90(62.1)	101(72.7)	0.057
Duration of Hospital Stay (Days) Median(IQR)	5(3–8)	4(3–7)	5(4–10)	< 0.001
CD4 T-lymphocytes count (cells/μL) median(IQR)	54(18–144)	41 (14–110)	86(25–220)	< 0.001
BMI Median(IQR)	19.2(17.0–21.5)	19.1(16.6–20.8)	19.2(17.3–21.8)	0.222
BMI ≤18.5	95(33.4)	48(33.1)	47(33.8)	0.901
On efavirenz based regimen	109(38.3)	48(33.1)	61 (43.9)	0.061
Haemoglobin g/dl mean(SD)	9.2(2.8)	8.6(2.4)	9.6(3.0)	0.030

Key: n = number of participants in category, *IQR* interquartile range, *SD* standard deviation, *BMI* Body Mass Index, *cART* combination Antiretroviral therapy, All values are stated as n(%) unless indicated otherwise. p-values of ≤ 0.05 were considered statistically significant

regression analysis, dichotomies of optimal/suboptimal and deficient/not deficient serum vitamin D status were evaluated but only results for suboptimal/optimal category are presented in Table 3.

Female patients had significantly higher median serum 25(OH) D concentration; 23.3 ng/ml (IQR 17.9–32.4) compared to males; 20.65 ng/ml (IQR15.0–30.3) ($p = 0.013$). Age > 50 years, CD4 < 200/μL, BMI ≤ 18.5, being cART-naive and being on non-EFV based- regimen were associated with marginally higher median serum 25(OH) D concentrations though none of these achieved statistical significance. None of these variables was associated with higher odds of vitamin D insufficiency or deficiency in univariate or multivariate logistic regression analysis (Table 3). Further univariate and multivariate logistic regression was also conducted using the same predictor variables but only for the HIV^+/PTB^+ patients. Still none of these variables were a significant predictor of vitamin D status.

Median 25(OH) D concentrations and PTB-related outcomes

Effect of VD status as a dichotomy of optimal or suboptimal on PTB status, duration of hospital stay, cause of death and survival at 8 weeks follow-up post enrolment, was determined using univariate logistic regression. A multivariate logistic regression model incorporating each of PTB status, duration of hospital stay, cause of death and survival at 8 weeks follow-up post enrolment in turn as dependent variables and VD status (≥30 or < 30 ng/ml), gender, age (≥50 or < 50 years), CD4 cell count (≥200 or < 200 cells/μL) and cART status (experienced or naïve) as the explanatory variables was fitted. The OR (95% CI) derived from logistic regression analyses of vitamin D status as an explanatory variable for each of the given PTB-related outcomes adjusted for the other explanatory variables are presented in Table 4.

In univariate analysis, patients with optimum serum 25(OH) D concentrations were 1.9 times (OR 1.91; 95% CI 1.1–3.2) more likely to be PTB^+ compared to those with serum 25(OH) D concentrations < 30 ng/ml. The OR decreased to 1.82 (95% CI 1.1–2.9) when a serum 25(OH) D concentration cut-off of 20 ng/ml was used.

During follow-up, 75 (28.3%) patients died whilst 19 (6.7%) had incomplete data of whom 4(1.4%) were lost to follow up. Those with incomplete mortality data had median serum 25(OH) D of 25.9 ng/ml (IQR18.9–32.4). Of the 75 deceased patients, 49(65.3%) died from a PTB-related cause. Median serum 25(OH) D concentration of

Table 2 Median 25(OH) D concentrations and vitamin D status

Variable	All $n = 284$	HIV^+/PTB^+ $n = 145$	HIV^+/PTB^- $n = 139$	p-value
Serum 25(OH) D ng/ml Median (IQR)	22.1 (16.4–31.5)	25.3 (18.0–33.7)	20.4 (14.6–26.9)	0.0003
Vitamin D Deficient	116(40.9)	49 (33.8)	67(48.2)	0.014
Vitamin D Insufficient	88(31)	46 (31.7)	42(30.2)	0.790
Optimal Vitamin D	80(28.2)	50(34.5)	30(21.6)	0.016
Severe vitamin D Deficiency	5 (1.8)	0(0)	5(3.6)	0.021

Key: Vitamin D deficient: 25(OH)D: < 20 ng/ml, Vitamin D insufficient: 25(OH) D: 20-29 ng/ml, Optimal Vitamin D 25(OH) D: ≥ 30 ng/ml, Severe Vitamin D Deficiency: 25(OH) D: < 10 ng/ml, n number of patients in each category. All values expressed as n(%) unless otherwise stated. p-values of ≤ 0.05 were considered statistically significant

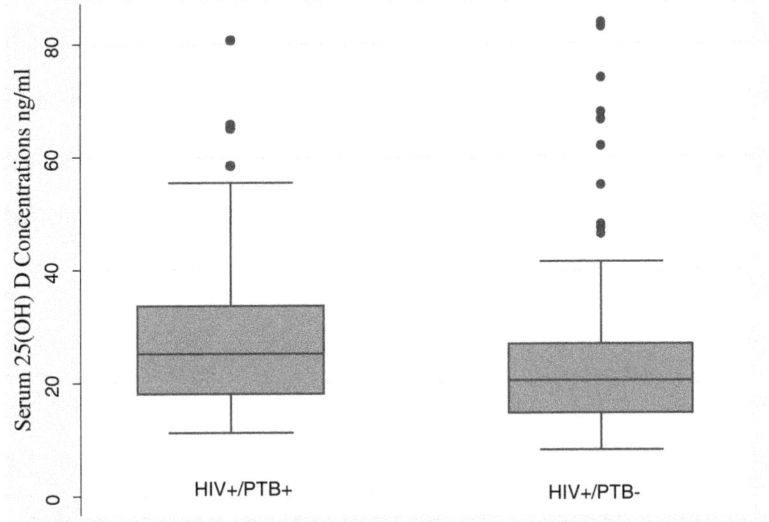

Fig. 1 Box and whisker plot showing the distribution of serum vitamin D concentrations by PTB status. Median serum 25(OH) D concentrations were significantly higher in HIV⁺/PTB⁺ group compared to HIV⁺/PTB⁻ group ($p = 0.0003$). Key: HIV+ = Human Immunodeficiency Virus positive, PTB+ = Pulmonary Tuberculosis positive, PTB- = Pulmonary Tuberculosis negative

patients who died from a PTB-related cause were higher but not significantly so compared to that of those who died from other causes ($p = 0.059$). Similarly, in univariate analysis patients that died from a PTB-related cause were 3.2 times more likely to have serum 25(OH) D levels ≥30 ng/ml compared to those that died from non-PTB related causes, but the difference was not statistically significant (OR3.19; 95% CI 0.9–10.7). None of the explanatory variables (VD status, gender, age, CD4 cell count or cART status) for the cause of death were

Table 3 Correlates of serum 25(OH) D levels

Variable	Serum 25(OH) D ng/ml Median(IQR)	*p*-value	Univariate Odds ratio (95%CI)	Multivariate Odds ratio (95%CI)
Gender				0.91(0.49–1.62)
Male	20.65 (15.0–30.3)	0.013	Referent	
Female	23.3 (17.9–32.4)		0.84 (0.49–1.42)	
Age				1.32(0.40–2.09)
≤ 50 years	18.91 (15.6–27.5)	0.142	Referent	
> 50 years	22.63 (16.6–32.9)		1.42 (0.7–2.9)	
CD4 Count				0.36 (0.11–1.17)
< 200/μL	22.65 (16.6–32.9)	0.127	0.69 (0.4–1.3)	
≥ 200	19.98 (15.6–28.8)		Referent	
BMI				0.61(0.27–1.38)
≤ 18.5	22.27 (16.6–33.6)	0.643	0.84 (0.5–1.5)	
> 18.5	21.98 (16.4–30.9)		Referent	
EFV-Based Regimen				0.87(0.32–2.34)
Yes	20.50 (15.1–33.1)	0.664	Referent	
No	21.81 (16.6–30.9)		0.97 (0.4–2.3)	
cART status				0.90(0.49–1.62)
Yes	20.84 (15.6–33.0)	0.244	Referent	
No	22.97 (16.9–30.6)		1.04 (0.6–1.8)	

Key: *IQR* interquartile range, *CI* confidence interval, *BMI* Body Mass Index, *EFV* efavirenz, *cART* combination antiretroviral therapy. *p*-values of ≤ 0.05 were considered statistically significant

Table 4 Association of serum 25(OH) D concentrations and outcomes in HIV-infected TB suspects

Variable	Serum 25(OH) D ng/ml Median(IQR)	*p*-value	Univariate Odds ratio (95%CI)	Multivariate Odds ratio[b] (95%CI)
PTB status $n = 284$				1.84 (1.1–3.2)
1. PTB^+ $n = 145$	25.3 (18.0–33.7)	0.0003	1.91 (1.1–3.2)	
2. PTB^- $n = 139$	20.4 (14.6–26.9)		Referent	
8-week outcome $n = 265$[a]				0.90 (0.5–1.7)
1. Alive $n = 190$	21.91 (16.9–31.1)	0.767	Referent	
2. Deceased $n = 75$	21.97 (15.8–31.7)		0.93 (0.5–1.7)	
Cause of Death $n = 75$				4.25 (1.1–16.2)
1. PTB $n = 49$	23.28 (16.6–34.8)	0.059	3.19(0.9–10.7)	
2. Other	18.47 (15.0–29.4)		Referent	
Hospital Stay $n = 245$[a]				0.87 (0.5–1.6)
1. ≤7 days $n = 179$	22.14 (17.0–30.7)	0.740	Referent	
2. > 7 days	22.10 (14.5–35.7)		0.89 (0.5–1.7)	

Key: *IQR* interquartile range, *CI* confidence interval, *PTB* pulmonary tuberculosis, *TB* tuberculosis. *p*-values of ≤ 0.05 were considered statistically significant. [a]some lost to follow up or incomplete data in records and [b]OR adjusted for binaries of gender, age (≥50 or < 50 years), CD4 cell count (≥200 or < 200 cells/μL) and cART status (experienced or naïve)

statistically significant in univariate logistic regression. However in multivariate analysis, patients that died from a PTB-related cause were 4.3 times more likely to have serum 25(OH) D concentration above ≥30 ng/ml; OR 4. 25 (95% CI1.1–16.2). Stepwise logistic regression analysis for predictors of cause of PTB related death, fitted a model with gender (OR 0.5; 95%CI 0.2–1.4), cART status (OR 0.39; 95%CI 0.1–1.1) and VD status (OR 3.89; 95%CI 1.1–13.8).

The patients that were recorded as deceased ($n = 75$) at the 8-week follow up time point were re-stratified by initial laboratory based PTB diagnosis. A statistically significantly higher median serum 25(OH) D concentration 24. 92 ng/ml (IQR 16.7–34.8) was observed in the PTB^+ group ($n = 38$) compared to the PTB^- group ($n = 37$) with 25(OH) D of 17.58 ng/ml (IQR 14.6–27.1); $p = 0.026$.

No significant differences were observed in median serum 25(OH) D concentrations between patients that died and those that were alive ($p = 0.77$) or those hospitalised for ≥7 days and those hospitalised for shorter durations ($p = 0.74$) after the 8 weeks follow up period.

Discussion

Our results contribute to a small but growing pool of studies that refute the commonly accepted hypothesis that lower serum 25(OH) D concentrations are associated with PTB [10, 15, 16, 19, 22]. In the present study, median serum 25(OH) D concentrations for both the HIV^+/PTB^+ and HIV^+/PTB^- groups were above the threshold for VDD but still below the cut-off for optimum serum 25(OH) D concentration. In addition, we observed significantly higher proportion of patients with optimum 25(OH) D concentrations in the HIV^+/PTB^+ group and significantly higher proportion of VDD patients in the HIV^+/PTB^- group.

Furthermore, patients with serum 25(OH) D concentrations above the optimum threshold were twice more likely to be PTB^+ compared to those with lower concentrations. Surprisingly, we observed no significant association between vitamin D status and all-cause mortality although in multivariate logistic regression analysis patients that died from a PTB-related cause were 4.3 times more likely to have serum 25(OH) D levels ≥30 ng/ml compared to those that died from non-PTB related causes.

Our findings though, are in discordance with the generally implied role of vitamin D in mycobacterial immunity that has been suggested by in vitro studies. In vitro studies suggest a role of 25(OH) D in control of MTB infection and by deduction, increased susceptibility in individuals with insufficient 25(OH) D levels. In the present study, HIV^+/PTB^+ patients had insufficient but significantly higher median serum 25(OH) D concentrations compared to HIV^+/PTB^- individuals.

Our observation of higher median serum 25(OH) D levels in HIV^+/PTB^+ participants compared to HIV^+/PTB^- patients whilst unexpected could be a consequence of active PTB and HIV-infection modulation. MTB and HIV-1gp120 peptides stimulate toll-like receptors 1/2 which in turn have been reported to induce CYP27B1 expression in infected macrophages in vitro [7] We speculate that if the same process occurs in vivo, the resultant accelerated production of 1,25(OH)D might in turn lead to increased mobilisation of 25(OH) D from adipose tissue and consequent elevation in circulation. Alternatively, HIV induced chronic inflammation characterised by tumour necrosis factor-alpha (TNF-α) overproduction, may result in renal 1α-hydroxylase impairment [23] leading to reduced parathyroid stimulatory effect on 1,25(OH)2D production thereby leading to accumulation of 25(OH) D in circulation.

We were unable to verify the assertion by Zeng et al., who in a meta-analysis concluded that only severe VDD (< 10 ng/ml) was associated with significant risk of active TB [11]. Five patients were severely vitamin D deficient in our study and interestingly all were PTB^- lending support to our observation of lack of association of VDD with PTB albeit the number is small.

The overall 40.9% prevalence of VDD in our study falls within the range of 29–73% reported in literature [24]. Although only an overall 28.2% of the patients had optimal serum 25(OH) D levels, the majority of these were HIV^+/PTB^+. In concordance with findings from a study conducted in Uganda [25], 66.2% of $HIV^+/\ PTB^+$ patients had serum 25(OH) D levels above 20 ng/ml but this is sharply contrasted by a study from Cape Town South Africa [26] that reported only 14% of $HIV^+/\ PTB^+$ patients with concentrations above 20 ng/ml. Such latitudinal-related differences in relative proportions of individuals with insufficient 25(OH) D concentrations among Black Africans from different countries could be attributed to the solar zenith angle that influences the efficiency of ultra violet induced cutaneous synthesis of vitamin D [27].

Correlates of serum vitamin D concentration

Females had significantly higher median serum 25(OH) D concentrations compared to males contrary to reports of association of male gender with higher serum vitamin D concentrations [28]. Other studies reported no significant differences by gender [29]. We speculate that higher median serum 25(OH) D concentrations in females might have been associated with wasting, the hallmark of both PTB and HIV [30]. Female patients in the present study had marginally higher BMI compared to males. The higher adiposity associated with lower serum 25(OH) D concentrations, may however imply more vitamin D being stored in adipose tissue hence enhanced release during wasting associated with HIV infection and/or active PTB.

Age, CD4+ T-lymphocyte count, BMI, cART status and EFV-based cART regimen were not associated with vitamin D status in univariate or multivariate analysis. Older age has been reported as a risk factor for VDD in an HIV-infected population [31] due to reduced dermal efficiency to synthesize vitamin D [32]. Our findings of no age association may be due to the relatively younger median age of our study patients.

Patients on cART had marginally insignificantly lower median 25(OH) D levels compared to cART-naïve. The association between VDD and cART is controversial. Although VDD has been associated with cART [29] other studies have reported lack of association [8] whilst others reported higher 25(OH) D levels in those on cART [33]. The modulation of vitamin D status by cART has largely been attributed to the effects of protease inhibitors and certain non-nucleoside reverse transcriptase inhibitors (NNRTIs) on vitamin D metabolism.

Similar to findings from another study [34], patients on an EFV-based cART regimen in the present study had marginally insignificantly lower median 25(OH) D levels. NNRTIs notably EFV, have been reported to accelerate 25(OH) D catabolism through the induction of the enzyme CYP24 which converts both 25(OH) D and the active form of vitamin D, 1,25(OH)D, to inactive metabolites [35]. EFV has also been reported to reduce the expression of cytochrome CYP2R1, which hydroxylates vitamin D3 and vitamin D2, an initial step in vitamin D activation [36]. Although the relatively shorter median duration since cART initiation in our study may plausibly contribute to the differences, the possibility of racial differences in the response to EFV cannot be ruled out. Indeed, lack of response to EFV has been reported for non-Caucasian patients [37]. We however, note the possible contribution of diminished power to detect any difference given the limited number of participants on cART and also those on an EFV-based regimen.

8-week mortality and 25 (OH) D concentrations

Hypovitaminosis D has been associated with poorer disease outcomes and higher risk of all-cause mortality in the general population as well as in both cART-experienced and naïve HIV-infected individuals [8, 31, 38]. In the present study, median 25(OH) D concentrations were not significantly different between patients that died within the 8-week follow up period and those that were still alive. In multivariate logistic regression analysis, patients that died from a PTB-related cause within 8 weeks had significantly higher odds of having optimal vitamin D status compared to those that were alive. This observation is concordant with the other findings reported in this study and could be explained in a similar manner.

We observed no significant difference in median 25(OH) D concentrations between patients admitted into hospital for at least 7 days and those that were admitted for longer. In concordance with current findings, Sherwood et al. reported no significant associations between 25(OH) D levels with mortality or length of hospitalisation [39]. Similarly, a study conducted in Tanzania observed no relationship between all-cause mortality and dichotomous outcomes of insufficient versus sufficient serum 25(OH) D concentrations although those with sufficient levels had a lower risk of death [11].

Limitations

The limitations of our study include (i) the cross sectional study design which precludes inference of causal relationships between serum 25(OH) D and PTB, (ii) possibility of reverse causation as 25(OH) D levels were measured when patients were already HIV and/or MTB infected, thus the temporal relationship between infection and vitamin D status could therefore not be established, (iii) stratification of patients into such substrata as cART regimen and cause of death could have diminished statistical power to detect any effect modification and (iv)the lack of consensus on the definitions of vitamin D status in literature also compromised the interpretation of findings across different studies.

Despite these limitations, our study has some strengths. The study sample size was relatively large and although unmatched for gender, age, proportion on cART, BMI and duration on cART, there were no significant differences between the two groups thus giving credence to our findings.

Conclusions

Our findings though at variance with the generally accepted association between serum vitamin D status and PTB, are in concordance with findings from a few other studies that report an association between high serum 25(OH) D concentrations and risk of PTB. It is possible that the reason for this observed variation could be genetic given the complex and diverse actions of vitamin D. Thus, genetic polymorphisms in the vitamin D receptor, or in the multiple enzymes involved in vitamin D metabolism, remain attractive candidates for further study.

Abbreviations

25(OH) D: 25 Hydroxyvitamin D; BMI: Body Mass Index; cART: Combination anti-retroviral therapy; CD4: Cluster of differentiation 4; CI: Confidence interval; EFV: Efavirenz; HIV: Human immunodeficiency virus; IQR: Interquartile range; LAM: Lipoarabinomannan; MRCZ: Medical research council of Zimbabwe; MTB: Mycobacterial tuberculosis; NNRTIs: Non-nucleoside reverse transcriptase inhibitors; OR: Odds ratio; PTB: Pulmonary tuberculosis; RCT: Randomised controlled trial; TB: Tuberculosis; VDD: Vitamin D deficiency; Xpert MTB RIF: GeneXpert *Mycobacteria tuberculosis* rifampicin

Acknowledgements

We thank the study participants from the RCT-LAM study for their participation in the parent study and for giving us permission to use their left-over archived specimens and data in the current study.

Funding

The authors gratefully acknowledge funding from the European and Developing Countries Trials Partnership (IP.0932040009), Southern Africa Consortium for Research Excellence and grant number 2U2RTW007367 from the Fogarty International Centre, National Institutes of Health, USA through the International Clinical, Operations, and Health Services Research Training Award for AIDS and TB. The funders played no role in the design of the study and collection, analysis, and interpretation of data and in writing the manuscript.

Authors' contributions

CM, LSZ, WBM and MWM conceived the study and its design. CM, MMC and DZM participated in the collection of clinical material and study participant recruitment. CM, DZM and KM conducted the laboratory tests. TB and CM performed data analysis. CM wrote the first draft with input from LSZ, WBM, MWM, DZM, KM, TB and MMC. All authors reviewed and approved the final version of the manuscript.

Competing interests

The authors declare that they have no competing interests.

Author details

[1]Department of Chemical Pathology, University of Zimbabwe, College of Health Sciences, P.O. Box A178, Avondale, Harare, Zimbabwe. [2]Department of Immunology, University of Zimbabwe, College of Health Sciences, P.O. Box A178, Avondale, Harare, Zimbabwe. [3]Biomedical Research and Training Institute, Harare, Zimbabwe. [4]Department of Obstetrics and Gynaecology, University of Zimbabwe, College of Health Sciences, P.O. Box A178, Avondale, Harare, Zimbabwe.

References

1. World Health Organization. Global tuberculosis report 2015. Geneva: World Health Organization; 2015. http://apps.who.int/iris/bitstream/10665/191102/9789241565059_eng.pdf. Accessed 29 Sept 2017
2. Adeiza MA, Abba AA, Okpapi JU. HIV-associated tuberculosis: a sub-saharan african perspective. Sub-Saharan Afr J Med. 2014;1:1.
3. Campbell GR, Spector SA. Vitamin D inhibits human immunodeficiency virus type 1 and Mycobacterium tuberculosis infection in macrophages through the induction of autophagy. PLoS Pathog. 2012; https://doi.org/10.1371/journal.ppat.1002689
4. Kamen DL, Tangpricha V. Vitamin D and molecular actions on the immune system: modulation of innate and autoimmunity. J Mol Med. 2010;88:441–50.
5. Holick MF. Deficiency of sunlight and vitamin D. BMJ. 2008;336:1318–9.
6. Lambert AA, Drummond MB, Mehta SH, Brown TT, Lucas GM, Kirk GD, et al. Risk factors for vitamin D deficiency among HIV-infected and uninfected injection drug users. PloS one. 2014; https://doi.org/10.1371/journal.pone.0095802.
7. Coussens AK, Martineau AR, Wilkinson RJ. Anti-inflammatory and antimicrobial actions of vitamin D in combating TB/HIV. Scientifica. 2014; https://doi.org/10.1155/2014/903680.
8. Shepherd L, Souberbielle JC, Bastard JP, Fellahi S, Capeau J, Reekie J, et al. Prognostic value of vitamin D level for all-cause mortality, and association with inflammatory markers, in HIV-infected persons. J Infect Dis. 2014;210: 234–43.
9. Mehta S, Giovannucci E, Mugusi FM, Spiegelman D, Aboud S, Hertzmark E, et al. Vitamin D status of HIV-infected women and its association with HIV disease progression, anemia, and mortality. PloS one. 2010; https://doi.org/10.1371/journal.pone.0008770.
10. Owolabi O, Agbla S, Owiafe P, Donkor S, Togun T, Sillah AK, et al. Elevated serum 25-hydroxy (OH) vitamin D levels are associated with risk of TB progression in Gambian adults. Tuberculosis. 2016;98:86–91.
11. Zeng J, Wu G, Yang W, Gu X, Liang W, Yao Y, et al. A serum vitamin D level< 25nmol/l pose high tuberculosis risk: a meta-analysis. PloS one. 2015; https://doi.org/10.1371/journal.pone.0126014.
12. Huang SJ, Wang XH, Liu ZD, Cao WL, Han Y, Ma AG, et al. Vitamin D deficiency and the risk of tuberculosis: a meta-analysis. Drug Des Devel Ther. 2017;11:91–102.
13. Daley P, Jagannathan V, John KR, Sarojini J, Latha A, Vieth R, et al. Adjunctive vitamin D for treatment of active tuberculosis in India: a randomised, double-blind, placebo-controlled trial. Lancet Infect Dis. 2015;15:528–34.
14. Tukvadze N, Sanikidze E, Kipiani M, Hebbar G, Easley KA, Shenvi N, et al. High-dose vitamin D3 in adults with pulmonary tuberculosis: a double-blind randomized controlled trial. Am J Clin Nutr. 2015;102:1059–69.
15. Friis H, Range N, Changalucha J, PrayGod G, Jeremiah K, Faurholt-Jepsen D, et al. Vitamin D status among pulmonary TB patients and non-TB controls: a cross-sectional study from Mwanza, Tanzania. PloS one. 2013; https://doi.org/10.1371/journal.pone.0081142.

16. Nielsen NO, Skifte T, Andersson M, Wohlfahrt J, Søborg B, Koch A, et al. Both high and low serum vitamin D concentrations are associated with tuberculosis: a case-control study in Greenland. Br J Nutr. 2010;104:1487–91.
17. Peter JG, Zijenah LS, Chanda D, Clowes P, Lesosky M, Gina P, et al. Effect on mortality of point-of-care, urine-based lipoarabinomannan testing to guide tuberculosis treatment initiation in HIV-positive hospital inpatients: a pragmatic, parallel-group, multicountry, open-label, randomised controlled trial. Lancet. 2016;387:1187–97.
18. Zijenah LS, Kadzirange G, Bandason T, Chipiti MM, Gwambiwa B, Makoga F, et al. Comparative performance characteristics of the urine lipoarabinomannan strip test and sputum smear microscopy in hospitalized HIV-infected patients with suspected tuberculosis in Harare Zimbabwe. BMC Infect Dis. 2016;16:20.
19. Conesa-Botella A, Goovaerts O, Massinga-Loembe M, Worodria W, Mazakpwe D, Luzinda K, et al. Low prevalence of vitamin D deficiency in Ugandan HIV-infected patients with and without tuberculosis. Int J Tuberc Lung Dis. 2012;16:1517–21.
20. Dawson-Hughes B, Heaney RP, Holick MF, Lips P, Meunier PJ, Vieth R. Estimates of optimal vitamin D status. Osteoporos Int. 2005;16:713–6.
21. Wejse C, Olesen R, Rabna P, Kaestel P, Gustafson P, Aaby P, et al. Serum 25-hydroxyvitamin D in a west African population of tuberculosis patients and unmatched healthy controls. Am J Clin Nutr. 2007;86:1376–83.
22. Musarurwa C, Zijenah LS, Duri DZ, Mateveke-Dangaiso K, Mhandire K, Chipiti MM, et al. Association of high serum vitamin D concentrations with active pulmonary TB in an HIV co-endemic setting, Harare Zimbabwe. BMC Infect Dis. 2017;17:142.
23. Mansueto P, Seidita A, Vitale G, Gangemi S, Iaria C, Cascio A. Vitamin D Deficiency in HIV Infection: Not Only a Bone Disorder. BioMed Res Int. 2015; https://doi.org/10.1155/2015/735615.
24. Dao CN, Patel P, Overton ET, Rhame F, Pals SL, Johnson C, et al. Low vitamin D among HIV-infected adults: prevalence of and risk factors for low vitamin D levels in a cohort of HIV-infected adults and comparison to prevalence among adults in the US general population. Clin Infect Dis. 2011;52:396–405.
25. Nansera D, Graziano FM, Friedman DJ, Bobbs MK, Jones AN, Hansen KE. Vitamin D and calcium levels in Ugandan adults with human immunodeficiency virus and tuberculosis. Int J Tuberc Lung Dis. 2011;15:1522.
26. Martineau AR, Timms PM, Bothamley GH, Hanifa Y, Islam K, Claxton AP, et al. High-dose vitamin D3 during intensive-phase antimicrobial treatment of pulmonary tuberculosis: a double-blind randomised controlled trial. Lancet. 2011;377:242–50.
27. Engelsen O. The relationship between ultraviolet radiation exposure and vitamin D status. Nutrients. 2010;2:482–95.
28. Al-Horani H, Abu Dayyih W, Mallah E, Hamad M, Mima, M, Awad R, et al. Nationality, Gender, Age, and Body Mass Index Influences on Vitamin D Concentration among Elderly Patients and Young Iraqi and Jordanian in Jordan. Biochem Res Int. 2016; https://doi.org/10.1155/2016/8920503.
29. Conesa-Botella A, Florence E, Lynen L, Colebunders R, Menten J, Moreno-Reyes R. Decrease of vitamin D concentration in patients with HIV infection on a non nucleoside reverse transcriptase inhibitor-containing regimen. AIDS Res Ther. 2010;7:40.
30. Wanke C, Kotler D. HIV wasting collaborative consensus committee. Collaborative recommendations: the approach to diagnosis and treatment of HIV wasting. J Acquir Immune Defic Syndr. 2004;37suppl:S284–8.
31. Viard JP, Souberbielle JC, Kirk O, Reekie J, Knysz B, Losso M, et al. Vitamin D and clinical disease progression in HIV infection: results from the EuroSIDA study. AIDS. 2011;25:1305–15.
32. Pilz S, Dobnig H, Nijpels G, Heine RJ, Stehouwer CD, Snijder MB, et al. Vitamin D and mortality in older men and women. Clin Endocrinol. 2009;71: 666–72.
33. Ramayo E, Gonzalez-Moreno MP, Macias J, Cruz-Ruíz M, Mira JA, Villar-Rueda AM, et al. Relationship between osteopenia, free testosterone, and vitamin D metabolite levels in HIV-infected patients with and without highly active antiretroviral therapy. AIDS Res Hum Retrovir. 2005;21:915–21.
34. Poowuttikul P, Thomas R, Hart B, Secord E. Vitamin D insufficiency/ deficiency in HIV-infected inner city youth. J Int Assoc Provid AIDS Care. 2014;13:438–42.
35. Schwartz JB, Moore KL, Yin M, Sharma A, Merenstein D, Islam T, et al. Relationship of vitamin D, HIV, HIV treatment, and lipid levels in the Women's interagency HIV study of HIV-infected and uninfected women in the United States. J Int Assoc Provid AIDS Care. 2014;13:250–9.
36. Cheng JB, Levine MA, Bell NH, Mangelsdorf DJ, Russell DW. Genetic evidence that the human CYP2R1 enzyme is a key vitamin D 25-hydroxylase. Proc Natl Acad Sci U S A. 2004;101:7711–5.
37. Havers F, Smeaton L, Gupte N, Detrick B, Bollinger RC, Hakim J, et al. 25-Hydroxyvitamin D insufficiency and deficiency is associated with HIV disease progression and virological failure post-antiretroviral therapy initiation in diverse multinational settings. J Infect Dis. 2014;210:244–53.
38. Sudfeld CR, Wang M, Aboud S, Giovannucci EL, Mugusi FM, Fawzi WW. Vitamin D and HIV progression among Tanzanian adults initiating antiretroviral therapy. PloS one. 2012; https://doi.org/10.1371/journal.pone.0040036.
39. Sherwood JE, Mesner OC, Weintrob AC, Hadigan CM, Wilkins KJ, Crum-Cianflone NF, et al. Vitamin D deficiency and its association with low bone mineral density, HIV-related factors, hospitalization, and death in a predominantly black HIV-infected cohort. Clin Infect Dis. 2012;55:1727–36.

24

2′-5′-Oligoadenylate synthetase 1 polymorphisms are associated with tuberculosis

Shouquan Wu[1], Yu Wang[1], Guo Chen[1,2], Miaomiao Zhang[1], Minggui Wang[1] and Jian-Qing He[1*]

Abstract

Background: 2′-5′-Oligoadenylate synthetase 1 (OAS1) plays an important role in inflammatory immune reactions. *OAS1* polymorphisms have been associated with increased susceptibility to various diseases. We investigated the association of polymorphisms in *OAS1* with tuberculosis (TB).

Methods: A total of 1215 TB cases and 1114 healthy controls were enrolled from two independent studies. Genotyping was conducted using the improved multiplex ligase detection reaction (iMLDR) method. Associations between *OAS1* polymorphisms (rs2240190, rs1131454, 10,774,671 and 11,066,453) and TB risk were established based on distributions of allelic frequencies using different genetic models.

Results: Significant association was observed between rs10774671, rs1131454 and TB. In the initial study, the G allele of rs10774671 was a significantly protective factor against TB ($P = 0.006$) and the genotype of GG differed significantly between TB patients and controls under the codominant model ($P = 0.008$) after Bonferroni correction. In the validation study, we also observed that the rs10774671 G allele ($P = 0.001$) and GG genotype ($P = 0.$ 001) were associated with TB. In addition, we found that the rs1131454 G allele ($P = 0.004$) and GG genotype ($P = 0.001$) were protective against TB in the Chinese Han population.

Conclusions: We report novel associations of polymorphisms in *OAS1* with TB in the Chinese Tibetan and Han populations. Similar studies in different populations and functional studies are warranted to confirm our results.

Keywords: Alleles, Tuberculosis, 2′-5′-Oligoadenylate synthetase 1, Polymorphism, Association study

Introduction

Tuberculosis (TB) is an infectious disease that constitutes a major global health problem. It is a major cause of morbidity and mortality globally, particularly in Asia and Africa, and ranks alongside human immunodeficiency virus (HIV) as a leading cause of death worldwide [1]. In 2017, an estimated 1.7 billion individuals were newly infected with the causative agent of TB [1]. However, only 5–15% of them will develop TB during their lifetime [2]. The outcome of TB infection is affected by many factors, such as malnutrition, co-infection with other pathogens, exposure to microbes and previous vaccination [3]. It was reported that host genetic factors play a crucial role in determining an individual's susceptibility to TB [4]. Recently, a number of genes potentially associated with TB susceptibility have been analysed in case-control studies.

Studies performed in mouse models and in patients indicate an important role of interferon (IFN) during TB infection [5, 6]. IFN-α, IFN-β and IFN-γ play significant immunomodulatory roles in the protection of the host against infections. As the main mediator of the type II immune response, IFN-γ is critical for controlling infections by intracellular pathogens, such as Mycobacteria [7]. Specifically, IFN-γ plays a vital role in resistance to *Mycobacterium tuberculosis* (*MTB*) by activating macrophages, monocytes and Th1 cells [8]. 2′-5′-oligoadenylate synthetases (OASs) are IFN-inducible enzymes that play vital roles in the innate immune response against viruses. The OAS family includes OAS1, OAS2, OAS3,

* Correspondence: jianqhe@gmail.com
[1]Department of Respiratory and Critical Care Medicine, West China Hospital, Sichuan University, No. 37, Guo Xue Alley, Chengdu 610041, Sichuan, People's Republic of China
Full list of author information is available at the end of the article

and OAS-like (OASL) protein. The *OAS1* gene encodes OAS1, which is an extensively characterized enzyme induced by IFNs [9]. Binding of IFNs to their specific receptors results in induction of *OAS1* gene expression [10]. OAS1 is activated by the presence of double-stranded RNA and stimulates the oligomerisation of ATP into 2′,5′-linked oligoadenylates (2-5A) [11]. 2-5A can bind to latent ribonuclease L (RNase L), which then dimerizes into the active form. This active form facilitates apoptosis [12], attenuates proliferation [13] and inhibits protein synthesis [13]. It is possible that polymorphisms in *OAS1* influence the expression of IFN-γ, the elimination of *MTB*, and ultimately affect the development of TB [14, 15].

Other OAS family members including OAS2, OAS3, and OASL also have been the focus of much research. OAS2 encodes the p69 and p71 IFN-induced isoforms [16]. OAS2 play an important role in the control of bacterial infection through direct interaction with pattern-recognition receptors. It also has immunomodulatory function through immune cell receptor interaction [16]. In terms of the ability to synthesize 2-5A, OAS3 shows higher activity than OAS1 [17]. OAS3 is specialized for binding long dsRNA. The major function of OAS3 during infection is to produce 2-5A activators of RNaseL [18]. In contrast to other OAS family members, OASL lacks any synthetic activity. OASL has the ability to regulate type I IFN responses when infected with pathogens. It has been suggested that OASL could act as a regulator in the control of antiviral innate immunity through IFN signalling [19].

Single-nucleotide polymorphisms (SNPs) can regulate *OAS1* function at multiple levels, including expression, alternative splicing and enzyme activity. So far, among the OAS gene cluster, *OAS1* polymorphisms have been the most studied and were reported to influence susceptibility to various diseases. For example, SNPs in *OAS1* have been identified as candidates for susceptibility to viral infections, such as West Nile virus [20], hepatitis C [21], Chikungunya [22], dengue [23] and measles [24]. Previous data also indicated that *OAS1* polymorphisms and haplotypes were potential risk factors for autoimmune conditions, including type 1 diabetes [25] and multiple sclerosis [26]. In addition, *OAS1* polymorphisms were reported to be associated with respiratory infection [27]. However, no previous studies have examined the association between *OAS1* and TB.

Collectively, these observations prompted us to propose the hypothesis that *OAS1* polymorphisms confer susceptibility to TB. The purpose of the study was to evaluate the prevalence of polymorphisms within the *OAS1* gene in TB cases and healthy controls from the Chinese Tibetan and Han populations.

Methods

Population study

The initial study comprised 613 patients with TB and 602 healthy controls recruited from the People's Hospital of the Aba Tibetan Autonomous Prefecture. In the independent validation study, we selected 571 TB cases and 543 healthy controls based on the same inclusion and exclusion criteria from the Chinese Han population. All subjects were unrelated ethnic Chinese.

The patients' selection criteria were: 1) written consent and agreement to participate the study; 2) having a diagnosis of TB; 3) age ≥ 18 years. The diagnosis of TB was based on sputum smear tests, sputum culture, clinical symptoms and radiological and histological pathologic examinations. Patients with HIV, hepatitis B or C, diabetes, immune-mediated disorders or other lung diseases were excluded from our study. Controls were individuals without history of TB and active TB infection that had undergone routine medical examination.

Informed consents were obtained from all individual participants included in the study. The study was approved by the ethical committee of the West China Hospital of Sichuan University.

SNP selection and genotyping

Tag SNPs in the study were downloaded from the Chinese Han in Beijing database of HapMap (http://hapmap.ncbi.nlm.nih.gov/index.html.en, HapMap Data Rel 27 Phase II + III, on NCBI B36 assembly, dbSNP b126) in a region stretching from 1000 base pairs upstream and 1000 base pairs downstream of *OAS1*; other SNPs of *OAS1* were also selected from previous studies [27, 28]. Tag SNPs were filtered according to the following criteria: (i) Hardy-Weinberg equilibrium (HWE) test $P \geq 0.05$; (ii) r^2 of pairwise linkage disequilibrium (LD) ≤ 0.8 and (iii) minor allele frequency (MAF) ≥ 0.05.

A sample of 5 ml of peripheral blood was obtained from each participant and placed in a test tube containing EDTA. We then isolated genomic DNA from the collected whole blood samples using a genomic DNA purification kit, in accordance with the manufacturer's instructions (Axygen Scientific Inc., Union City, CA, USA). Genotyping was conducted using PCR and the improved multiple ligase detection reaction (iMLDR). Five percent of samples were re-genotyped to verify the initial results.

Statistical analysis

HWE and the differences in sex between the case and control were evaluated by the Chi-squared test. Unpaired *t*-tests were used to evaluate the significance of differences in age between the case and control groups. Genotype and allele frequencies of SNPs in the TB group vs. those in the control group were calculated by logistic regression. As the genetic determinants of TB were age- and gender-dependent [29, 30], logistic regression was used to adjust for gender and age. Odds ratio (OR) and 95% confidence interval (95% CI) were examined to estimate the magnitude of the risk. LD and haplotype analyses were conducted using the SHEsis online software platform (http://analysis.bio-x.cn). A 2-sided P value of less than 0.05 was considered statistically significant and P values were conservatively Bonferroni-corrected for multiple comparisons. Power calculation was performed ($\alpha = 0.05$) by Quanto software (version 1.2.4, May 2009). The power of the two cohorts to detect relative risks (RR) of 2.0, 3.0 and 4.0 using the four SNPs studied under an allele genetic model were estimated by the Quanto software and are listed in Table S1. The two cohorts have reasonable power (> 80%) to detect genetic factors with RR 2.0 and above under the allele model in all four SNPs (Table S1). Gene-gene interaction was detected using the multifactor dimensionality reduction (MDR) software and MDR permutation testing module (http://www.epistasis.org and http://sourceforge.net/projects/mdr/files/mdrpt). We performed an eQTL analysis by using the GTEx Portal database (https://gtexportal.org/home/). All analyses were conducted using the Statistical Package for the Social Sciences (SPSS; SPSS Inc., Chicago, IL, USA), version 19.0.

Genotype data of rs10774671 in the Han Chinese in Beijing (CHB) were obtained from the HapMap project and whole-genome Expression data were obtained from the Gene Expression Omnibus of PubMed. rs10774671 genotype data were downloaded from the 1000 Genomes Browser (https://www.ncbi.nlm.nih.gov/variation/tools/1000genomes/). DNA samples were collected from participants living in the residential community at Beijing Normal University. As a result, a total of 40 individuals provided genotypic data of rs10774671. We then used the mRNA data obtained from lymphoblastoid cell lines (extracted from Gene Expression Omnibus of Pubmed, accession number GSE6536) to analyze the associations between rs10774671 and *OAS1* mRNA expression levels [31].

Results

Demographic characteristics of the study groups

In the initial study, the number of cases was 613 (male = 392; female = 221) and the controls was 602 (male = 392; female = 210). The validation cohort comprised 584 cases (male = 299; female = 285) and 543 controls (male = 266; female = 277). The mean age was 34.53 ± 14.54 years for the case group and 34.63 ± 13.85 years for the control group in the initial study. There were no significant differences between the case and control groups regarding age and sex ($P > 0.05$) in this cohort. However, the mean age was significantly different between cases (mean age = 36.50 ± 15.49) and controls (mean age = 39.35 ± 15.13) in the validation cohort ($P = 0.002$).

Analysis of HWE and association of *OAS1* SNPs with TB

A total of four SNPs (rs2240190, rs1131454, 10,774,671 and 11,066,453) were selected for analysis. Two of these four were tag SNPs (rs1131454 and rs10774671). All four SNPs did not deviate from HWE. The MAFs of SNPs were more than 0.05. Table 1 provides basic information on the four SNPs in our study.

The allele frequencies in the two groups are shown in Table 2. The genotype frequencies of the *OAS1* polymorphisms under different genetic models are summarized in Table 3. In the initial cohort, a significant association was only detected in the allele frequency of rs10774671 and the G allele acted as a protective factor against TB ($P = 0.006$, OR = 0.74, 95% CI: 0.59–0.92). Compared with the AA genotype, the frequency of the GG genotype of rs10774671 polymorphism in the case group significantly differed from the controls under the codominant model (GG vs. AA: $P = 0.008$, OR = 0.41, 95% CI: 0.21–0.80), suggesting that rs10774671 decreased the risk of TB.

To verify the results of the Tibetan population, we analyzed an independent population of Chinese Han individuals. We found that rs10774671 was also significantly associated with TB in the Chinese Han population. Compared with allele A, the G allele was more common in the control group ($P = 0.001$, OR = 0.72, 95% CI: 0.59–0.87). We also found that the GG genotype was a protective factor against TB under codominant (GG VS.

Table 1 Characteristics of the 4 SNPs in *OAS1* in the present study

SNP	Position	Region	Tibetan population		Han population	
			MAF	HWE	MAF	HWE
rs2240190 (C > A)	113,346,127	Intron 1	0.190	0.975	0.190	0.783
rs1131454 (A > G)	113,348,870	Exon 3	0.406	0.973	0.379	0.924
rs10774671 (A > G)	113,357,193	Exon 7 splice acceptor site	0.237	0.294	0.210	0.819
rs11066453 (A > G)	113,365,621	Intron 7	0.136	0.807	0.132	0.848

Abbreviation: *SNP* single nucleotide polymorphism, *MAF* minor allele frequency, *HWE* Hardy Weinberg equilibrium

Table 2 Allele distribution of *OAS1* polymorphisms in the two populations

SNP	Tibetan population				Han population			
	Cases, n (%)	Controls, n (%)	$P^{\#}$	OR[#](95%CI)	Cases, n (%)	Controls, n (%)	$P^{\#}$	OR[#](95%CI)
rs2240190(C > A)								
C	941(76.8)	954(79.2)			918(81.0)	864(80.0)		
A	285(23.2)	250(20.8)	0.128	1.16(0.96–1.41)	216(19.0)	216(20.0)	0.556	0.94(0.76–1.16)
rs1131454(A > G)								
A	778(63.5)	726(60.3)			704(62.1)	610(56.5)		
G	448(36.5)	478(39.7)	0.110	0.88(0.74–1.03)	430(37.9)	470(43.5)	0.004*	0.78(0.66-0.93)
rs10774671(A > G)								
A	1051(85.7)	984(81.6)			896(79.0)	793(73.4)		
G	175(14.3)	222(18.4)	0.006*	0.74(0.59-0.92)	238(21.0)	287(26.6)	0.001*	0.72(0.59-0.87)
rs11066453 (A > G)								
A	1171(95.5)	1124(93.4)			984(86.8)	937(86.8)		
G	55(4.5)	80(6.6)	0.022	0.66(0.47–0.94)	150(13.2)	143(13.2)	0.807	1.03(0.81–1.32)

SNP single nucleotide polymorphism, *CI* confidence interval, *OR* odds ratio
[#]adjusted by sex and age
*Bonferroni correction was performed with $p \le 0.0125$ (0.05/4) considered significant

AA: $P = 0.001$, OR = 0.40, 95% CI: 0.23–0.69) and recessive (GG VS. AA+GA: $P = 0.005$, OR = 0.46, 95% CI: 0.27–0.79) models (Table 4). In addition, rs1131454 was associated with TB susceptibility in the validation study. Compared with the control group, the TB group had lower proportions of the G allele ($P = 0.004$, OR = 0.78, 95% CI: 0.66–0.93) and GG genotype (codominant model: GG vs. AA, $P = 0.001$, OR = 0.52, 95% CI: 0.36–0.76; recessive model: GG vs. AA+GA, $P = 0.002$, OR = 0.59, 95% CI: 0.42–0.82).

Linkage disequilibrium and haplotype analyses

Information on LD for these four SNPs in the Chinese Tibetan population is shown in Fig. 1. LD among these four SNPs in the *OAS1* gene was evaluated by the LD test using r^2, which confirmed that these SNPs were not in LD ($r^2 < 0.5$). No haplotypes were associated with TB in the two studies (Table 4).

Gene–gene interactions

rs2240190, rs1131454 and rs10774671 formed the best gene-gene interaction model with a testing balanced accuracy of 57.61% and cross-validation consistency of 10/10. It was confirmed statistically significant using 1000-fold permutation testing ($P = 0.001$).

eQTL and gene expression analysis for rs10774671

eQTL analysis using the GTEx Portal database showed significant eQTL effects of rs10774671 ($P < 0.001$) on *OAS1* expression in whole blood from 369 individuals. The 40 CHB were divided into three groups according to rs10774671genotypic data. In brief, 15 CHB had the AA genotype, 20 had the GA genotype and 5 had the GG genotype. As shown in Fig. 2, GEO2R analysis revealed that the rs10774671 polymorphism was associated with *OAS1* expression levels after adjustment for multiple comparisons ($P < 0.001$).

Discussion

In China, the ethnic Tibetan population is more likely to be infected with TB than the Han population [32, 33]. It is possible that host genetic difference is one of the bases of TB susceptibility. In this study, four SNPs in *OAS1* (rs2240190, rs1131454, 10,774,671 and 11,066,453) were investigated in Chinese Han and Chinese Tibetan patients with TB. Our data showed, for the first time, that the G allele and the GG genotype of rs10774671 in *OAS1* were associated with TB in the two populations.

OAS1 is an enzyme that plays an important role in innate antiviral defence [34]. This enzyme is activated by the presence of double-stranded or single-stranded RNA with a secondary structure and catalyses the oligomerisation of ATP into 2-5A [35]. These processes activate latent RNase L, which degrades viral and cellular RNA and blocks protein synthesis. In accordance with this function, human OAS1 mainly affects susceptibility to viral infections [35, 36]. Given the importance of the OAS1 protein, SNPs in the *OAS1* gene may affect susceptibility to infectious diseases. In the present study, we demonstrated that polymorphisms in *OAS1* were associated with TB. It is unclear why the heightened antiviral enzyme activity in individuals was associated with TB, but this association may be explained as follows. One explanation is that the major role of the OAS proteins is as immune regulators in innate immunity, although previous studies indicated that they also play important

Table 3 Association between genotype of *OAS1* and TB in the two populations

SNP	Genetic model	genotype	Tibetan population				Han population			
			Case, n (%)	Controls, n (%)	$P^{\#}$	OR[#](95%CI)	Case, n (%)	Controls, n (%)	$P^{\#}$	OR[#](95%CI)
rs2240190 (C > A)	Codominant	CC	361(58.9)	383(63.6)	–	1.00	368(64.9)	343(63.5)		
		CA	219(35.7)	188(31.2)	0.084	1.24(0.97–1.58)	182(32.1)	178(33.0)	0.659	0.94(0.73–1.22)
		AA	33(5.4)	31(5.1)	0.567	1.16(0.70–1.94)	17(3)	19(3.5)	0.637	0.87(0.44–1.69)
	Dominant	AA+CA	252(41.1)	219(36.3)	0.084	1.23(0.97–1.55)	199(35.1)	197(36.5)	0.595	0.94(0.73–1.20)
		CC	361(58.9)	383(63.6)	–	1.00	368(64.9)	343(63.5)		
	Recessive	AA	33(5.4)	31(5.1)	0.819	1.06(0.64–1.76)	17(3)	197(36.5)	0.673	0.87(0.44–1.69)
		CC + CA	580(94.6)	571(94.9)	–	1.00	550(73.4)	521(96.5)		
rs1131454 (A > G)	Codominant	AA	246(40.1)	230(38.2)	–	1.00	205(36.2)	170(31.5)		
		GA	286(46.7)	266(44.2)	0.971	1.01(0.79–1.28)	294(51.9)	270(50.0)	0.353	0.88(0.68–1.15)
		GG	81(13.2)	106(17.6)	0.054	0.71(0.51–1.01)	68(12.0)	100(18.5)	0.001*	0.52(0.36-0.76)
	Dominant	GG + GA	367(59.9)	372(61.8)	0.484	0.92(0.73–1.16)	362(42.0)	370(68.5)	0.067	0.79(0.61–0.02)
		AA	246(40.1)	230(38.2)	–	1.00	205(36.2)	170(31.5)		
	Recessive	GG	81(13.2)	106(17.6)	0.037	0.72(0.52–0.98)	68(12.0)	100(18.5)	0.002*	0.59(0.42-0.82)
		AA+GA	522(86.8)	496(82.4)	–	1.00	499(88.0)	440(81.5)		
rs10774671 (A > G)	Codominant	AA	451(73.6)	409(68.0)	–	1.00	351(61.9)	294(92.4)		
		GA	149(24.3)	164(27.2)	0.148	0.83(0.64–1.07)	194(34.2)	205(38.0)	0.053	0.78(0.61–1.00)
		GG	13(2.1)	29(4.8)	0.008*	0.41(0.21-0.80)	22(3.9)	41(7.6)	0.001*	0.40(0.23-0.69)
	Dominant	GG + GA	162(26.4)	193(32.0)	0.032	0.76(0.59–0.98)	216(28.4)	246(45.6)	0.007	0.72(0.56–0.91)
		AA	451(73.6)	409(68.0)	–	1.00	351(61.9)	294(92.4)		
	Recessive	GG	13(2.1)	29(4.8)	0.013	0.43(0.22–0.83)	22(3.9)	41(7.6)	0.005*	0.46(0.27-0.79)
		AA+GA	600(97.9)	573(95.2)	–	1.00	545(96.1)	499(92.4)		
rs11066453 (A > G)	Codominant	AA	558(91.0)	525(87.2)	–	1.00	426(75.1)	408(75.6)		
		GA	55(9.0)	74(12.3)	0.060	0.70(0.49–1.02)	132(23.3)	121(22.4)	0.550	1.09(0.82–1.45)
		GG	0(0)	3(0.5)	–	–	9(1.6)	11(2.0)	0.592	0.78(0.32–1.92)
	Dominant	GG + GA	55(9.0)	77(12.8)	0.035	0.68(0.47–0.97)	141(20.2)	132(24.4)	0.649	1.07(0.81–1.41)
		AA	558(91.0)	525(87.2)	–	1.00	426(75.1)	408(75.6)		
	Recessive	GG	0(0)	3(0.5)	–	–	9(1.6)	132(24.4)	0.558	0.77(0.31–1.87)
		AA+GA	613(100)	599(99.5)	–	–	558(98.4)	529(98.0)		

SNP single nucleotide polymorphism, *CI* confidence interval, *OR* odds ratio

[#]adjusted by sex and age

*Bonferroni correction was performed with $p \leq 0.0125$ (0.05/4) considered significant

Table 4 Haplotype analyses in the Tibetan population

	Tibetan population				Han population			
Haplotype	Cases, n (%)	Controls, n (%)	P	OR	Cases, n (%)	Controls, n (%)	P	OR
AGAA	198 (16.1)	162 (13.5)	0.038	1.27(1.01–1.59)	132(11.4)	113(10.4)	0.454	1.11 (0.85–1.45)
AGGA	53 (4.3)	80 (6.6)	0.018	0.65(0.46–0.93)	74(6.4)	94(8.7)	0.043	0.72(0.53–0.99)
CAAA	690 (56.3)	640 (53.2)	0.035	1.19(1.01–1.40)	538(46.4)	459(42.5)	0.052	1.18(1.00–1.40)
CAAG	54 (4.4)	78 (6.5)	0.034	0.68(0.48–0.97)	150(12.9)	142(13.1)	0.926	0.99(0.77–1.27)
CGAA	75 (6.1)	94 (7.8)	0.153	0.80(0.58–1.09)	60(5.2)	69(6.4)	0.227	0.80(0.56–1.15)
CGGA	121 (9.9)	141 (11.7)	0.207	0.85(0.66–1.10)	190(16.4)	193(17.9)	0.357	0.90(0.72–1.12)
Other[a]	35 (2.9)	9 (0.7)	–		15(1.4)	11(0.9)		

CI confidence interval, *OR* odds ratio
[a]Those lowest frequency threshold (LFT) < 0.03 were pooled in this part
Bonferroni correction was performed with p ≤ 0.008 (0.05/6) considered significant
For each haplotype, alleles are arranged in order of rs2240190, rs1131454, 10,774,671 and 11,066,453

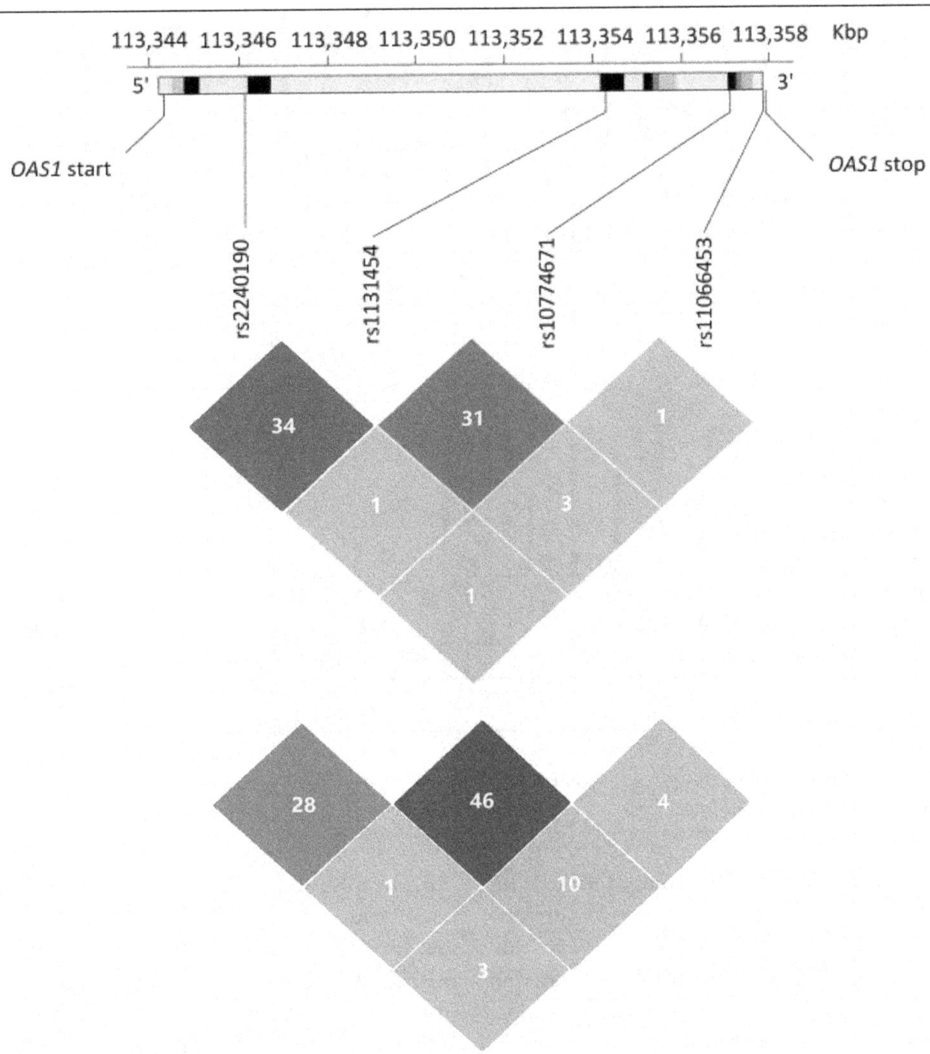

Fig. 1 Genomic structure, localization and LD of the genotyped polymorphisms within *OAS1* in both Tibetan (above) and Han (below) populations. The figure shows the genomic structure and localization of the genotyped polymorphisms in *OAS1* retrieved from the HapMap database. In the upper panel, the black and grey boxes represent exons, and light grey ones represent introns. Locations of the four genotyped SNPs are indicated by the connecting line. In the lower panel LD (r^2 value) estimates corresponding to all pairs of SNPs are shown.

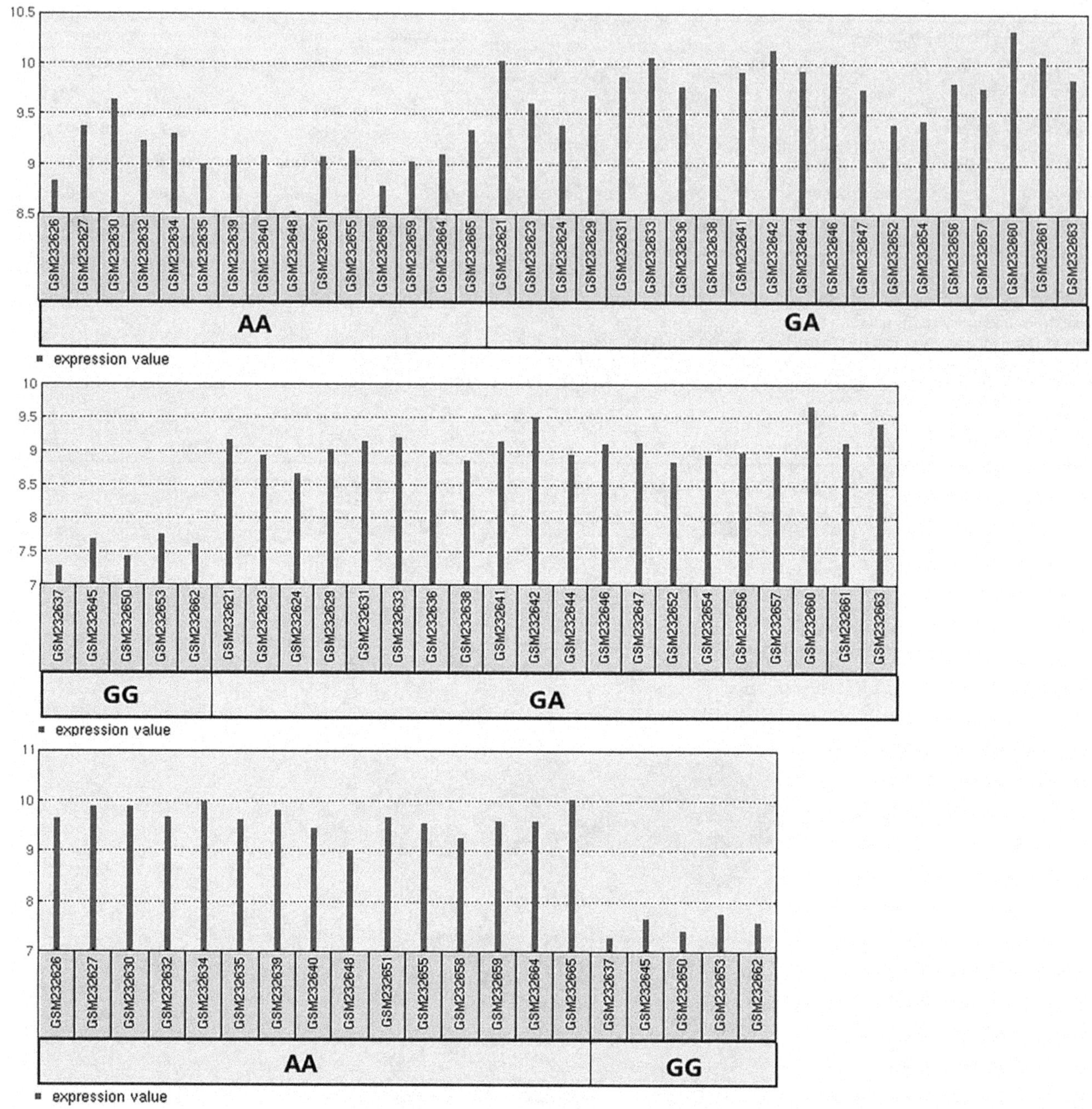

Fig. 2 OAS1 mRNA expression levels among the different genotypes of rs10774671. The black bars represent fold change. The black bars below show all sample identifiers annotated by GSM numbers

roles in other cellular functions. The role of OAS1 in immune-related diseases has been shown by a number of association studies [25, 26]. It is well known that the immune response against TB plays a critical role in the progression of *MTB* infection. Another explanation is that the *OAS1* gene affects susceptibility to TB through the type II IFN pathway [14, 15]. Type II IFN (IFN-γ) is critical for host defence against certain bacterial and parasitic pathogens [37]. IFN-γ can activate infected host macrophages to inhibit the replication of *MTB* directly [38]. In addition, OAS gene expression was regulated by both type I and type II IFNs [39]. A previous study suggested that IFN-γ could increase the levels of OAS mRNA [40]. Furthermore, *OAS1* gene up-regulation was observed in several gene expression signatures that differentiated active TB from latent TB infection [41, 42]. It was also established that there was a prominent correlation between OAS expression and TB [14]. Moreover, data from Noguchi et al. revealed the potential role of *OAS1* polymorphisms in respiratory infection [27].

Therefore, we assume that the polymorphism in the *OAS* gene may be associated with the risk of TB infection through the type II IFN pathway.

As a functional *OAS1* polymorphic marker, rs10774671 was reported to be associated with disease/viral infection [36, 43]. rs10774671 is located at the last nucleotide of intron 6 in *OAS1*, which acts as a splice-acceptor site for exon 7. The G allele was demonstrated to allow splicing to occur leading to the production of a p46 form with high enzymatic OAS activity [20]. The rs10774671 A allele usually prevents splicing at this site and thus splicing happens further downstream, resulting in the p48 and p52 forms associated with low OAS enzymatic activity. rs10774671 could also control other splice variants of OAS including p42 and p44 [20]. In addition, the HapMap genotypic data (Fig. 2) of rs10774671 suggested that individuals with GG genotype had lower expression levels than those with AA and GA genotypes. However, rs10774671 GG genotype was reported to be associated with the highest enzyme activity of OAS1 in unstimulated lymphocytes [44]. The inconsistent results between mRNA expression and enzyme activity may attribute to the reason that gene expressions at the transcriptional and translational levels might be different. Our data were partly consistent with these observations, in that the G allele and GG genotype had significant protective effects against TB, whereas the AG genotype was not associated with TB. Furthermore, this result was validated in the Chinese Han population. Considering the aforementioned functional effects of rs10774671 on phenotypes, we speculate that rs10774671 could alter *OAS1* expression levels precluding the type I IFN pathway resulting in a protective response.

In order to detect whether two or more SNPs interact either directly or indirectly to change TB risk separate from their independent effects, we conducted a gene-gene interaction analysis. We did not find any significant differences in single SNP analysis between cases and controls groups for rs2240190, rs1131454 and 11,066,453. However, rs2240190, rs1131454 and rs10774671 formed the best gene-gene interaction model. This result was consistent with the phenomenon that most diseases including TB are caused by multiple factors and gene-gene or gene-environment interactions are characteristic of the genetic factors. In addition, we also conducted a haplotype analysis which was based on the association between a polymorphism and the ancestral haplotype [45]. However, inconsistent with the gene-gene interaction result, there was no significant association between haplotypes and TB. Since the haplotype analysis approach was used for analyzing haplotype effects at numerous closely linked loci, and the gene-gene interaction analysis could be used for analyzing the unlinked loci [46, 47]. We speculate the discrepant results are likely attributable to different methods.

rs2240190 is located in intron 1 and it may have an alternative splicing regulatory effect, based on the Functional Single Nucleotide Polymorphism database [48]. To the best of our knowledge, no previous studies investigated the association between rs2240190 and disease. Only one study suggested that this genetic polymorphism was not in LD with rs10774671 [27]. rs1131454 (formerly rs3741981), in the evolutionarily conserved exon 3, is nonsynonymous (the G → A transition results in a G → S amino acid change). This polymorphic locus is close to the dsRNA binding domain of all OAS1 isoforms. In general, the AA, GA and GG genotypes of rs1131454 lead to low, intermediate and high OAS1 enzyme activity, respectively [44]. This polymorphic locus was demonstrated to be functional in the progression of the severe acute respiratory syndrome [49]. In our study, we demonstrated that the G allele and GG genotype were associated with TB in the Han population.

Genome-wide association studies with longitudinal data found that rs11066453 was a significant disease susceptibility locus, as confirmed by the Health Examination cohort [50]. Furthermore, the rs11066453 polymorphism was strongly related to *OAS1* mRNA expression levels in Epstein–Barr virus infection [51], and the monoallelically expressed *OAS1* gene was also significantly associated with the gamma-glutamyltransferase level [28]. This strong association of the *OAS1* gene that contains the rs11066453 polymorphism in the development and progression of human diseases may be due to it affecting *OAS1* expression. However, inconsistent with these findings, there was no significant association with TB susceptibility detected in the present study.

There are several limitations in our study. First, lack of data regarding the association between other genes in the OAS cluster and TB limited our understanding of genetic mechanisms regulating the pathogenesis of TB. Second, our study lacked clinical information for the Tibetans, which limited the analysis of the association with clinical characteristics. Finally, functional validation of the included SNPs was not carried out. As a result, the true causal allele underlying the genetic association result is still unknown.

In conclusion, we were the first to investigate the association between *OAS1* polymorphisms and TB in the Chinese Tibetan population and validated the results in an independent cohort. We found that rs10774671, located in the *OAS1* gene region is associated with susceptibility to TB in Tibetans and may act as a protective factor against TB, which was validated in the Chinese Han population. In addition, we also found that rs1131454 was a protective factor against TB in the Chinese Han population. rs2240190, rs1131454 and rs10774671 formed the best gene-gene interaction model in MDR analysis and may be considered as one of the multiple contributors to the progress of this complicated disease. However, in order to get more detailed mechanistic insight into the pathway of how OAS1 may act on TB, there is a need for further research in this field. Similar studies in different populations, gene-environment interactions analysis and functional studies are warranted to confirm and reinforce our results.

Abbreviations

CI: Confidence interval; HIV: Human immunodeficiency virus; HWE: Hardy-Weinberg equilibrium; IFN: Interferon; iMLDR: Improved multiple ligase detection reaction; LD: Pairwise linkage disequilibrium; MAF: Minor allele frequency; MDR: Multifactor dimensionality reduction; MTB: *Mycobacterium tuberculosis*; OAS1: 2'-5'-oligoadenylate synthetase 1; OR: Odds ratio; RNase L: Ribonuclease L; RR: Relative risks; SNPs: Single-nucleotide polymorphisms; TB: Tuberculosis

Acknowledgements

The authors are grateful for all the cases and the controls who volunteered for participating in the study.

Funding

This work was supported in part by the National Natural Science Foundation of China (Beijing, China) Grants 81870015, 81072432. This funding supported the costs of the design of the study and collection, analysis, and interpretation of data and in writing the manuscript.

Authors' contributions

All authors read and approved the final manuscript. Conceived and designed the experiments: JQH. Performed the experiments: YW SQW GC. Analyzed the data: SQW JQH. Contributed reagents/materials/analysis tools: MMZ MGW. Wrote the paper: SQW JQH. Obtained ethical permission for the use of blood when taking samples: YW SQW JQH.

Ethics approval and consent to participate

The study was approved by the ethical committee of the West China Hospital of Sichuan University (the NO.131 file). The ethical approval is as follows. All participants in both groups voluntarily joined this study with written informed consents. A sample of 5 ml of peripheral blood was obtained from each participant.

All procedures performed in studies involving human participants were in accordance with the ethical standards of the institutional and/or national research committee and with the 1964 Helsinki declaration and its later amendments or comparable ethical standards.

Consent for publication

Not applicable.

Competing interests

The authors declare that they have no conflict of interest.

Author details

[1]Department of Respiratory and Critical Care Medicine, West China Hospital, Sichuan University, No. 37, Guo Xue Alley, Chengdu 610041, Sichuan, People's Republic of China. [2]Division of Geriatrics, Sichuan Provincial People's Hospital, Chengdu, Sichuan, China.

References

1. World Health Organization (2018). Global tuberculosis report 2018. http://www.who.int/tb/publications/global_report/en/ (accessed Sep 26, 2018).
2. Comstock GW, et al. The prognosis of a positive tuberculin reaction in childhood and adolescence. Am J Epidemiol. 1974;99(2):131–8.
3. van de Vosse E, et al. Human genetics of intracellular infectious diseases: molecular and cellular immunity against mycobacteria and salmonellae. Lancet Infect Dis. 2004;4(12):739–49.
4. Newport MJ, et al. A mutation in the interferon-gamma-receptor gene and susceptibility to mycobacterial infection. N Engl J Med. 1996;335(26):1941–9.
5. Manca C, et al. Virulence of a Mycobacterium tuberculosis clinical isolate in mice is determined by failure to induce Th1 type immunity and is associated with induction of IFN-alpha /beta. Proc Natl Acad Sci U S A. 2001;98(10):5752–7.
6. de Paus RA, et al. Inhibition of the type I immune responses of human monocytes by IFN-alpha and IFN-beta. Cytokine. 2013;61(2):645–55.
7. van de Vosse E, et al. Genetic deficiencies of innate immune signalling in human infectious disease. Lancet Infect Dis. 2009;9(11):688–98.
8. Flynn JL, et al. An essential role for interferon gamma in resistance to Mycobacterium tuberculosis infection. J Exp Med. 1993;178(6):2249–54.
9. Hovnanian A, et al. The human 2',5'-oligoadenylate synthetase locus is composed of three distinct genes clustered on chromosome 12q24.2 encoding the 100-, 69-, and 40-kDa forms. Genomics. 1998;52(3):267–77.
10. Sadler AJ, Williams BR. Interferon-inducible antiviral effectors. Nat Rev Immunol. 2008;8(7):559–68.
11. Hovanessian AG, Justesen J. The human 2'-5'oligoadenylate synthetase family: unique interferon-inducible enzymes catalyzing 2'-5' instead of 3'-5' phosphodiester bond formation. Biochimie. 2007;89(6–7):779–88.
12. Domingo-Gil E, Esteban M. Role of mitochondria in apoptosis induced by the 2-5A system and mechanisms involved. Apoptosis. 2006;11(5):725–38.
13. Yaffe A, et al. Inhibition of 2-5A synthetase expression by antisense RNA interferes with interferon-mediated antiviral and antiproliferative effects and induces anchorage-independent cell growth. Cell Growth Differ. 1996;7(8):969–78.
14. Leisching G, et al. OAS1, 2, and 3: significance during active tuberculosis? J Infect Dis. 2018;217(10):1517–21.
15. Leisching G, et al. The association of OASL and type I Interferons in the pathogenesis and survival of intracellular replicating bacterial species. Front Cell Infect Microbiol. 2017;7:196.
16. Justesen J, et al. Gene structure and function of the 2'-5'-oligoadenylate synthetase family. Cell Mol Life Sci. 2000;57(11):1593–612.
17. Ibsen MS, et al. The 2'-5'-oligoadenylate synthetase 3 enzyme potently synthesizes the 2'-5'-oligoadenylates required for RNase L activation. J Virol. 2014;88(24):14222–31.
18. Li Y, et al. Activation of RNase L is dependent on OAS3 expression during infection with diverse human viruses. Proc Natl Acad Sci U S A. 2016;113(8):2241–6.
19. Dunn GP, et al. The immunobiology of cancer immunosurveillance and immunoediting. Immunity. 2004;21(2):137–48.
20. Lim JK, et al. Genetic variation in OAS1 is a risk factor for initial infection with West Nile virus in man. PLoS Pathog. 2009;5(2):e1000321.
21. Zhao Y, et al. Evaluate the relationship between polymorphisms of OAS1 gene and susceptibility to chronic hepatitis C with high resolution melting analysis. Clin Exp Med. 2013;13(3):171–6.
22. Chaaithanya IK, et al. Association of Oligoadenylate Synthetase Gene Cluster and DC-SIGN (CD209) gene polymorphisms with clinical symptoms in Chikungunya virus infection. DNA Cell Biol. 2016;35(1):44–50.
23. Thamizhmani R, Vijayachari P. Association of dengue virus infection susceptibility with polymorphisms of 2'-5'-oligoadenylate synthetase genes: a case-control study. Braz J Infect Dis. 2014;18(5):548–50.
24. Haralambieva IH, et al. Genetic polymorphisms in host antiviral genes: associations with humoral and cellular immunity to measles vaccine. Vaccine. 2011;29(48):8988–97.
25. Tessier MC, et al. Type 1 diabetes and the OAS gene cluster: association with splicing polymorphism or haplotype? J Med Genet. 2006;43(2):129–32.
26. Fedetz M, et al. OAS1 gene haplotype confers susceptibility to multiple sclerosis. Tissue Antigens. 2006;68(5):446–9.
27. Noguchi S, et al. Differential effects of a common splice site polymorphism on the generation of OAS1 variants in human bronchial epithelial cells. Hum Immunol. 2013;74(3):395–401.

28. Park YM, et al. Genome-wide detection of allelic gene expression in hepatocellular carcinoma cells using a human exome SNP chip. Gene. 2014; 551(2):236–42.
29. Hall NB, et al. Polymorphisms in TICAM2 and IL1B are associated with TB. Genes Immun. 2015;16(2):127–33.
30. Sabri A, et al. Association study of genes controlling IL-12-dependent IFN-gamma immunity: STAT4 alleles increase risk of pulmonary tuberculosis in Morocco. J Infect Dis. 2014;210(4):611–8.
31. Chen C, et al. A rare variant at 11p13 is associated with tuberculosis susceptibility in the Han Chinese population. Sci Rep. 2016;6:24016.
32. He S, et al. Association of IL4, IL6, and IL10 polymorphisms with pulmonary tuberculosis in a Tibetan Chinese population. Oncotarget. 2018;9(23):16418–26.
33. Wang L, et al. The fifth national tuberculosis epidemiological survey in 2010. Chin J Antituber. 2012;34(8):485–508.
34. Schneider WM, et al. Interferon-stimulated genes: a complex web of host defenses. Annu Rev Immunol. 2014;32:513–45.
35. Tsutsui-Takeuchi M, et al. Roles of retinoic acid-inducible gene-I-like receptors (RLRs), toll-like receptor (TLR) 3 and 2′-5′ oligoadenylate synthetase as viral recognition receptors on human mast cells in response to viral infection. Immunol Res. 2015;61(3):240–9.
36. Liu X, et al. A functional variant in the OAS1 gene is associated with Sjogren's syndrome complicated with HBV infection. Sci Rep. 2017; 7(1):17571.
37. Boehm U, et al. Cellular responses to interferon-gamma. Annu Rev Immunol. 1997;15:749–95.
38. MacMicking JD, et al. Immune control of tuberculosis by IFN-gamma-inducible LRG-47. Science. 2003;302(5645):654–9.
39. Zhou A, et al. Interferon action and apoptosis are defective in mice devoid of 2′,5′-oligoadenylate-dependent RNase L. EMBO J. 1997;16(21):6355–63.
40. Corrias MV, et al. Induction of 2.5 OAS gene expression and activity is not sufficient for IFN-gamma-induced neuroblastoma cell differentiation. Int J Cancer. 1995;62(2):223–9.
41. Berry MP, et al. An interferon-inducible neutrophil-driven blood transcriptional signature in human tuberculosis. Nature. 2010; 466(7309):973–7.
42. Ottenhoff TH, et al. Genome-wide expression profiling identifies type 1 interferon response pathways in active tuberculosis. PLoS One. 2012; 7(9):e45839.
43. Bader El Din NG, et al. Impact of OAS1 exon 7 rs10774671 genetic variation on liver fibrosis progression in Egyptian HCV genotype 4 patients. Viral Immunol. 2015;28(9):509–16.
44. Bonnevie-Nielsen V, et al. Variation in antiviral 2′,5′-oligoadenylate synthetase (2′5′AS) enzyme activity is controlled by a single-nucleotide polymorphism at a splice-acceptor site in the OAS1 gene. Am J Hum Genet. 2005;76(4):623–33.
45. Gabriel SB, et al. The structure of haplotype blocks in the human genome. Science. 2002;296(5576):2225–9.
46. Thornton-Wells TA, et al. Genetics, statistics and human disease: analytical retooling for complexity. Trends Genet. 2004;20(12):640–7.
47. Cordell HJ, et al. Case/pseudocontrol analysis in genetic association studies: a unified framework for detection of genotype and haplotype associations, gene-gene and gene-environment interactions, and parent-of-origin effects. Genet Epidemiol. 2004;26(3):167–85.
48. Lee PH, Shatkay H. F-SNP: computationally predicted functional SNPs for disease association studies. Nucleic Acids Res. 2008;36(Database issue):D820–4.
49. Hamano E, et al. Polymorphisms of interferon-inducible genes OAS-1 and MxA associated with SARS in the Vietnamese population. Biochem Biophys Res Commun. 2005;329(4):1234–9.
50. Lee Y, et al. On the analysis of a repeated measure design in genome-wide association analysis. Int J Environ Res Public Health. 2014;11(12):12283–303.
51. Kim YJ, et al. Large-scale genome-wide association studies in east Asians identify new genetic loci influencing metabolic traits. Nat Genet. 2011; 43(10):990–5.

Yield of close contact tracing using two different programmatic approaches from tuberculosis index cases

Carla Loredo[1], Michelle Cailleaux-Cezar[1], Anne Efron[2], Fernanda Carvalho Queiroz de Mello[1] and Marcus Barreto Conde[1,3*]

Abstract

Background: Being a contact of a pulmonary tuberculosis (TB) case is a risk factor for active and latent TB. The objective of this study is to determine the contact tracing yield using two different programmatic definitions of close contact in the city of Rio de Janeiro, Brazil.

Methods: This is a retrospective quasi-experimental study. Data were obtained by reviewing the medical records from TB index cases and their close contacts admitted to the Outpatient TB Clinic of the Institute of Thoracic Diseases, University of Rio de Janeiro. From January 2001 to December 2004, a close contact was defined as an individual who shared an enclosed space with a TB index case for a total period of ≥ 100 hours, whereas from January 2005 to December 2008 the definition of close contact was changed to an individual who shared an enclosed space with a TB index case ≥ 4 hours a week. The primary outcome of this study was newly diagnosed pulmonary TB cases and the secondary outcome was the prevalence of latent TB infection (LTBI) among close contacts during both periods.

Results: From 2001–2004, 810 close contacts from 257 index cases were evaluated and the prevalence of active TB and LTBI were 2% (16/810) and 62% (496/794), respectively. From 2005–2008, 1,310 close contacts from 369 index cases were identified and the prevalence of active TB and LTBI were 2.7% (35/1,310) and 69% (877/1,275), respectively. There was not a statically significant difference in the detection of active TB ($p = 0.3$) between the 2 time periods, but the detection of LTBI was significant higher ($p = 0.003$). The number needed to screen (contacts/new cases) decreased from 50 to 37 and the number need to contact trace (index cases/new cases) decreased from 16 to 10 from 2001–2004 to 2005–2008.

Conclusion: In conclusion, the findings of this study suggest that the less conservative definition of TB close contacts (sharing space ≥ 4 h/week) can be a helpful tool for increasing the rate of diagnosis for newly active pulmonary TB cases and for the detection of LTBI among contacts of active pulmonary TB cases.

Keywords: Tuberculosis, Contact, Diagnosis, Latent tuberculosis

* Correspondence: marcusconde@hucff.ufrj.br
[1]Institute of Thoracic Diseases of Federal University of Rio de Janeiro, Rio de Janeiro, Brazil
[3]Hospital Universitário Clementino Fraga Filho, Cidade Universitária, Rua Professor Rodolpho Paulo Rocco n° 255, 6° andar, Rio de Janeiro 21941-913, Brazil
Full list of author information is available at the end of the article

Background

It is internationally recognized that children under five years of age and persons living with human immunodeficiency virus (PLHIV) who were exposed to infectious cases of tuberculosis (TB) must be evaluated for active TB and considered for treatment of latent TB infection (LTBI) once active TB is excluded [1,2]. In Brazil, since 2009, the recommendation has been that close contacts of an infectious TB case, despite their age and HIV status, must be investigated for active TB and LTBI [3,4]. However, the different definitions utilized for the term "close contact of TB" can make the yield of contact tracing irregular among different settings [3,5-7]. In the Outpatient TB Clinic of the Institute of Thoracic Diseases (IDT) of the Federal University of Rio de Janeiro (UFRJ), Brazil, all contacts of TB index cases who shared and enclosed space for ≥ 100 hours in total used to be defined as a close contact and eligible to be investigated for active TB and for LTBI. However, in 2005, the TB Clinic of IDT/UFRJ reduced the exposure time for TB contacts from 100 total hours to ≥ 4 hours a week. This new definition for "close contacts" was based on the definition utilized by the Tuberculosis Trial Consortium (TBTC) from Center for Diseases Control and Prevention for the Study 26 Protocol (www.clinicaltrials.gov; NCT00164450), a clinical trial of 9 months of daily Isoniazid (INH) *versus* 12 weeks of weekly Rifapentine/INH for the prevention of TB. The Federal University of Rio de Janeiro (UFRJ) in collaboration with Johns Hopkins University was one of TBTC sites for Study 26 [8].

The purpose of this study was to compare the yield of contact tracing between the close contact definition utilized during the period of 2001–2004 (sharing space with an index case ≥ 100 hours total) with the definition utilized in the period 2005–2008 (sharing space with an index case ≥ 4 hours per week). Our hypothesis was that the change in the operational definition of a close contact to 4 hours/week would increase the detection of news cases of active TB and LTBI and reduce the number needed to contact trace (NNS).

Methods

Design

This is a quasi-experimental study with internal comparison.

Setting

This study was conducted in the Outpatient TB Clinic of the IDT/UFRJ, a referral center for TB treatment and for TB Clinical Trials (former site 29, Hopkins-Brazil, from the Tuberculosis Trial Consortium of Center for Diseases Control and Prevention) in Rio de Janeiro, Brazil. The incidence rate of TB in Rio de Janeiro city during the first period of the study ranged from 94/100,000 (2001) to 85/100,000 habitants (2004) and during the second period it ranged from 80/100,000 (2005) to 70/100,000 habitants (2008) [9].

Subject selection and data collection

The chart number of all TB cases and their contacts that were admitted to the TB Clinic of IDT/UFRJ between April 1st, 2001 to December 30th, 2008 were obtained from the register book. A data collection instrument was pre-tested and modified during a pilot study conducted in December 2008 with 20 charts (data not shown). The following data were recorded from the chart review: results from acid fast bacilli (AFB); TB culture; tuberculin skin test (TST); chest X ray (CXR); demographic data (sex, age); smoking status; alcohol consumption; use of illicit drugs; presence of diabetes; prior TB treatment; institutionalization (prison, shelter, or nursing home) within last 3 years; and HIV status (patients were tested for HIV only if active TB had been diagnosed; contacts were not tested for HIV). All contacts of a TB index case that were evaluated for LTBI and/or active TB in the Outpatient TB Clinic of IDT/UFRJ were enrolled in this study. Exclusion criteria were subjects with unavailable records, contacts with prior active TB treatment, missing results from the HIV test (index cases only), AFB, TST or culture and those with contaminated culture for *Mycobacterium tuberculosis* recorded in the chart.

As per the TB Clinic routine, during the interview in which the TB treatment is prescribed to an index case, a health care worker (HCW) explained to the patient the definition of a close contact (which was different on depending of the period evaluated, 2001–2004 or 2005–2008). Following this explanation, the HCW provided a printed invitation for close contacts ≥ 15 years old who were identified during the interview to attend a lecture conducted weekly in the TB Clinic. Because the Outpatient TB Clinic is an adult Clinic, the HCW instructed the index case to take all close contacts under 15 years of age to the Pediatric Outpatient Clinic of the University. The weekly lecture about TB was presented by a nurse who explained to all close contacts concepts about latent TB infection, active TB, diagnosis and treatment. After the lecture all contacts were invited to have a TST. Contacts with a positive TST or documented conversion as well as those with respiratory symptoms underwent a physical examination and had a CXR performed. Symptomatic subjects and/or those with altered CXR were instructed to provide two unsupervised sputum specimens for smear and *Mycobacterium tuberculosis* culture testing. Subjects with abnormal CXRs who were unable to provide sputum spontaneously underwent sputum induction with hypertonic saline solution. The TST was administered using the Mantoux technique and was read by a trained and certified (degree of intra-reader reliability > 95% and inter-reader reliability ≥ 80%) HCW. All testing was performed using purified protein derivative (PPD), RT23 (0.1 ml = 2 TU) (Staten Serum Institute, Copenhagen, Denmark) [10].

Ethical approval

The study was approved by the Federal University of Rio de Janeiro Ethics Committee in July 2008.

Definitions

Participants who reported smoking at least 100 cigarettes in their lifetime and who, at the time of survey, were smoking at least one day a week were defined as a current smoker; respondents who reported smoking less than 100 cigarettes in their lifetime and who, at the time of the survey, did not smoke at all were defined as former smoker; respondents who reported never having smoked any cigarette were defined as never smoking. Alcohol abuse was defined as daily consumption of at least 30 grams of alcohol for men and 24 grams for women. The definition of a close TB contact from 2001–2004 were all contacts of TB index cases who shared an enclosed space for ≥ 100 hours total. The definition of a close TB contact from 2005–2008 was those who shared an enclosed space ≥ 4 hours per week with a TB index case. A positive TST and conversion to a positive test were defined according to criteria of the American Thoracic Society and the Centers for Disease Control and Prevention [10,11]. LTBI cases were defined as a close contact with a positive TST or with a documented conversion. Confirmed active TB was defined as growth of *M. tuberculosis* in culture from respiratory specimen.

Statistical methods

The primary outcome was newly diagnosed pulmonary TB during both periods (2001–2004 and 2005–2008). We also calculated the number of contacts needed to screen (NNS) to find one new case of active TB and the number need to contact trace (NNCT) [12,13]. The NNS is calculated by dividing the number of contacts screened by the number of new cases diagnosed [12]. The NNCT is calculated as the number of index cases divided by the number of new active TB cases [13]. The secondary outcome was the prevalence of LTBI among contacts during both periods (2001–2004 and 2005–2008).

Statistical analysis

The Chi square test was used in the analysis of dichotomous variables and Fisher's exact test was used when appropriate. The odds ratio (OR) of the association between independent variables and outcomes with 95% confidence interval (CI) was calculated. A p-value <0.05 was considered statistically significant. The results were analyzed using IBM SPSS Statistics 20.

Results

Over a 92-month period, 806 patients with active pulmonary TB were admitted to the Outpatient TB Clinic of IDT/UFRJ. All medical records were reviewed and 180 active TB cases were excluded because the AFB results were unknown (n = 13), the M.tb culture results were missing or contaminated (n = 45), HIV status was unknown (n = 25) or the culture for *Mycobacterium tuberculosis* was negative (n = 97). From 626 active TB index cases included in the analysis (257 from 2001–2004 and 369 from 2005–2008), 2,979 contacts (1,090 from 2001–2004 and 1,889 from 2005–2008) were identified. Flow-charts showing the evaluation of contacts stratified by the AFB of the index case in both periods of study are presented in Figures 1 and 2. In the period from 2001–2004 (contacts shared ≥ 100 hours total) 810 contacts were evaluated. Two per cent (16/810) of those contacts were diagnosed as a newly active TB cases (detection rate of 1,975/100000) and 62% (496/794) as having LTBI. In the period from 2005–2008 (contacts shared ≥ 4 hours/week) 1,310 contacts were evaluated and 2.7% (35/1.310) had a diagnosis of active TB (detection rate of 2,442/100,000 habitants) and 69% (877/1,275) were diagnosed with LTBI. There was not a statically significant difference in the detection of active TB (16/810 or 2% *versus* 35/1310 or 2.7%, $p = 0.3$) between the 2 time periods, but the detection of LTBI was significant higher (496/794 or 62% *versus* 877/1275 or 69%, $p = 0.003$). However, the NNS for a newly diagnosed TB case decreased from 50 in the period from 2001–2004 to 37 in the period from 2005–2008. The same occurred with the NNCT, decreasing from 16 in the first period to 10 in the second. The characteristics of the study population are shown in Table 1. There were statistically significant differences between both samples in some variables, with slightly more males, household contacts, smokers and cases of diabetes in the first period (2001–2004). The association of different variables to the diagnosis of active TB and LTBI among contacts in both periods studied is presented in Tables 2 and 3, respectively. There was a statistically significant association between smoking and newly diagnosed active TB in the sample during the second period as well as those living in poor areas (slums) (Table 2). There was an association between a positive AFB in the index case and the diagnosis of LTBI in samples from both time periods. Smoking and alcohol abuse were associated with the diagnosis of LTBI only in the second period.

Discussion

Our findings confirm the importance of screening for active TB and LTBI among adult close contacts of TB cases with no known additional risk factors in a setting with a moderate incidence of TB. The prevalence rate of

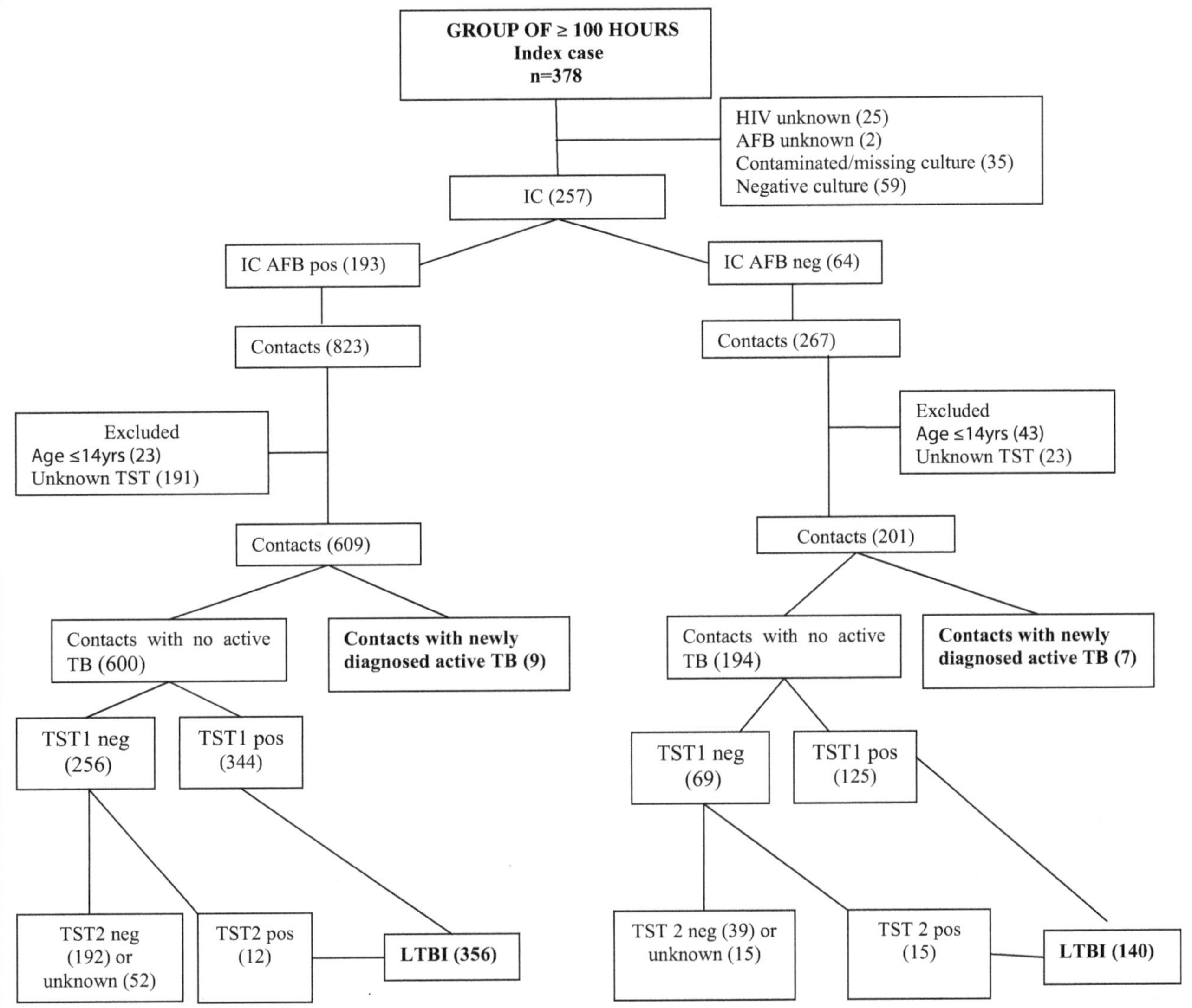

Figure 1 Contact evaluation of period 2001–2004.

newly diagnosed TB cases among contacts in 2001–2004 (2%; 1,975/100,000 habitants) and in 2005–2008 (2.7%; 2,442/100,000 habitants) was similar to the prevalence of active TB reported by a meta-analysis (41 articles included in a systematic review) that determine the yield of contact investigation in resource limited settings and found a prevalence of 2.3% (95% CI 2.1–2.5) for bacteriological confirmed active TB cases [14]. Our findings were also similar to those found in a more recent meta-analysis that included 70 studies from low and middle-income settings in which the prevalence of microbiologically proven TB among contacts was 3.1 (95% CI 2.2–4.4) [15]. Although the prevalence rates are similar, it should be noted that the definitions of "contact" varied considerably between the studies analyzed in both meta-analyses. Interestingly, the prevalence of newly diagnosed TB cases (2.7%, 35/1,310) among close contacts in the second period of the present study was the same prevalence of TB cases (2.7%, 15/542) among respiratory symptomatic patients with cough for one week or more who sought care in a Primary Health Center, as reported in a study conducted in the same city of Rio de Janeiro [16]. It should be pointed out that the passive case finding among respiratory symptomatic subjects spontaneously attending Primary Health facilities is the current strategy for TB case finding in Brazil. Furthermore, with exception of few reference Centers for TB like the TB Clinic of IDT/UFRJ, investigation for active TB among close contacts is not routinely conducted, although it is suggested in the National Program of TB [4].

Although the total number of contacts identified during the 2005–2008 (n = 1,310) was higher than in 2001–2004 (n = 810), the NNS for newly diagnosed TB (50 *versus* 37) and the NNCT (16 *versus* 10) decreased from

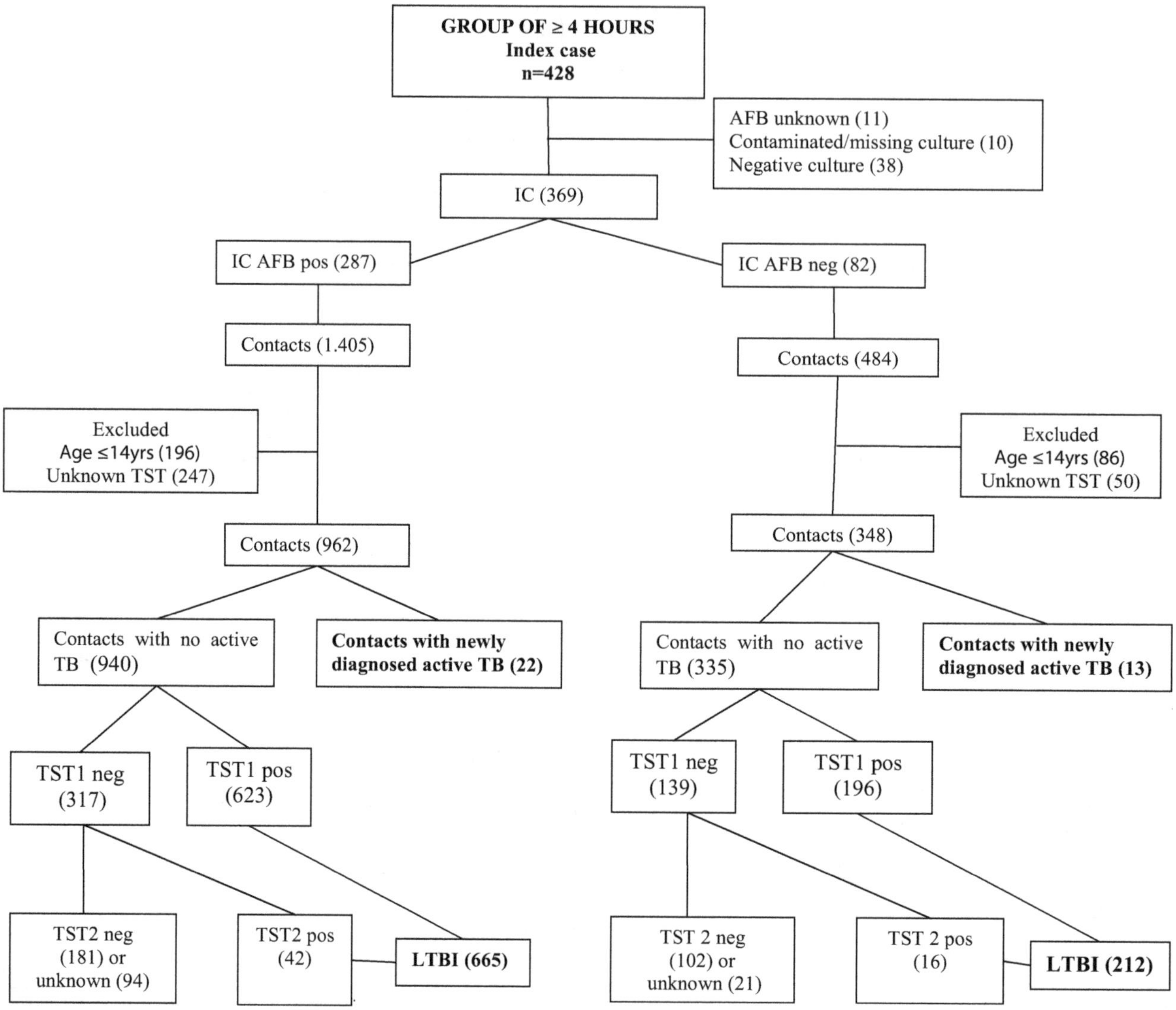

Figure 2 Contact evaluation of period 2005–2008.

the first to the second period. A review recently published by the World Health Organization (WHO) summarizes the weighted average NNS to find one case of TB in different risk groups in different epidemiological situations [2]. In settings with moderate incidence (30–100 new cases/100,000 inhabit) like Rio de Janeiro city, the average NNS (40; ranging 7–355) was 20% lower than the NNS found in the first period (NNS = 50) and similar to the NNS found in the second period of our study (NNS = 37). The significant reduction in the NNS in the second period may suggest that the less conservative definition of "close contact" applied during this period may be more effective in identifying new cases of TB than the definition of "close contact" used in the first period of this study.

The only variable associated with a new diagnosis of active TB among contacts in both periods was "living in a slum" and variables associated with LTBI were an AFB positive index case, smoking and alcohol abuse (Tables 2 and 3). Interestingly the AFB of the index case and the variable "living in same house" were not associated with active TB diagnosis. On the other hand, in our sample, a positive AFB smear in the index case in both periods, as well as smoking and alcohol abuse in the second period were identified as independent factors associated with the prevalence of LTBI. Smoking and alcohol abuse have been associated with LTBI in specific high risk groups such as adult prisoners, nursing home residents and immigrants from countries with high prevalence of TB disease [17-20]. In fact, a meta-analysis showed that smoking ($p < 0,001$, OR = 2.1 95% CI 1.4 -3.1) and alcohol abuse ($p = 0.001$ OR = 4.7 95% CI 1.8-9.8) were independent factors associated with LTBI [21]. A study conducted by Rose and colleagues evaluated the prevalence of LTBI among 1,590 contacts of pulmonary TB

Table 1 Demographic characteristics of the study population stratified by period

		Period		
Characteristics		**2001-2004 n = (810)**	**2005-2008 n = (1310)**	***p value***
Age (mean ± DP)		38 (±16)	37 (±15)	0.2
Gender	Male	513 (63.6%)	762 (58.4%)	0.02
	Female	297 (36.4%)	548 (41.6%)	
Index case AFB positive	yes	609 (75. 2%)	962 (73. 4%)	0.3
	no	201 (24. 8%)	348 (26. 6%)	
Index case HIV positive	yes	4(0. 4%)	5 (0.3%)	0.9
	no	801 (99. 6%)	1284 (99. 7%)	
Contact households	yes	634 (78. 3%)	785 (59. 9%)	<0.001
	no	176 (21. 7%)	525 (40. 1%)	
Smoking	yes	82 (10.2%)	94 (7,2%)	0.01
	no	722 (89.8%)	1210 (92,8%)	
Use of injectable drugs	yes	2 (0. 2%)	12 (0.9%)	0.1
	no	801 (99.8%)	1286 (99. 1%)	
Use of non-injectable drugs	yes	17 (2.1%)	23 (1.8%)	0.6
	no	786 (97.9%)	1281 (98.2%)	
Residing in poor areas(slum)	yes	121 (16.0%)	216 (18.2%)	0.2
	no	635 (84.0%)	971 (81.8%)	
Prisoners/previous hospitalization	yes	28 (3.5%)	36 (2.8%)	0.4
	no	776 (96.5%)	1267 (97.2%)	
Diabetes *mellitus*	yes	22 (2.7%)	16 (1.2%)	0. 01
	no	783 (97.3%)	1294 (98.8%)	
Alcohol abuse	yes	19 (2. 4%)	45 (3.4%)	0.2
	no	786 (97. 6%)	1262 (96.5%)	
Use of immunosuppressive drugs	yes	4 (0. 5%)	4 (0.3%)	0.4
	no	801 (99.5%)	1299 (99.7%)	

Statistical test used for all variables was Chi-square, except for comparing age mean (Student).

patients and found that a higher prevalence of LTBI was associated with AFB positivity and "living in same house" group [7]. However, while the AFB of the index case was associated with LTBI among younger contacts, intimacy of exposure was the variable associated with LTBI among contacts older than 30 years [7]. Furthermore, a study conducted in Pakistan (1961) also found similar prevalence of LTBI (60% *versus* 61%) among contacts of index cases with AFB positive (531 contacts/100 cases) and AFB negative smears (460 contacts/100 cases) [22].

The prevalence of LTBI in both samples of our study (62% and 69%) were greater than the prevalence of LTBI among contacts reported by a study conducted in Botswana and a meta-analysis of studies conducted in low–middle income countries (45.3; 95% CI 40.6–50,1 and 51.4% ; 95% CI 50.6–52,2) [13,14].

The higher level of TB incidence (94/100,000) during the first period of the study (2001–2004) when compared to the second period of the study (2005–2008) could correspond to higher rates of disease transmission which potentially generated a larger population of latently infected individuals that could have eventually resulted in the higher yield of contact-tracing in the second period of the study. However, the incidence rate of TB in years prior (1997–2000) to the study was even higher (110/100,000) and the detection rate of active TB and LTBI during the second period of the study was higher than during the first one [9]. This suggests that the higher level of detection of active and latent TB in the second period of study was the consequence of the less conservative approach used in this period of the study than the impact of higher TB incidence rate in the first period of study.

This study has important limitations. Although the setting is a clinical research site, this is a retrospective study and the evaluation of study subjects and the data collection were conducted under pragmatic clinical 'non-study' conditions. The allocation of contacts in both groups (enclosed space with a TB index

Table 2 Variables associated with newly diagnosed active TB cases in both periods

Period							
2001-2004				2005-2008			
Variables (n)	**Contacts with newly diagnosed active TB case(n = 16)**	***p* value**	**OR (CI 95%)**	**Variables (n)**	**Contacts with newly diagnosed active TB case (n = 35)**	***p* value**	**OR (CI 95%)**
Index case AFB positive (n =193)	9 (56.2%)	0.1	0,4 (0.1-1.1)	Index case AFB positive (n = 287)	22 (62.9%)	0.2	0,6 (0.3-1.2)
Household contact (n = 620)	14 (87.5%)	0.5	1,9 (0.4-8.7)	Household contact (n = 761)	24 (68.6%)	0.3	1,4 (0.7-3.0)
Smoking contact (n = 81)	1 (6.2%)	0.9	0,5 (0.07-4.4)	Smoking contact (n = 88)	6 (17.1%)	0.04	2,7 (1.1-6.8)
Contacts living in poor areas (slum) (n = 111)	10 (62.5%)	<0.001	9.4 (3.3-26.5)	Contacts living in poor areas (slum) (n = 205)	11 (36.7%)	0.01	2,6 (1.2-5.7)
Contacts prisoners/previous hospitalization (n = 26)	2 (12.5%)	0.1	4,1 (0.9-19.3)	Contacts prisoners/previous hospitalization (n = 35)	1 (2.9%)	0.6	1.0 (0.1-7.7)

Excluded from the table are injecting drug use, use of non-injectable drugs, diabetes "mellitus", and use of immunosuppressive drugs because no contact was diagnosed with TB. Statistical test used was Chi-square.

case for ≥ 100 hours/total period or ≥ 4 hours/week) was not random. However, to our knowledge, this is the first manuscript comparing pragmatically two different definitions of "close contact". There was an important loss (20-25%) of subjects (index cases and contacts) in both periods. However, the sample studied is still notable and allows important conclusions and analysis. The design of the study does not allow the assessment of the exact duration of exposure (in hours) related to the highest detection of LTBI or newly active TB. However in clinical practice, an individual who has 4 h/week of exposure to a pulmonary TB patient could have a total of 100 h of exposure if the exposure to index case occurred over 7 months. So, this study analyzed the impact of an operational change (definition of exposure to an active pulmonary TB patient) and not the duration of exposure (in hours) itself. Our study population only included close contacts ≥ 15 years old. Based on this, the real prevalence of close contacts can be underestimated. The index cases of our sample were, mostly subjects enrolled in Clinical Research trials of TB in our TB Clinic and were people from the community and with no initially known risk factors for TB. The study findings are restricted to the data domain in terms of

Table 3 Variables associated with latent TB infection (LTBI) in both periods

2001-2004				2005-2008			
Variables (n)	**Contacts with LTBI (n = 496)**	***p* value**	**OR (CI 95%)**	**Variables (n)**	**Contacts with LTBI (n = 877)**	***p* value**	**OR (CI 95%)**
Index case AFB positive (n = 193)	356 (71.8%)	0.001	0.5 (0.3-0.7)	Index case AFB positive (n = 287)	665 (75.8%)	<0.001	1.7 (1.3–2.3)
Index case HIV positive (n = 4)	12 (2.4%)	0.2	0.4 (0.1-1.3)	Index case HIV positive (n = 5)	16 (1.8%)	0.1	0.4 (0.1–1.1)
Household contact (n = 620)	387 (78%)	0.7	0.9 (0.6-1.3)	Household contact (n = 761)	547 (62.4%)	0.07	1.2 (0.9-1.6)
Smoking contact (n = 81)	54 (10.9%)	0.8	1.0 (0.6-1.8)	Smoking contact (n = 88)	82 (9.4%)	<0.001	9.5 (2.9 – 30.5)
Contacts living in poor areas (slum) (n = 111)	71 (15.5%)	0.6	1.1 (0.7-1.8)	Contacts living in poor areas (slum) (n = 205)	141 (17.7%)	0.9	0.9 (0.6-1.3)
Contacts prisoners/previous hospitalization (n = 26)	22 (4.5%)	0.1	2.6 (0.8-7.6)	Contacts prisoners/previous hospitalization (n =35)	20 (2.3%)	0.3	0.6 (0.2-1.3)
Contacts with alcohol abuse (n = 18)	13 (2.6%)	0.9	1.2 (0.4-3.4)	Contacts with alcohol abuse (n = 45)	44 (5%)	<0.001	14.9 (2.0-109)

Excluded from the table are injecting drug use, use of non-injectable drugs, diabetes "mellitus" and use of immunosuppressive drugs because no contact was diagnosed with LTBI. Statistical test used was Chi-square.

population demographics as well as TB incidence rate and further analysis may be required to expand the domain of results to a more generalized setting.

Conclusions

The findings of this study suggest that the change in the operational definition of a close contact to 4 hours/week increased the detection of news cases of active TB and LTBI, as well as decreased TB NNS (from 50 to 37) and NNCT (from 16 to 10) for active TB case. New studies including cost effectiveness are needed in order to confirm the effectiveness of this strategy

Competing interests

The authors declare that they have no competing interests.

Authors' contributions

CL participated in the study design of the study, carried out the data collection, performed the statistical analysis and drafted the manuscript. MCC participated of the statistical analysis and helped to draft the manuscript. AE participated in the study design of the study and helped to draft the manuscript. FCQM participated of the statistical analysis and helped to draft the manuscript. MBC conceived and coordinated the study, participated in the study design and of its statistical analysis and helped to draft the manuscript. All authors read and approved the final version of the manuscript.

Acknowledgements

The authors thank to the health care workers of the Outpatient TB Clinic of the Institute of Thoracic Diseases (IDT) of the Federal University of Rio de Janeiro (UFRJ) and to all patients. MBC was supported by the Conselho Nacional de Desenvolvimento Científico e Tecnológico (CNPq; PQ-2; 311162/2014-17). This MS was also supported by the Johns Hopkins University Center for AIDS Research (1P30AI094189).

Author details

[1]Institute of Thoracic Diseases of Federal University of Rio de Janeiro, Rio de Janeiro, Brazil. [2]Center for Tuberculosis Research, Johns Hopkins University, Baltimore, Maryland, USA. [3]Hospital Universitário Clementino Fraga Filho, Cidade Universitária, Rua Professor Rodolpho Paulo Rocco n° 255, 6° andar, Rio de Janeiro 21941-913, Brazil.

References

1. World Health Organization: *Guidelines for intensified case-finding and isoniazid preventive therapy for people living with HIV in resource constrained settings.* Geneva: Department of HIV/AIDS, Stop TB Department; 2011. http://whqlibdoc.who.int/publications/2011/9789241500708_eng.pdf.
2. World Health Organization: **Systematic screening for active tuberculosis: principles and Recommendations.** Geneva: World Health Organization (WHO); 2013. (WHO/HTM/TB/2013.04). http://apps.who.int/iris/bitstream/10665/84971/1/9789241548601_eng.pdf.
3. Conde MB, Melo FAF, Marques AM, Cardoso NC, Pinheiro VG, Dalcin PT, Machado Junior A, Lemos AC, Netto AR, Durovni B, Sant'Anna CC, Lima D, Capone D, Barreira D, Matos ED, Mello FC, David FC, Marsico G, Afiune JB, Silva JR, Jamal LF, Telles MA, Hirata MH, Dalcolmo MP, Rabahi MF, Cailleaux-Cesar M, Palaci M, Morrone N, Guerra RL, Dietze R, *et al*: **III Brazilian Thoracic Association Guidelines on tuberculosis.** *J Bras Pneumol* 2009, **35:**1018–1048.
4. Ministério da Saúde do Brasil: **Manual de Recomendações para o Controle da Tuberculose no Brasil.** Brasília: Ministério da Saúde do Brasil; 2011. http://portal.saude.gov.br/portal/arquivos/pdf/manual_de_recomendacoes_tb.pdf.
5. Jasmer RM, Nahid P, Hopewell PC: **Clinical practice. Latent tuberculosis infection.** *N Eng J Med* 2002, **347:**1860–1866.
6. Small PM, Fujiwara PI: **Management of tuberculosis in the United States.** *N Eng J Med* 2001, **345:**189–200.
7. Rose CE, Zerbe GO, Lantez SO, Bailey WC: **Establishing Priority during investigation of tuberculosis contacts.** *Int J Tuberc Lung Dis* 1979, **119:**603–609.
8. Sterling TR, Villarino ME, Borisov AS, Shang N, Gordin F, Bliven-Sizemore E, Hackman J, Hamilton CD, Menzies D, Kerrigan A, Weis SE, Weiner M, Wing D, Conde MB, Bozeman L, Horsburgh R Jr, Chaisson RE: **Three Months of Rifapentine and Isoniazid for Latent Tuberculosis Infection.** *N Engl J Med* 2011, **365**(23):2155–2166.
9. Portal da Saúde [homepage on the Internet]: **TUBERCULOSE - Casos confirmados notificados no Sistema de Informação de Agravos de Notificação - SINAN Net.** Brasília: Ministério da Saúde do Brasil; 2013. http://dtr2004.saude.gov.br/sinanweb/tabnet/dh?sinannet/tuberculose/bases/tubercbrnet.def.
10. American Thoracic Society: **Target tuberculin testing and treatment of latent tuberculosis infection.** *Am J Respir Crit Care Med* 2000, **161:**221–247.
11. Center for Diseases Control: **Guidelines for the investigation of contacts of persons with infections tuberculosis.** Atlanta: Center for Diseases Control and Prevention (CDC); 2002. http://www.cdc.gov/mmwr/pdf/rr/rr5415.pdf.
12. Kranzer K, Houben RM, Glynn JR, Bekker LG, Wood R, Lawn SD: **Yield of HIV-associated tuberculosis during intensified case finding in resource-limited settings: a systematic review and meta-analysis.** *Lancet Infect Dis* 2010, **10:**93–102.
13. Puryear S, Seropola G, Ho-Foster A, Arscott-Mills T, Mazhani L, Firth J, Goldfarb DM, Ncube R, Bisson GP, Steenhoff AP: **Yield of contact tracing from pediatric tuberculosis index cases in Gaborone Botswana.** *Int J Tuber Lung Dis* 2013, **17**(8):1049–1055.
14. Morrison J, Pai M, Hopewell PC: **Tuberculosis and latent tuberculosis infection in close contacts of people with pulmonary tuberculosis in low-income and middle-income countries: a systematic review and meta-analysis.** *Lancet Infect Dis* 2008, **8**(6):359–368.
15. Fox GJ, Barry SE, Britton WJ, Marks GB: **Contact investigation for tuberculosis: a systematic review and meta-analysis.** *Eur Respir J* 2013, **41:**140–156.
16. Bastos LG, Fonseca LS, Mello FC, Ruffino-Netto A, Golub JE, Conde MB: **Prevalence of pulmonary tuberculosis among respiratory symptomatic subjects in an out-patient primary health unit.** *Int J Tuberc Lung Dis* 2007, **11**(2):156–160.
17. Anderson RH, Sy FS, Thompson S, Addy A: **Cigarette smoking and tuberculin skin test conversion among incarcerated adults.** *Am J Prev Med* 1997, **13**(3):175–181.
18. Nisar M, Williams CS, Ashby D, Davies PD: **Tuberculin testing in residential homes for the elderly.** *Thorax* 1993, **48:**1257–1260.
19. Plant AJ, Wartkins RE, Gushualak B, Rouke TO, Jones W, Streeton J, Sang D: **Predictores of tuberculin reactivity among prospective Vietnamese migrants: The effect of smokimg.** *Epidemiol Infect* 2002, **128:**37–45.
20. Solsona J, Caylà JA, Nadal J, Bedia M, Mata C, Brau J, Maldonado J, Milà C, Alcaide J, Altet N, Galdós-Tangüis H: **Screening for tuberculosis upon admission to shelters and free-meal services.** *Eur J Epidemiol* 2001, **17:**123–128.
21. Slama K, Chiang CY, Enarson DA, Hassmiller K, Fanning A, Gupta P, Ray C: **Tobacco and tuberculosis: A quantitative Systematic review and meta-analysis.** *Int J Tuberc Lung Dis* 2007, **11:**1049–1061.
22. Yad MI: **Observations on the examination of contacts of tuberculosis patients - a 15 year study (1953–67).** *Bull Int Union Tuberc* 1974, **49**(suppl 1):261–266.

26

Comparison of same day diagnostic tools including Gene Xpert and unstimulated IFN-γ for the evaluation of pleural tuberculosis

Richard Meldau[1], Jonny Peter[1], Grant Theron[1], Greg Calligaro[1], Brian Allwood[1], Greg Symons[1], Hoosain Khalfey[1], Gina Ntombenhle[1], Ureshnie Govender[1], Anke Binder[1], Richard van Zyl-Smit[1] and Keertan Dheda[1,2*]

Abstract

Background: The accuracy of currently available same-day diagnostic tools (smear microscopy and conventional nucleic acid amplification tests) for pleural tuberculosis (TB) is sub-optimal. Newer technologies may offer improved detection.

Methods: Smear-microscopy, adenosine deaminase (ADA), interferon gamma (IFN-γ), and Xpert MTB/RIF [using an unprocessed (1 ml) and centrifuged (~20 ml) sample] test accuracy was evaluated in pleural fluid from 103 consecutive patients with suspected pleural TB. Culture for *M.tuberculosis* and/or histopathology (pleural biopsy) served as the reference standard. Patients were followed prospectively to determine their diagnostic categorisation.

Results: Of 93 evaluable participants, 40 had definite-TB (reference positive), 5 probable-TB (not definite but treated for TB) and 48 non-TB (culture and histology negative, and not treated for TB). Xpert MTB/RIF sensitivity and specificity (95% CI) was 22.5% (12.4 - 37.6) and 98% (89.2 - 99.7), respectively, and centrifugation did not improve sensitivity (23.7%). The Xpert MTB/RIF internal positive control showed no evidence of inhibition. Biomarker specific sensitivity, specificity, PPV, and NPVs were: ADA (48.85 IU/L; rule-in cut-point) 55.3% (39.8 - 69.9), 95.2% (83.9 - 98.7), 91.4 (73.4 - 95.4), 69.7% (56.7 - 80.1); ADA (30 IU/L; clinically used cut-point) 79% (63.7 - 89), 92.7% (80.6 - 97.5), 91.0 (73.4 - 95.4), 82.7% (69.3 - 90.1); and IFN-γ (107.7 pg/ml; rule-in cut-point) 92.5% (80.2 - 97.5), 95.9% (86.1 - 98.9), 94.9% (83.2 - 98.6), 93.9% (83.5 - 97.9), respectively (IFN-γ sensitivity and NPV better than Xpert [$p < 0.05$] and rule-in ADA [$p < 0.05$]).

Conclusion: The usefulness of Xpert MTB/RIF to diagnose pleural TB is limited by its poor sensitivity. IFN-γ is an excellent rule-in test and, compared to ADA, has significantly better sensitivity and rule-out value in a TB-endemic setting.

Keywords: Tuberculosis, Diagnosis, Xpert MTB/RIF, Interferon gamma, Adenosine deaminase, Pleural fluid

Background

Tuberculosis (TB) remains a global health problem, with an estimated 1.4 million deaths and 8.7 million new cases reported in 2011 [1]. Pulmonary TB is the most common form of TB, with extrapulmonary TB (EPTB) accounting for ~15% of cases, but this estimate increases to ~50% in high HIV prevalence settings [2]. Pleural TB, a common form of EPTB, remains a common problem for physicians practising in high, intermediate and low TB burden settings, particularly where there are large immigrant populations. The diagnosis of pleural TB is challenging due to the paucibacillary nature of biological samples, and the need for diagnostic confirmation using invasive, expensive, and time consuming procedures such as blind pleural biopsy, imaging-guided-pleural biopsy, and medical or surgical thoracoscopy [3].

Proxy markers such as adenosine deaminase (ADA), an enzyme that catalyzes the conversion of adenosine and deoxyadenosine to inosine and deoxyinosine has

* Correspondence: keertan.dheda@uct.ac.za
[1]Lung Infection and Immunity Unit, Division of Pulmonology & UCT Lung Institute, Department of Medicine, University of Cape Town, Cape Town, South Africa
[2]Institute of Infectious Diseases and Molecular Medicine, University of Cape Town, Cape Town, South Africa

been widely studied [4]. ADA testing is relatively easy, inexpensive and rapid, with pooled sensitivity and specificity estimates of 92% and 90%, respectively, across different prevalence settings depending on the cut-point used [4]. Interferon gamma (IFN-γ), an inflammatory cytokine secreted from macrophages and CD4 (+) T cells in response to *M. tuberculosis* infection, and that tends to concentrate in the pleural space, has been shown to be an alternative biological marker for pleural TB diagnosis with pooled sensitivity and specificity estimates of 89% and 97%, respectively [5]. In high TB/HIV burden settings the performance was shown to be even better: sensitivity 97% and specificity 100% [6].

More recently the Xpert MTB/RIF assay, a fully automated quantitative real-time hemi-nested PCR, was introduced into high burden settings and is able to detect *M. tuberculosis* within 2 hours and also provide information about rifampicin susceptibility [7]. The assay has been validated using sputum samples and recently endorsed by the WHO as a rapid test for both smear-positive and smear-negative (paucibacillary) respiratory samples [8,9]. However, there are limited data about the Xpert MTB/RIF assay using pleural fluid [10-17] and thus the usefulness of this assay in the context of pleural TB remains unclear. Limitations of previously published work include the relatively small number of patients with pleural TB (usually quoted as part of a larger series of patients with EPTB), a paucity of biopsy-proven or culture positive samples as a gold standard, the lack of comparative analysis with other commonly used biomarkers, and a lack of attention to the technical factors that could impact Xpert MTB/RIF performance, including PCR inhibition, level of detection, and correlation with bacterial load. Furthermore, there are also limited data from high TB and HIV prevalence settings.

To address these knowledge gaps we prospectively evaluated the performance of the Xpert MTB/RIF assay, and other same-day diagnostic biomarkers, using pleural fluid obtained from patients with suspected pleural TB from Cape Town in South Africa.

Methods

Patient recruitment, characterization and routine laboratory tests

Consecutive patients with suspected pleural TB, including any symptoms including cough, fever, night sweats, loss of weight, haemoptysis and chest pain, and features consistent with a pleural effusion on chest x-ray, were prospectively recruited from Groote Schuur, Somerset and Victoria Hospitals in Cape Town, South Africa, over a three year period from October 2009 to September 2012. The University of Cape Town Human Research Ethics Committee approved the study, and all patients provided written informed consent for study participation and pleural biopsy.

Routine TB diagnostic work up (pleural fluid analysis, sputum for microscopy and culture, when available, and lymph node or other organ biopsy) was performed by the referring physician. Although not routine, a closed pleural biopsy using an Abrams needle was performed by a study physician trained in this procedure to improve patient categorization. All biopsies were performed after aspiration of pleural fluid. Patients were offered voluntary HIV testing. Pleural fluid samples were collected for routine biochemical and cytological analysis (protein, albumin, ADA, glucose, cell differential, cytology), concentrated fluorescence smear microscopy, and liquid culture for *M. tuberculosis* using the MGIT 960 (Becton Dickinson, Sparks, Maryland) with the remaining fluid used for Xpert MTB/RIF and IFN-γ analysis. Pleural biopsy samples were sent for histology and liquid culture. Adenosine deaminase activity in pleural fluid was determined by colorimetric technique by the National Health Laboratory Services, using the user-defined method on a Roche Cobas Integra (Roche Diagnostics Ltd, Switzerland). Pleural fluid ADA levels greater than 30 U/L, in keeping with local guidelines and clinical practice, were reported as suggestive of pleural TB [18,19].

Given the limitations of a single pleural fluid TB culture for confirming a diagnosis, patients were categorised as follows: *Definite*-TB: patients with at least one positive *M. tuberculosis* culture by liquid culture (in either pleural fluid, biopsy or sputum) and/or caseating granulomatous inflammation suggestive of TB on histological examination of pleural biopsy tissue, and with improvement on anti-TB treatment (all patients in this category received anti-TB treatment); *Probable*-TB: patients not meeting the criteria for definite-TB but with a clinical-radiological picture suggestive of TB and who were treated for TB with clinical response (all patients in this category received anti-TB treatment); *Non*-TB: patients for whom no microbiological or histological evidence of *M. tuberculosis* could be found, and/or for whom an alternative diagnosis was available. These patients at presentation and on follow-up did not receive anti-TB treatment.

All the laboratory staff performing the requested tests, including Xpert MTB/RIF and IFN-γ measurement, were blinded to all microbiological and clinical information.

IFN-γ measurement

Interferon gamma (IFN-γ) concentrations were measured in pleural fluid supernatant in duplicate using the InterGam Ultrasensitive Rapid Immuno-suspension Assay (IRISA; Antrum Biotech, Cape Town, South Africa; limit of detection = 5 to 10 pg/ml). Pleural fluid supernatant was prepared by centrifuging pleural fluid at 3000×g for 15 min to remove any unwanted debris.

Xpert MTB/RIF assay

A 1 ml aliquot of raw pleural fluid and a 1 ml aliquot of concentrated (centrifuged) pleural fluid from each patient was diluted with 2 ml of the Xpert MTB/RIF sample buffer. The 1 ml concentrated pleural fluid aliquot was prepared by centrifugation of a median (IQR) of 20 (10-20) ml pleural fluid at 3000×g for 15 min, with the supernatant discarded and the pellet made up to 1 ml with phosphate buffer solution. The pleural fluid and sample buffer solutions were then mixed vigorously and incubated at room temperature for 15 min, with further mixing halfway through the incubation. A 2 ml volume of the diluted samples was then transferred to an Xpert MTB/RIF cartridge and run on the GeneXpert (Cepheid, Dx System Version 4.0c) machine. The limit of detection was determined in duplicate by spiking 0, 50, 75, 100 and 150 H37Rv CFU to 1 ml aliquots of pleural fluid from subjects confirmed not to have TB, before dilution with sample buffer and subsequent Xpert MTB/RIF analysis. This experiment was repeated twice. Inhibition was evaluated by comparing the PCR cycle-threshold (C_T) values of the internal positive control (lyophilized *Bacillus atrophaeus* subsp. *globigii* spores) from unconcentrated and concentrated samples.

Statistical analysis

Categorical variables were compared using the χ^2 test and continuous variables were compared using Student's t-test where appropriate, with Mann-Whitney used for non-parametrically distributed continuous variables. Correlations were analyzed using the Spearman coefficient for non-parametrically distributed variables. Diagnostic accuracy, including 95% confidence intervals, was assessed using sensitivity, specificity, positive predictive value (PPV), negative predictive value (NPV) (Open Epi, Version 2.3.1) and area under the receiver operator curve (AUROC) in definite-TB and non-TB groups (Graphpad Prism, Version 5.03).

Results

A total of 103 patients with pleural effusion and suspected TB were enrolled. Ten patients were excluded from the final analysis: three had incomplete clinical data and seven were on anti-TB treatment for more than 48 hours prior to the samples being taken (see Figure 1 for patient flow and test results available).

Clinical and demographic data

Forty subjects were confirmed to have definite-TB, 48 non-TB and 5 participants probable-TB (not meeting diagnostic criteria but receiving TB treatment). The subjects with non-TB effusions had a spectrum of malignant and non-malignant diagnoses including: lymphoma, adenocarcinoma, small cell carcinoma, and parapneumonic effusion. Of the 65 subjects consenting to HIV testing, 17% (11) were positive. Clinical and demographic data are summarized in Table 1.

Performance outcomes of IFN-γ

IFN-γ levels were evaluated in 93 patients (40 definite-TB, 5 probable-TB and 48 non-TB). Median (IQR) IFN-γ levels were approximately 100 times higher in definite-TB compared to non-TB effusions: 131.8 (131.8-162.7) versus 0.57 (0.0-5.71) pg/ml, $p < 0.0001$ (Figure 2). A receiver operating characteristic (ROC) curve derived rule-in cut point of 107.7 pg/ml was used to determine the sensitivity and specificity (95% CI) (Figure 3). Table 2 compares the diagnostic accuracy of the IFN-γ with other same-day diagnostics in definite-TB versus non-TB groups. IFN-γ sensitivity was unaffected by the inclusion of probable- with definite-TB patients (see Additional file 1: Table S1 in the online supplementary data), and diagnostic accuracy was not significantly different in HIV-infected compared to uninfected patients (see Additional file 1: Table S2 in the online supplementary data).

Performance outcomes of pleural fluid ADA

Adenosine deaminase levels were measured in 84 patients. Median (IQR) ADA levels were 5 times higher in definite-TB compared to non-TB effusions: 51.7 (35.2-62.1) versus 11.5 (7.1-18.8) U/L, $p < 0.0001$. Using a clinical cut point of >30 U/L (South African national standard [18]), the sensitivity (95%CI), specificity, NPV and PPV were 79.0% (63.7-89.0), 92.7% (80.6-97.5), 82.7% (69.3-91.0) and 91.0% (73.4-95.4), respectively (Table 2). Relevant values using the rule-in cut-point (at least 95% specificity) are shown in Table 2. The ROC and scatter plot of ADA are shown in Figures 2 and 3.

Grouping the probable TB with the definite-TB group reduced the sensitivity to 74.5% but the specificity remained unchanged, when using the clinically used cut point of >30 U/L. A similar trend occurred when using the rule-in cut point of 48.85 U/L (see Additional file 1: Table S1 in the online supplementary data). HIV status had no significant impact on the ADA diagnostic accuracy (see Additional file 1: Table S3 in the online supplementary data).

Performance outcome for Xpert MTB/RIF assay including inhibition and detection threshold

Xpert MTB/RIF was performed on 93 participants. Xpert MTB/RIF detected 9 out 40 subjects with definite-TB. The sensitivity (95%CI) and specificity using 1 ml of unprocessed pleural fluid was 22.5% (12.4, 37.6) and 98.0% (89.2, 99.7) respectively. Xpert MTB/RIF sensitivity

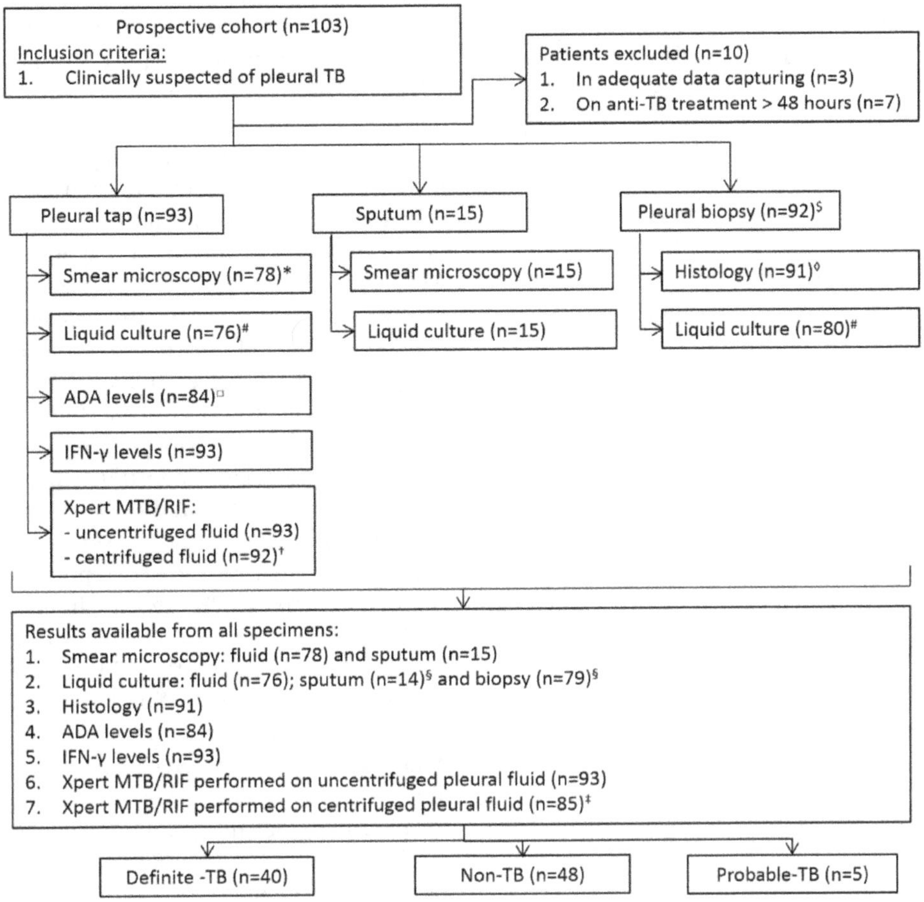

Figure 1 Patient flow and test results available for final diagnoses. [$]biopsy not performed (n = 1); *no fluid smear requested (n = 15); [#]liquid culture not requested, pleural fluid (n = 17) and pleural biopsy (n = 12); [§]indeterminate liquid culture: contamination (n = 1) and sample rejected (n = 1); [◊]histology not requested (n = 1); [□]ADA measurements not requested (n = 9); [†]sample lost during processing (n = 1), [‡]indeterminate Xpert MTB/RIFF result (n = 7).

and specificity did not improve when a concentrated (centrifuged) pleural fluid samples was used ($p = 0.90$, Table 3). However, the number of indeterminate results generated in concentrated compared to unprocessed pleural fluid samples was higher 7/92 vs. 0/93 ($p < 0.05$). Table 2 compares the diagnostic accuracy of Xpert MTB/RIF and other same-day diagnostics. Of note, Xpert MTB/RIF pleural fluid testing detected one rifampicin-resistant result that was confirmed by liquid culture to be a true-positive MDR-TB case.

Spiking raw pleural fluid demonstrated that the Xpert MTB/RIF assay was able to reliably detect ≥75 CFU per millilitre of pleural fluid (Figure 4a). No significant difference was seen between unprocessed and concentrated pleural fluid internal probe amplifications with median C_T values of (95% CI) of 27.6 (27.5, 28.5) and 27.4 (27.6, 28.9), respectively. The median time-to-positivity (TTP) (IQR) for pleural fluid and pleural biopsy culture were 28.0 days (23.3-31.1) and 19.0 days (17.7-24.6), respectively (data not shown). No correlation was observed between C_T values and TTP from pleural fluid liquid culture, however, there was a correlation (Spearman $r = 0.93$, $p = 0.02$) between C_T values and the TTP from pleural biopsy culture.

In contrast to the findings with ADA and IFN-γ, when subjects were stratified by HIV status, Xpert MTB/RIF had a higher sensitivity in HIV infected versus uninfected persons [50% (21.6-78.5) vs. 9.1% (2.6-27.9), $p = 0.031$ (see Additional file 1: Table S4 in the online supplementary data). A similar trend was seen when comparing pleural fluid and biopsy culture as reference standard (see Additional file 1: Table S5 in the online supplementary data).

Xpert MTB/RIF in combination with ADA or IFN-γ did not significantly improve the diagnostic accuracy when compared to ADA or IFN-γ alone (Table 2).

Discussion

Given that a reliable same-day diagnostic tool for pleural TB is lacking, we prospectively evaluated and compared

Table 1 Baseline characteristics of the definite tuberculosis (TB) and non-TB patients

	Definite-TB	Non-TB	p-value
Patients (n)	40	48	
Age (yrs)	39 (29,55)	61 (54,69)	<0·0001#
Sex			
Male	24 (60%)	29 (60.4%)	
Female	16 (40%)	19 (39.6%)	
Race			
White	1 (2.5%)	5 (10.4%)	
Black	28 (70%)	9 (18.8%)	<0.0001*
Mixed	11 (27.5%)	34 (70.8%)	<0.0001*
HIV Status			
HIV-infected	8 (20%)	1 (2.0%)	<0.05*
HIV uninfected	22 (55%)	29 (60.4%)	
Refused testing	4 (10%)	3 (6.3%)	
Unknown	6 (15%)	15 (31.3%)	
History of Previous TB			
Yes	6 (15%)	5 (10.4%)	
No	31 (77.5%)	39 (81.3%)	
Unknown	3 (7.5%)	4 (8.3%)	
BCG Status			
Yes	20 (50%)	25 (52.1%)	
No	10 (25%)	5 (10.4%)	
Unknown	10 (25%)	18 (37.5%)	
Current smoker			
Yes	7 (17.5%)	18 (37.5%)	<0.05*
No	32 (80%)	26 (54.1%)	<0.05*
Unknown	1 (2.5%)	4 (8.3%)	

Data are presented as median (IQR) or n (%) or yrs (IQR). *BCG*: bacilli Calmette-Guerin. #: unpaired t-test; *: Chi-squared test.

the use of ADA, IFN-γ and Xpert MTB/RIF using pleural fluid from patients with suspected TB. Our key findings were (i) Xpert MTB/RIF had poor sensitivity and this was neither the result of a sub-optimal level of detection compared to other types of biological samples nor increased PCR inhibition, (ii) Xpert MTB/RIF sensitivity was not improved by concentrating larger volumes of pleural fluid, (iii) ADA and IFN-γ are good rule-in tests for TB pleural effusions but the higher sensitivity of IFN-γ would be preferable over ADA for rule-in, particularly in low-burden settings where a high INF-γ level is unlikely to be due to cancer, (iv) the excellent rapid rule-out value of IFN-γ, compared to ADA, is of particular clinical usefulness in high burden settings as it could be used to prompt a search for an alternative diagnosis and hence medical or surgical biopsy. The sheer burden of disease and resource constraints, including lack of skilled operators, in high burden settings means that a routine biopsy-based approach cannot be undertaken. Moreover, the majority of patients suspected with pleural TB were unable to produce sputum.

The Xpert MTB/RIF assay, which can simultaneously detect the presence of *M. tuberculosis* and rifampicin resistance in sputum specimens, has shown great promise in the rapid diagnosis of TB, with an average sensitivity and specificity of 90.4% and 98.4%, respectively [8]. It has also improved the rapid diagnosis of pulmonary TB (sensitivity of ~68%) in smear-negative patients and recently been endorsed by the Scientific and Technical Advisory Board of the WHO for use in paucibacillary samples [9,20]. However, there are hardly any data about Xpert performance in pleural fluid. Published studies have generally been performed in low burden settings as a laboratory exercise reporting yields in samples from extra-pulmonary sites, and only reported on a handful of patients with TB pleural effusion [10,12-16]. This may explain the high sensitivity reported in these studies (range 58% to 100%) and high specificities (87% to 100%) [10-16]. Recently Friedrich and co-workers in a selected cohort found that 20 out of 25 patients had confirmed TB and that Xpert sensitivity was 25% [11]. We have confirmed these findings in a larger unselected cohort and further interrogated the technical performance of the assay. The level of detection was ≥75 colony forming units per ml, and there was no evidence of PCR inhibition using the internal positive control. Centrifugation of pleural fluid made little difference. The time to positivity data (median > 28 days) confirms the low organism load within the pleural space compared to pleural tissue. Indeed, there was a trend to shorter time to positivity in liquid culture from samples that were culture positive/Xpert positive compared to those that were culture positive/Xpert negative (data not shown). Collectively, these data confirm the notion that pleural TB is a paucibaciliary disease and thus concentration/centrifugation of at least 20 ml of pleural fluid makes little difference to diagnostic yield. Xpert performed better in HIV-infected individuals, which may reflect a higher organism load in the pleural fluid [21].

In high burden settings such as South Africa, a high ADA level is frequently used to guide initiation of anti-TB therapy [4,5]. In this study, although ADA levels were 5 times higher in TB patients than in non-TB patients, using the laboratory accepted cut-point in Cape Town (30 U/L) roughly 20% of TB patients would have been missed and 1 in 10 incorrectly started on anti-TB therapy. Despite the inability of ADA to definitively confirm *M. tuberculosis*, it is a low cost and relatively rapid (same day) assay and has a high PPV when disease prevalence is high [22]. In low prevalence settings, however, PPV is too low to be clinically useful. Indeed, a recent meta-analysis of 63 studies including 2796 pleural TB

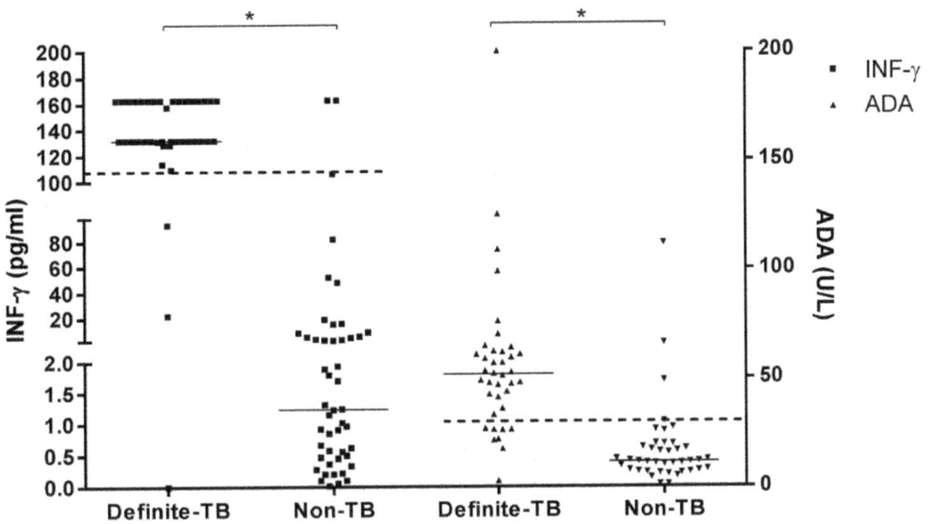

Figure 2 Scatter plot of interferon gamma (IFN-γ) and adenosine deaminase (ADA) using pleural fluid from patients with TB and non-TB pleural effusions. *: $p < 0.0001$ (Mann-Whitney). See Additional file 1: Table S6 in the online supplementary data for final diagnosis of non-TB patients with ADA and/or IFN-γ levels above cut points.

patients and 5297 non-TB patients reported the sensitivity of ADA to be 92% and specificity 90% at a cut-point of 41.9 U/L (median cut-point in the pooled studies, which each used a different cut-point) [4]. Thus, 1 in 10 patients would be over diagnosed with TB. The specificity of ADA may be improved if the proportion of lymphocytes is taken into account as was recently shown [22]. However, this is not universally helpful as about ~25% of TB pleural effusions , may be neutrophil predominant [23].

Interferon gamma, similarly, was significantly higher in TB (100 fold) compared to non-TB patients. Using an ROC curve-determined cut-point of 107.7 pg/ml, only 3 definite-TB patients were missed. By contrast, Xpert sensitivity, like pleural fluid culture (~40%) [2], was poor

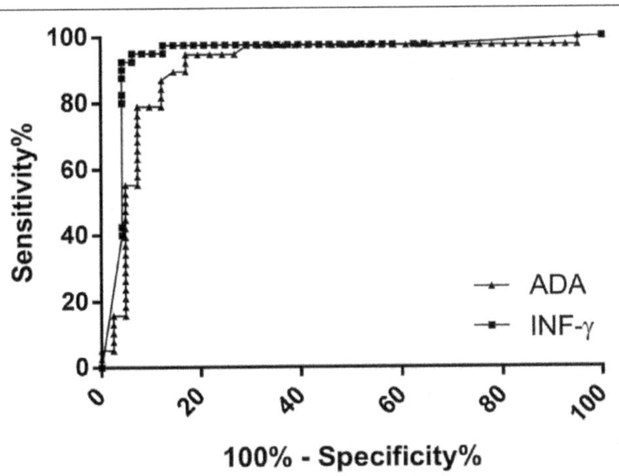

Figure 3 Area under the receiver operator characteristic (ROC) curves for interferon gamma (IFN-γ) and adenosine deaminase (ADA) were 0.94 and 0.91, respectively.

and therefore additional tools are required for optimal diagnosis when a non-biopsy approach is used. Thus, a 'one size fits all' approach with Xpert is inappropriate. Although closed pleural biopsy has a high diagnostic yield it is often unavailable in resource-poor settings, and even when available the large numbers of cases preclude routine biopsy in district general hospitals. In this study we have confirmed our previous findings, and those of others, that IFN-γ is both a highly accurate rule-in and rule-out diagnostic test for pleural TB [6,24-26], however it must be accepted that the 107.7 pg/ml cut point was generated using the current cohort and further prospective testing is required to confirm the high sensitivity and specificity. Although it can be easily measured by a commercially available ELISA-kit, it is not routinely performed due to the high cost and the kits only being available in a 96 well format, which lead to a considerable wastage of unused wells [27]. Interestingly, of the only two non-TB patients that had elevated IFN-γ, one patient had an empyema, which is known to cause elevated IFN-γ and is a contra-indication to using the test, and the other patient was lost to follow-up and thus the true TB status was unclear. A previous study from our group demonstrated a similar accuracy (sensitivity 97% specificity 98%) [6]. An obvious drawback is the lack of susceptibility data, but in resource-poor settings culture confirmation with susceptibility can follow if there is a poor response to treatment. In any event a culture isolate or positive NAAT would be required to determine susceptibility- the yield of both are low in pleural TB. It would have been interesting to perform Xpert on the pleural tissue biopsies but technically this was not feasible due to the limited

Table 2 Per patient diagnostic accuracy of Xpert MTB/RIF, IFN-γ, and ADA for the diagnosis pleural tuberculosis

Assay	Definite-TB vs. Non TB					
	Sensitivity% (95% CI)	Specificity% (95% CI)	PPV% (95% CI)	NPV% (95% CI)	+LR (95% CI)	-LR (95% CI)
Xpert MTB/RIF	22.5% *#□$£ (12.4, 37.6) 9/40	98% (89.2, 99.7) 47/48	90% (59.6, 98.3) 9/10	60.3% †◊•▪ (49.2, 70.4) 48/78	10.8 (1.43, 81.65)	0.79ç°¤§¿ (0.67, 0.94)
IFN-γ	92.5%*O (80.2, 97.5) 37/40	95.9% (86.1, 98.9) 46/48	94.9% (83.2, 98.6) 37/39	93.9%†∞ (83.5, 97.9) 46/49	22.20 (5.70, 86.46)	0.08çð (0.03, 0.23)
ADA (Clinical cut point)	79% Δ#× (63.7, 89) 30/38	92.7% (80.6, 97.5) 38/41	91% (73.4, 95.4) 30/33	82.7% ‡◊ (69.3, 91.0) 38/46	10.79 (3.59, 32.47)	0.23° (0.12, 0.42)
ADA (Rule-in cut point)	55.3% □O×€¥ (39.8, 69.9) 21/38	95.2% (83.9, 98.7) 39/41	91.4% (73.3, 97.6) 21/23	69·7% ∞⌂ (56.7, 80.1) 39/56	11.33 (2.85, 45.1)	0.47¤ðþ (0.33, 0.67)
Xpert MTB/RIF followed by IFN-γ if MTB/RIF-negative	92.5%$€ (80.2, 97.5) 37/40	93.8% (83.2, 97.9) 45/48	92.5% (80.2, 97.5) 37/40	93.8%•⌂ (83.2, 97.9) 45/48	14.80 (4.93, 44.43)	0.08§þ (0.03, 0.24)
Xpert MTB/RIF followed by ADA (clinical cut-point) if MTB/RIF-negative	81.6%£¥ (66.6, 90.8) 31/38	92.7% (80.6, 97.5) 38/41	91.2% (77.1, 97) 31/34	84.5%▪ (71.3, 92.3) 38/45	11.15 (3.70, 33.49)	0.20¿ (0.10, 0.39)
p-value	*; #; $ and £: $p < 0.0001$ O; □; ×; € and ¥: $p < 0.05$			† and •: $P < 0.0001$ ◊; ∞; ▪ and ⌂: $p < 0.05$		ç; °; ¤; §; ¿; ð and þ: non overlapping CI

A positive *MTB* (*Mycobacterium tuberculosis*) fluid culture and/or positive *MTB* biopsy culture and/or histology in keeping with *MTB* infection used as a reference. *PPV*: positive predictive value, *NPV*: negative predictive value, *+LR*: positive likelihood ratio, *-LR*: negative likelihood ratio, *CI*: confidence interval, *IFN-γ*: interferon gamma, *ADA*: adenosine deaminase. *IFN- γ* cut point of 107.7 pg/ml determined by ROC. ADA clinical cut point of 30 U/L is used for clinical decision-making at Groote Schuur hospital. Rule-in ADA cut point of 48.85U/l determined by ROC.
Superscript symbols: *; #; $; £; O; □; ×; €; ¥; †; •; ◊; ∞; ▪; ⌂; ç; °; ¤; §; ¿; ð and þ were used to indicate which groups were being compared for statistical analysis.

Table 3 Per patient diagnostic accuracy of Xpert MTB/RIF assay using centrifuged and uncentrifuged pleural fluid to diagnose pleural tuberculosis

Assay	Definite-TB vs. Non-TB			
	Sensitivity% (95% CI)	Specificity% (95% CI)	PPV% (95% CI)	NPV% (95% CI)
Pleural fluid (uncentrifuged)	22.5% (12.4, 37.6) 9/40	98% (89.2, 99.7) 48/48	90% (59.6, 98.3) 9/10	60.3% (49.2, 70.4) 48/78
Centrifuged pellet	23.7% (13.0, 39.3) 9/38	100% (91.7, 100) 42/42	100% (70.1, 100) 9/9	59.2% (48.2, 70.3) 42/71
p-value	ns*	ns*	ns*	ns*

A median volume of 20 ml of pleural fluid was centrifuged at 3000 × g for 15 min with the pellet resuspended in sterile PBS, followed by Xpert *MTB/RIF*. A positive *MTB* (*Mycobacterium tuberculosis*) fluid culture and/or positive MTB biopsy culture and/or histology in keeping with MTB infection used as a reference. *PPV*: positive predictive value, *NPV*: negative predictive value, *CI*: confidence interval, *: Chi squared.

amount of tissue and potential for tube blockage in the machine when solid material is used. However this may not have improved the diagnostic accuracy, in a recent study, Xpert was unable to detect any TB cases and more indeterminate results occurred when performed on finely ground pleural tissue [17].

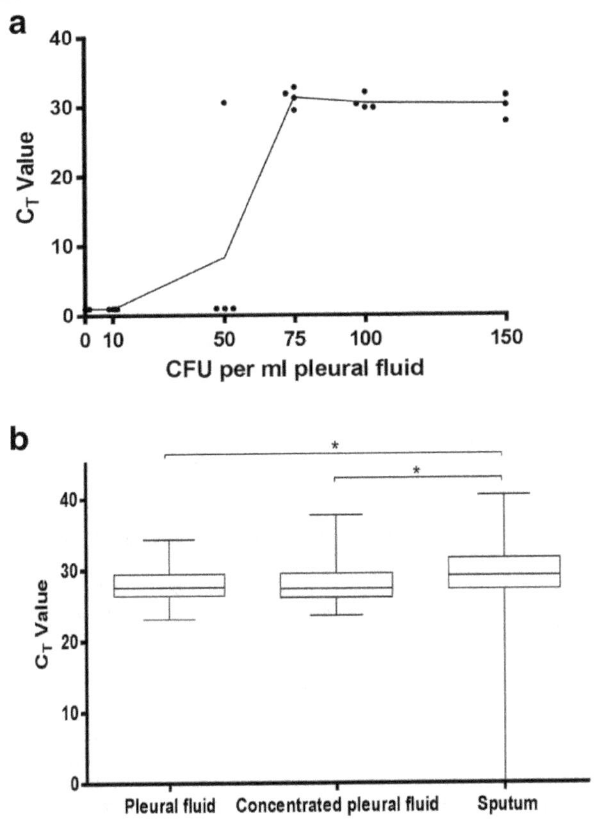

Figure 4 The determination of the: a) limit of detection of Xpert MTB/RIF and b) analysis of possible inhibition of Xpert MTB/RIF internal probe in pleural fluid samples. a) To determine the limit of detection, known amounts of colony forming units of stock H37Rv were added to 1 ml aliquots of pleural fluid in duplicate for two repeat experiments. **b)** CT values for Xpert MTB/RIF internal probe are represented as box and whiskers (min and max) for pleural fluid, concentrated pleural fluid (20 ml pellet resuspended in 1 ml) and sputum. *: $p < 0.0001$ (Mann-Whitney).

Affordability and cost effectiveness remains an important consideration in resource poor TB endemic countries. A comprehensive cost effectiveness analysis was beyond the scope of this paper, and we were unable to perform a simple cost analysis given the lack of a clinically validated commercially available unstimulated interferon gamma assay. Although the GeneXpert MTB/RIF assay is now being rolled out in many TB endemic countries [28], as we have demonstrated, sensitivity is largely sub-optimal [6,29]. Although ADA is widely available, specificity may also be also sub-optimal, as we and others have previously demonstrated. Nevertheless, it remains a widely available relatively low cost test. Diagnosing drug-resistant pleural TB also merits cost consideration. However, the GeneXpert MTB/RIF assay has a poor sensitivity in this context and thus whatever diagnostic modality is used (unstimulated interferon gamma, ADA, or GeneXpert MTB/RIF) pleural tissue or fluid culture is still required for susceptibility testing. There is an urgent need to make available a commercially and clinically validated, relatively rapid, single patient use assay for the measurement of unstimulated interferon gamma levels in pleural fluid and other forms of EPTB.

There are several limitations of our study. There were a low proportion of HIV-infected patients and several patients with unknown HIV status. However, HIV prevalence rates in TB patients in the Western Cape Province of SA are known to be lower than in the rest of the country [30], and patients often refuse testing. We only centrifuged 20 ml of fluid. However, we were limited by available sample, particularly when effusions were loculated. Moreover, a recent paper has showed that increasing the pleural fluid volume to 100 ml does not improve culture yields, despite improving the time to positivity [21]. The conclusions drawn here apply to high TB and HIV burden settings and, for the sake of external validity, require confirmation in other settings. However, given that HIV increases the concentration of organisms in pleural fluid and that the upper limit of the Xpert sensitivity (95% CI) was 37% suggests that Xpert is unlikely to perform well in any setting when using pleural fluid. We did not evaluate the potential impact on morbidity and length of hospital stay of ADA, IFN-γ and Xpert compared to empiric treatment based on laboratory analysis alone (lymphocyte predominance), however, this would have require a randomized design and up to ~25% of TB effusions are known to be neutrophil predominant [23]. The confidence intervals of the sensitivity estimates for interferon gamma and the GeneXpert MTB/ RIF assay are not ideal and therefore our findings should be confirmed using larger sample numbers and from different parts of the world.

Conclusion

The clinical usefulness of Xpert-MTB/RIF to diagnose pleural TB is limited by its poor sensitivity. By contrast, IFN-γ is an excellent rule-in test and, compared to ADA, has significantly better sensitivity and rule-out value in a high HIV prevalence setting. The high NPV of IFN-γ, compared to ADA, is particularly useful to clinicians as it prompts further work-up and tissue biopsy in patients who are unlikely to have TB, however further prospective testing is required.

Additional file

Additional file 1: Table S1. Per patient diagnostic accuracy of Xpert MTB/RIF, IFN-γ, and ADA for the diagnosis pleural tuberculosis. **Table S2.** Per patient diagnostic accuracy of IFN-γ for the diagnosis of pleural tuberculosis, stratified by HIV status. **Table S3.** Per patient diagnostic accuracy using ADA for the diagnosis of pleural tuberculosis, stratified by HIV status. **Table S4.** Per patient diagnostic accuracy of the Xpert MTB/ RIF assay, stratified by HIV status. **Table S5.** Per sample diagnostic accuracy of the XpertMTB/RIF assay for the diagnosis of pleural tuberculosis, using either fluid or biopsy culture as reference standard. Stratified by HIV status. **Table S6.** Non-TB patients with ADA and/or INF-γ levels above specified cut points.

Competing interests

KD, UG and GT have performed consultancy work for Antrum Biotech (Pty) Ltd, a UCT co-owned spin-off company, and kits for the study were donated by the company. However, Antrum Biotech played no role in study design, data analysis or its publication. Similarly, KD has been the recipient of grant funding from FIND Diagnostics, who also donated Xpert MTB/RIF cartridges to carry out the study but FIND played no role in study design, data analysis or its publication.

Authors' contributions

Concept and design, KD, RM, GT, JP. Laboratory experiments, RM, AB. Analysis and interpretation, RM, RvZS, JP, GC, GS, GN, BA, HK. Drafting the manuscript for important intellectual content, KD, RM, RvZS, GT, JP, UG. All authors read and approved the final manuscript.

Acknowledgements

This work was supported by the South African National Research Foundation (SARChI; KD), and the European and Developing Countries Clinical Trials Partnership (EDCTP; TB-NEAT and TESA; KD and GT).

References

1. World Health Organization: WHO: *Global Tuberculosis Report 2012.* Geneva, Switzerland: WHO; 2012:100.
2. Light RW: **Update on tuberculous pleural effusion.** *Respirology* 2010, **15**(3):451–458.
3. Koegelenberg CF, Diacon AH: **Pleural controversy: close needle pleural biopsy or thoracoscopy-which first?** *Respirology* 2011, **16**(5):738–746.
4. Liang QL, Shi HZ, Wang K, Qin SM, Qin XJ: **Diagnostic accuracy of adenosine deaminase in tuberculous pleurisy: a meta-analysis.** *Respir Med* 2008, **102**(5):744–754.
5. Jiang J, Shi HZ, Liang QL, Qin SM, Qin XJ: **Diagnostic value of interferon-gamma in tuberculous pleurisy: a metaanalysis.** *Chest* 2007, **131**(4):1133–1141.
6. Dheda K, van Zyl-Smit RN, Sechi LA, Badri M, Meldau R, Meldau S, Symons G, Semple PL, Maredza A, Dawson R, Wainwright H, Whitelaw A, Vallie Y, Raubenheimer P, Bateman ED, Zumla A: **Utility of quantitative T-cell responses versus unstimulated interferon-{gamma} for the diagnosis of pleural tuberculosis.** *Eur Respir J* 2009, **34**(5):1118–1126.
7. Theron G, Peter J, van Zyl-Smit R, Mishra H, Streicher E, Murray S, Dawson R, Whitelaw A, Hoelscher M, Sharma S, Pai M, Warren R, Dheda K: **Evaluation of the Xpert MTB/RIF assay for the diagnosis of pulmonary tuberculosis in a high HIV prevalence setting.** *Am J Respir Crit Care Med* 2011, **184**(1):132–140.
8. Chang K, Lu W, Wang J, Zhang K, Jia S, Li F, Deng S, Chen M: **Rapid and effective diagnosis of tuberculosis and rifampicin resistance with Xpert MTB/RIF assay: a meta-analysis.** *J Infect* 2012, **64**(6):580–588.
9. World HealthOrganization: *Report of the Tenth Meeting WHO Strategic and Technical Advisory Group for Tuberculosis (STAG-TB).* Geneva: World Health Organization; 2010:27–29.
10. Causse M, Ruiz P, Gutierrez-Aroca JB, Casal M: **Comparison of two molecular methods for rapid diagnosis of extrapulmonary tuberculosis.** *J Clin Microbiol* 2011, **49**(8):3065–3067.
11. Friedrich SO, von Groote-Bidlingmaier F, Diacon AH: **Xpert MTB/RIF assay for diagnosis of pleural tuberculosis.** *J Clin Microbiol* 2011, **49**(12):4341–4342.
12. Hillemann D, Rusch-Gerdes S, Boehme C, Richter E: **Rapid molecular detection of extrapulmonary tuberculosis by the automated GeneXpert MTB/RIF system.** *J Clin Microbiol* 2011, **49**(4):1202–1205.
13. Miller MB, Popowitch EB, Backlund MG, Ager EP: **Performance of Xpert MTB/RIF RUO assay and IS6110 real-time PCR for Mycobacterium tuberculosis detection in clinical samples.** *J Clin Microbiol* 2011, **49**(10):3458–3462.
14. Moure R, Martin R, Alcaide F: **Effectiveness of an integrated real-time PCR method for detection of the Mycobacterium tuberculosis complex in smear-negative extrapulmonary samples in an area of low tuberculosis prevalence.** *J Clin Microbiol* 2012, **50**(2):513–515.
15. Tortoli E, Russo C, Piersimoni C, Mazzola E, Dal Monte P, Pascarella M, Borroni E, Mondo A, Piana F, Scarparo C, Coltella L, Lombardi G, Cirillo DM: **Clinical validation of Xpert MTB/RIF for the diagnosis of extrapulmonary tuberculosis.** *Eur Respir J* 2012, **40**(2):442–447.
16. Vadwai V, Boehme C, Nabeta P, Shetty A, Alland D, Rodrigues C: **Xpert MTB/RIF: a new pillar in diagnosis of extrapulmonary tuberculosis?** *J Clin Microbiol* 2011, **49**(7):2540–2545.
17. Christopher DJ, Schumacher SG, Michael JS, Luo R, Balamugesh T, Duraikannan P, Pollock NR, Pai M, Denkinger CM: **Performance of Xpert (R) MTB/RIF on pleural tissue for the diagnosis of pleural tuberculosis.** *Eur Respir J* 2013, **42**(5):1427–1429.
18. Blake J, Berman P: **The use of adenosine deaminase assays in the diagnosis of tuberculosis.** *S Afr Med J* 1982, **62**(1):19–21.
19. Boonyagars LKS: **Use of Adenosine Deaminase for the Diagnosis of Tuberculosis: A Review.** *J Infect Dis Antimicrob Agents* 2010, **27**:8.
20. Steingart KR, Sohn H, Schiller I, Kloda LA, Boehme CC, Pai M, Dendukuri N: **Xpert (R) MTB/RIF assay for pulmonary tuberculosis and rifampicin resistance in adults.** *Cochrane Database Syst Rev* 2013, **1**:1–29.
21. von Groote-Bidlingmaier F, Koegelenberg CF, Bolliger CT, Chung PK, Rautenbach C, Wasserman E, Bernasconi M, Friedrich SO, Diacon AH: **The yield of different pleural fluid volumes for Mycobacterium tuberculosis culture.** *Thorax* 2013, **68**(3):290–291.
22. Garcia-Zamalloa A, Taboada-Gomez J: **Diagnostic accuracy of adenosine deaminase and lymphocyte proportion in pleural fluid for tuberculous pleurisy in different prevalence scenarios.** *PloS one* 2012, **7**(6):e38729.
23. McGrath EE, Warriner D, Anderson PB: **Pleural fluid characteristics of tuberculous pleural effusions.** *Heart Lung* 2010, **39**(6):540–543.

24. Hiraki A, Aoe K, Eda R, Maeda T, Murakami T, Sugi K, Takeyama H: **Comparison of six biological markers for the diagnosis of tuberculous pleuritis.** *Chest* 2004, **125**(3):987–989.
25. Liu YC, Shin-Jung Lee S, Chen YS, Tu HZ, Chen BC, Huang TS: **Differential diagnosis of tuberculous and malignant pleurisy using pleural fluid adenosine deaminase and interferon gamma in Taiwan.** *J Microbiol Immunol Infect* 2011, **44**(2):88–94.
26. Wang H, Yue J, Yang J, Gao R, Liu J: **Clinical diagnostic utility of adenosine deaminase, interferon-gamma, interferon-gamma-induced protein of 10 kDa, and dipeptidyl peptidase 4 levels in tuberculous pleural effusions.** *Heart Lung* 2012, **41**(1):70–75.
27. Sharma SK, Banga A: **Pleural fluid interferon-gamma and adenosine deaminase levels in tuberculosis pleural effusion: a cost-effectiveness analysis.** *J Clin Lab Anal* 2005, **19**(2):40–46.
28. Theron G, Zijenah L, Chanda D, Clowes P, Rachow A, Lesosky M, Bara W, Mungofa S, Pai M, Hoelscher M, Dowdy D, Pym A, Mwaba P, Mason P, Peter J, Dheda K: **Feasibility, accuracy, and clinical effect of point-of-care Xpert MTB/RIF testing for tuberculosis in primary-care settings in Africa: a multicentre, randomised, controlled trial.** *Lancet* 2014, **383**(9915):424–435.
29. Maartens G, Bateman ED: **Tuberculous pleural effusions: increased culture yield with bedside inoculation of pleural fluid and poor diagnostic value of adenosine deaminase.** *Thorax* 1991, **46**(2):96–99.
30. Mayosi BM, Wiysonge CS, Ntsekhe M, Volmink JA, Gumedze F, Maartens G, Aje A, Thomas BM, Thomas KM, Awotedu AA, Thembela B, Mntla P, Maritz F, Blackett KN, Nkouonlack DC, Burch VC, Rebe K, Parish A, Sliwa K, Vezi BZ, Alam N, Brown BG, Gould T, Visser T, Shey MS, Magula NP, Commerford PJ: **Clinical characteristics and initial management of patients with tuberculous pericarditis in the HIV era: the Investigation of the Management of Pericarditis in Africa (IMPI Africa) registry.** *BMC Infect Dis* 2006, **6**:2.

27

Oral intake of phenylbutyrate with or without vitamin D_3 upregulates the cathelicidin LL-37 in human macrophages: a dose finding study for treatment of tuberculosis

Akhirunnesa Mily[1†], Rokeya Sultana Rekha[1,2†], S M Mostafa Kamal[3], Evana Akhtar[1], Protim Sarker[1,2], Zeaur Rahim[1], Gudmundur H Gudmundsson[4], Birgitta Agerberth[2] and Rubhana Raqib[1*]

Abstract

Background: We earlier showed that 4-phenylbutyrate (PB) can induce cathelicidin LL-37 expression synergistically with 1,25-dihydroxyvitamin D_3 in a lung epithelial cell line. We aimed to evaluate a therapeutic dose of PB alone or in combination with vitamin D_3 for induction of LL-37 expression in immune cells and enhancement of antimycobacterial activity in monocyte-derived macrophages (MDM).

Methods: Healthy volunteers were enrolled in an 8-days open trial with three doses of PB [250 mg (Group-I), 500 mg (Group-II) or 1000 mg (Group-III)] twice daily (b.d.) together with vitamin D_3 {5000 IU once daily (o.d.)}, PB (500 mg b.d.) (Group-IV) or vitamin D_3 (5000 IU o.d.) (Group-V), given orally for 4 days. Blood was collected on day-0, day-4 and day-8; plasma was separated, peripheral blood mononuclear cells (PBMC), non-adherent lymphocytes (NAL) and MDM were cultured. LL-37 transcript in cells and peptide concentrations in supernatant were determined by qPCR and ELISA, respectively. In plasma, 25-hydorxyvitamin D_3 levels were determined by ELISA. MDM-mediated killing of *Mycobacterium tuberculosis (Mtb)* (H37Rv) was performed by conventional culture method.

Results: MDM from Group-II had increased concentration of LL-37 peptide and transcript at day-4, while Group-I showed increased transcript at day-4 and day-8 compared to day-0 ($p < 0.05$). Both Group-I and -II exhibited higher levels of transcript on day-4 compared to Group-III and Group-V ($p < 0.035$). Increased induction of peptide was observed in lymphocytes from Group-II on day-4 compared to Group-I and Group-IV ($p < 0.05$), while Group-IV showed increased levels on day-8 compared to Group-I and Group-III ($p < 0.04$). Intracellular killing of *Mtb* on day-4 was significantly increased compared to day-0 in Group-I, -II and -V ($p < 0.05$).

Conclusion: The results demonstrate that 500 mg b.d. PB with 5000 IU o.d. vitamin D_3 is the optimal dose for the induction of LL-37 in macrophages and lymphocytes and intracellular killing of *Mtb* by macrophages. Hence, this dose has potential application in the treatment of TB and is now being used in a clinical trial of adults with active pulmonary TB (NCT01580007).

Keywords: Innate immunity, Antimicrobial peptides, Monocyte derived macrophages, *Mycobacterium*

* Correspondence: rubhana@icddrb.org
[†]Equal contributors
[1]International Centre for Diarrheal Disease Research, Bangladesh (icddr,b), Mohakhali, Dhaka 1212, Bangladesh
Full list of author information is available at the end of the article

Background

Tuberculosis (TB), caused by *Mycobacterium tuberculosis* (*Mtb*), is a predominant public health problem worldwide and responsible for about 3 million deaths annually [1]. The prevalence of TB is increasing due to the spread of antibiotic-resistant strains of *Mtb* [2,3]. The deleterious consequences of co-infection with HIV is the emergence of XDR (extremely drug resistance) cases in Africa and other countries in recent years [4]. Advances in anti-tuberculous therapies and alternative treatment strategies are urgently required for the treatment of TB patients and exposed individuals at high risk of developing TB [5,6].

Antimicrobial peptides (AMPs) are important effectors of the innate defense system [7]. AMPs can limit growth and virulence properties of microbes directly or indirectly by enhancing the host immune system. Induction of endogenous AMP expression by administration of extrinsic compounds may be an attractive approach for alternative therapy in combating infectious diseases. Cathelicidins [8] and Defensins [9] and are major classes of AMPs, in mammals LL-37 is the only human cathelicidin and is expressed by both circulating white blood cells and epithelial surfaces including lungs [10].

The active form of vitamin D_3 was shown to regulate the production of AMPs, i.e. cathelicidin LL-37, which plays an important role in the innate immune defense against infections including TB [11,12]. These studies have encouraged many investigators to initiate vitamin D trials in TB patients with renewed enthusiasm [5,13-15] (NCT01130311; NCT00507000; NCT00366470; NCT00677339; NCT00918086). In a systemic review and meta-analysis of observational studies, evidence of an association with vitamin D_3 deficiency and active TB was demonstrated [16].

Our group has earlier shown that cathelicidin is downregulated in the mucosal epithelia during acute diarrhea [17,18] and in infection with *Neisseria gonorrhea* [19]. We showed that the downregulation of the rabbit cathelicidin (CAP-18) in the large intestine can be counteracted by oral treatment with sodium butyrate, a short chain fatty acid and phenylbutyrate (PB), an analogue of butyrate in experimental model of shigellosis [17,20]. PB further counteracted the downregulation of CAP-18 in the lung and tracheal epithelia through systemic effects [20]. We further demonstrated that PB can induce LL-37 expression synergistically with 1,25-dihydroxyvitamin D_3 at both protein and mRNA levels in a lung epithelial cell line [21]. It is thus likely that oral supplementation with PB will boost innate immunity in the lung mucosa by increasing expression of innate defense proteins. A dose of PB corresponding to that used for rabbits [20] for induction of cathelicidin was calculated by allometric scaling for use in adults. The calculations suggested that an effective dose for a 60 kg human would be approximately 600 mg of PB twice daily.

Our aim in this study was to determine the optimal dose of PB with or without vitamin D_3 in adults for induction of LL-37 in immune cells and increase in functional capacity of macrophages in killing of *Mtb*. Thus, healthy adult volunteers were treated with different doses of PB and in combination with a defined concentration of vitamin D_3.

Methods

Study design

Healthy participants (age range 18 to 55 yrs; n = 15) working at International Centre for Diarrheal Disease Research, Bangladesh (icddr,b) and National Institute of the Diseases of the Chest and Hospital (NIDCH), Dhaka, Bangladesh were recruited in this study. The study was approved by the Ethical Review Committee of icddr,b. Informed consent was obtained from the participants after explaining the nature and purpose of the study. Individuals were excluded if they had symptoms or clinical signs of infection, e.g. fever or diarrhea within the last 2–3 months, if taking corticosteroids, diuretics, or supplementary vitamin D_3 (either alone or as part of a multivitamin preparation). The volunteers were asked to abstain from taking any vitamins or supplements for at least two weeks prior to and during the study period. There were five groups, each consisting of 3 participants. Groups-I, -II and -III received the following doses respectively: 250 mg, 500 mg or 1 g of PB b.d. plus 5000 IU vitamin D_3 o.d. for 4 consecutive days. Group-IV received 500 mg PB b.d. and Group-V received 5000 IU vitamin D_3 o.d. for 4 consecutive days. All healthy volunteers were followed for another 4 days after the treatment to monitor possible side effects. Four-phenylbutyrate (Tributyrate) and the placebo tablet were obtained from Fyrklövern Scandinavia AB, Mönsterås, Sweden; vitamin D_3 (Vigantol oil) and the placebo oil were obtained from Merck KGaA, Darmstadt, Germany. The healthy volunteer trial was conducted to determine an optimal dose for the clinical trial in TB patients (NCT01580007).

Blood collection and cell culture

Peripheral blood was collected at 3 time points (day-0, day-4 and day-8) from each participant (25 mL/individual). Peripheral blood mononuclear cells (PBMCs) were isolated from whole blood by Ficoll-Hypaque density gradient centrifugation and plasma was collected and stored at −20°C for later measurement of 25-hydroxyvitamin D_3, calcium, (serum glutamate pyruvate transaminase (SGPT; liver function marker) and creatinine (kidney function marker). The PBMC pellet was washed and suspended in a culture medium containing 10% autologous plasma in RPMI-1640, 1% L-glutamine, 1% sodium pyruvate, 0.5% amphotericin B and 1% penicillin-streptomycin (Gibco, Grand Island, NY, USA) and plated in two parallel 4-well tissue culture plates (NUNC, Roskilde, Denmark). One tissue culture plate was utilized for analyses of LL-37 peptide and transcript and the other plate was used for macrophage-mediated *Mtb* killing assay.

PBMCs were counted and incubated in culture plates for 3 days. Thereafter, supernatant containing the non-adherent cells (mostly lymphocytes, 80-90%) was removed, centrifuged to collect the clear supernatant which was the extracellular fluid (ECF) of PBMC. The non-adherent lymphocytes were treated with saponin for 10 minutes, centrifuged and supernatant collected as intracellular fluid (ICF) from lymphocytes. Supernatant and cell pellet were stored for further analysis. The remaining adherent cells in the culture plate were MDM, which were harvested and treated with saponin. After centrifugation, supernatant (ICF) and cells were stored until further analysis. RNALater (Qiagen GmbH, Hilden, Germany) was added to the cell pellet for RNA extraction. In another experiment, one part of PBMC was stimulated ex vivo with Bacille Calmette-Guerin, (BCG, 10 μg/mL: Japan BCG Laboratory, Tokyo, Japan) for 3 days, supernatant containing the non-adherent cells was removed, centrifuged to collect the clear supernatant which was the ECF of BCG stimulated PBMC.

Vitamin D_3, calcium, albumin, SGPT and creatinine in plasma

In plasma, 25-hydroxyvitamin D_3 was measured by a commercial ELISA kit (IDS, Fountain Hills, Arizona, USA) that determines 25-hydroxyvitamin D_3 (100%), 25-hydroxyvitamin D_2 (75%) and 24,25-dihydroxyvitamin D_3 (≥100%). Calcium, albumin and creatinine were assessed by Roche automated clinical chemistry analyzer, Hitachi 902. Serum glutamate-pyruvate transaminase (SGPT) was measured by Beckman-Coulter AU680 (Japan).

LL-37 ELISA

LL-37 levels in ICF of macrophage and lymphocyte lysates as well as in ECF of PBMC and BCG stimulated PBMC were measured by ELISA. Duplicate samples were tested and concentrations were calculated using a standard curve generated from synthetic LL-37 (Innovagen, Lund, Sweden). Brief procedure of ELISA is as follow. Polystyrene microtiter plates (Maxisorp by NUNC, Naperville, IL, USA) were coated with monoclonal anti-LL-37 [22] (5 μg/ml) in carbonate buffer (15 mM sodium carbonate, 35 mM sodium bicarbonate and 0.02% sodium azide [pH 9.6]) and incubated overnight at 4°C. After washing, non-specific binding was blocked with 0.1% gelatin in tris-buffered saline (pH 7.5) for 1 hour at RT. Standards and samples were then added and incubated overnight at 4°C. Biotinylated rabbit anti-LL-37 (1 μg/mL) (Innovagen) was added and incubated for 2 h at room temperature (RT), followed by the incubation with Streptavidin-alkaline phosphatase conjugate (Chemicon, Melbourne, Australia) for another 2 h at RT. Four-methylumbelliferyl phosphate was used as substrate (Molecular Probes, Europe BV, Leiden, The Netherlands) and fluorescence was measured at an excitation wavelength of 360 nm and emission wavelength of 450 nm.

Quantitative real time RT-PCR amplification of LL-37 mRNA

RNA was extracted from macrophages and lymphocytes utilizing RNeasy Mini kit as described by the manufacturer (Qiagen GmbH). cDNA was synthesized using Superscript III First-Strand Synthesis System (Invitrogen, Grand Island, NY, USA). The CAMP gene encoding transcript LL-37 relative to the housekeeping 18S rRNA was measured in triplicate from the cDNA samples by real-time quantitative RT-PCR using CFX96 Real-Time PCR Detection Systems (Bio-Rad,) and the 18 s rRNA–housekeeping gene kit (Applied Biosystems, Foster City, CA, USA). The sequences of forward and reverse primers for LL-37 transcript were 5'-TCACCAGAGGATTGTGACTTCAA-3' and 5'-TGAGGGTCACTGTCCCCATAC-3', respectively (Primer Express; Applied Biosystems). The results were analyzed by using the relative standard method [19].

Macrophage mediated killing of *Mycobacterium tuberculosis*

MDM in the culture plates were infected with previously prepared log phased *Mtb* H37Rv strain (from Tuberculosis Research Center, Chennai, India) in culture medium without antibiotics [23]. Initially 3 different multiplicity of infection (MOI; 1:10; 1:25 and 1:50) were tested and the ratio of 1:25 was found to be the optimal MOI, resulting in a clear bacterial killing. After 2 hours of exposure the culture plates were washed 3 times with warm RPMI to remove the extracellular bacteria and the infected MDM were cultured for three additional days in a medium with autologous plasma and antibiotics (penicillin-streptomycin, amphotericin B) (Gibco). Thereafter, the cells were lysed with 0.3% saponin-PBS and vigorous pipetting to collect viable intracellular *Mtb*. The lysates were cultured on Middle Brook 7H11 agar medium supplemented with 10% Middle Brook OADC (oleic acid, albumin, dextrose and catalase) enrichment (Becton Dickinson, Sparks, MD, USA). Bacterial viability was calculated by counting colony forming units (CFU) on agar plates after 21–28 days of culture at 37°C. Before initiation of any intervention, the day-0 MDM-mediated killing served as the control for all groups.

Statistical analysis

Statistical analyses were performed using SigmaStat 3.1 for Windows (Systat Software Inc., Point Richmond, CA, USA) and SPSS 17.0 for Windows (SPSS Inc, Chicago, Illinois, USA). Results were expressed as mean with standard deviation. Sex and age was matched for each group.

Data distribution patterns were checked by using scatter plots, and normality and homogeneity of variances were checked by descriptive statistics. Two-way repeated measure ANOVA was performed when both the sphericity and normality of the data was met. When condition for sphericity was violated or normality of data failed, one Way Analysis of Variance (ANOVA) was performed followed by the Tukey multiple comparison test for between groups and within group variables. Kruskal-Wallis ANOVA on Ranks was performed when data was not normally distributed. Analysis of Co-variance was performed when data at entry level was significantly different. P-values < 0.05 were considered significant.

Results

Plasma levels of vitamin D_3 and calcium

The average of 25-hydroxyvitamin D_3 levels in plasma increased in all groups except for Group-IV (treated with only PB). However, the increase was not significant (Figure 1). Sex and age was matched for each group. Similarly, no changes were observed in albumin-adjusted calcium levels during the study period in any of the groups (data not shown).

SGPT level before treatment was normal in all healthy volunteers except for one male volunteer in Group-I, who had 66.49 IU/L that was above the normal upper range of 56 IU/L. However, the SGPT level (12.08 IU/L) declined on day-4 to normal level. None of the volunteers showed any increase in SGPT level after ingestion of PB alone or in combination with vitamin D_3 on day-4 or −8 (Additional file 1: Table S1).

Synergistic effects of PB and vitamin D_3 on LL-37 expression in macrophages

Significant differences in concentration of MDM derived LL-37 transcripts and peptides were observed within days. A significant increase in both peptide (p = 0.05) and transcript (p = 0.011) was noted in Group-II in day-4 compared to day-0 (Table 1 and 2). Group-I showed significantly higher levels of LL-37 transcript but not peptide at day-4 (p = 0.015) and day-8 (p = 0.042) compared to day-0. Group-IV showed a marginal increase in LL-37 transcript levels on day-4 compared to day-0 (p = 0.07) (Table 1).

When comparing between groups, Group-I and Group-II exhibited significantly higher levels of LL-37 transcript on day-4 compared to Group-III (p = 0.025 and p = 0.03 respectively) and Group-V (p = 0.03 and p = 0.035 respectively) (Table 1). Furthermore, Group-II showed higher levels of peptide compared to Group-IV (p = 0.01) (Table 2).

PB and vitamin D_3 induce LL-37 expression in lymphocytes

Lymphocyte-derived LL-37 transcript did not show any significant induction within days (Table 3). However, LL-37 peptide induction on day-4 was significantly higher in Group-II compared to Group-I (p = 0.03) and Group-IV (p = 0.05) (Table 4). Group-IV showed increased production of peptide on day-8 compared to Group-III (p = 0.03) and Group-I (p = 0.04).

No effects of PB and vitamin D_3 on LL-37 expression in PBMC

There was no significant induction of LL-37 production in ECF of total PBMC within days or between groups.

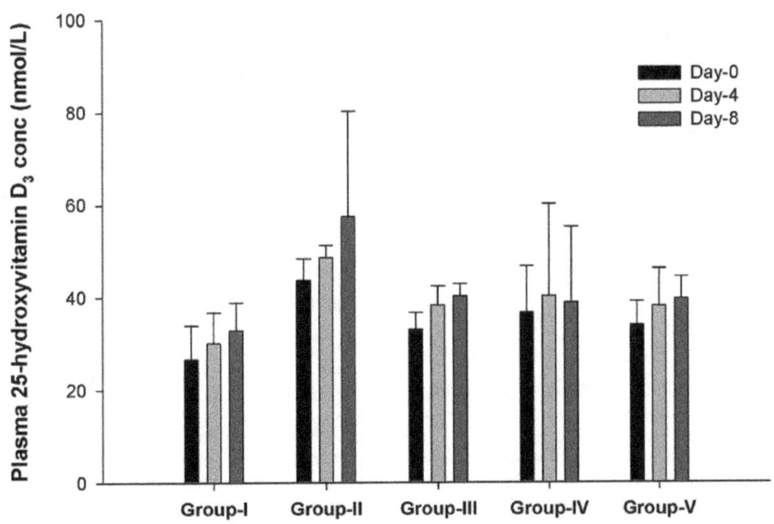

Figure 1 Plasma 25-hydroxyvitamin D_3 concentration in healthy adults before and after supplementation. Group-I: 250 mg PB b.d. + 5000 IU vitamin D_3 o.d.; Group-II: 500 mg PB b.d. + 5000 IU vitamin D_3 o.d.; Group-III: 1000 mg PB b.d. + 5000 IU vitamin D_3 o.d.; Group-IV: 500 mg PB b.d.; Group-V: 5000 IU vitamin D_3 o.d. PB: Phenylbutyrate. b.d.: twice daily. o.d. : once daily. Data were analyzed by One-way ANOVA.

Table 1 Expression of LL-37 transcript in monocyte-derived macrophages from healthy adults before and after supplementation

		LL-37 transcript (copy no.)		
		Day-0	Day-4	Day-8
Group-I	MDM	9.68 ± 9.0	64.37 ± 19.03[a 1,2]	21.61 ± 18.71[b]
Group-II	MDM	16.24 ± 1.77	62.42 ± 19.56[c 3,4]	38.25 ± 15.65
Group-III	MDM	10.94 ± 2.01	10.40 ± 16.19	41.05 ± 52.30
Group-IV	MDM	8.71 ± 4.64	33.87 ± 16.76	13.42 ± 9.57
Group-V	MDM	10.13 ± 5.41	11.54 ± 12.90	8.74 ± 6.27

Note: Group-I: 250 mg PB b.d. + 5000 IU vitamin D_3 o.d.; Group-II: 500 mg PB b.d. + 5000 IU vitamin D_3 o.d.; Group-III: 1000 mg PB b.d. + 5000 IU vitamin D_3 o.d.; Group-IV: 500 mg PB b.d.; Group-V: 5000 IU vitamin D_3 o.d.. Data expressed as Mean ± Standard Deviation. One Way Analysis of Variance (ANOVA) method was used for statistical analysis. Differences are significant, when $p < 0.05$. Difference between, [a]day-4 and day-0 within Group-I (p = 0.01); [b]day-8 and day-0 within Group-I (p = 0.04); [c]day-4 and day-0 within Group-II (p = 0.01); [1]Group-I and -III within day-4 (p = 0.02); [2]Group-I and -V within day-4 (p = 0.034); [3]Group-II and -III within day-4 (p = 0.031); [4]Group-II and -V within day-4 (p = 0.035). *PB*, Phenylbutyrate; *MDM*, Monocyte-derived macrophages; *b. d.*, Twice daily; *o.d.*, Once daily.

Stimulation of PBMC with live BCG also did not show any remarkable increase in LL-37 release in the ECF (0.53 ± 0.17 ng/10^6 PBMC) compared to the ECF of unstimulated PBMC (0.50 ± 0.17 ng/10^6 PBMC) (p = 0.92).

PB and/or vitamin D_3 mediate enhanced killing of *Mtb ex vivo*

Group-II demonstrated significantly higher intracellular killing of *Mtb* by MDM at day-4 (p = 0.027) compared to day-0. Group-I and -V exhibited a significant increase in intracellular killing on day-4 ($p < 0.001$ and p = 0.019 respectively) and day-8 ($p < 0.001$ and p = 0.051 respectively) compared to day-0 (Figure 2). The other Groups did not show any increase in the killing activity of MDM (Figure 2).

Table 2 Expression of LL-37 peptide in monocyte-derived macrophages from healthy adults before and after supplementation

		LL-37 level in ICF (ng/million cells)		
		Day-0	Day-4	Day-8
Group-I	MDM	0.52 ± 0.06	0.72 ± 0.28	0.68 ± 0.19
Group-II	MDM	0.33 ± 0.02	1.22 ± 0.49[a 1]	0.36 ± 0.05
Group-III	MDM	0.28 ± 0.00	0.27 ± 0.02	0.27 ± 0.02
Group-IV	MDM	0.15 ± 0.02	0.13 ± 0.02	0.16 ± 0.02
Group-V	MDM	0.21 ± 0.08	0.20 ± 0.05	0.23 ± 0.09

Note: Group-I: 250 mg PB b.d. + 5000 IU vitamin D_3 o.d.; Group-II: 500 mg PB b.d. + 5000 IU vitamin D_3 o.d.; Group-III: 1000 mg PB b.d. + 5000 IU vitamin D_3 o.d.; Group-IV: 500 mg PB b.d.; Group-V: 5000 IU vitamin D_3 o.d. Data expressed as Mean ± Standard Deviation. One Way Analysis of Variance (ANOVA) method was used for statistical analysis. Kruskal-Wallis ANOVA on Ranks was performed when the data was not normally distributed; analysis of Co-variance was performed when significant difference was found at entry level. Differences are significant, when $p < 0.05$. Difference between, [a]day-4 and day-0 within Group-II (p = 0.02); [1]Group-II and -III within day-4 (p = 0.034). *ICF*, Intracellular fluid; *PB*, Phenylbutyrate; *MDM*, Monocyte-derived macrophages; *b.d.*, Twice daily; *o.d.*, Once daily.

Table 3 Expression of LL-37 transcript in non-adherent lymphocytes in healthy adults before and after supplementation

		LL-37 transcript (copy no.)		
		Day-0	Day-4	Day-8
Group-I	NAL	9.60 ± 2.80	19.5 ± 7.65	7.46 ± 5.00
Group-II	NAL	29.57 ± 6.17	54.43 ± 16.48	38.25 ± 20.66
Group-III	NAL	19.33 ± 8.21	30.00 ± 10.60	20.00 ± 5.01
Group-IV	NAL	14.78 ± 3.08	18.68 ± 5.92	19.12 ± 10.33
Group-V	NAL	9.18 ± 2.39	23.30 ± 14.58	20.71 ± 7.45

Note. Group-I: 250 mg PB b.d. + 5000 IU vitamin D_3 o.d.; Group-II: 500 mg PB b.d. + 5000 IU vitamin D_3 o.d.; Group-III: 1000 mg PB b.d. + 5000 IU vitamin D_3 o.d.; Group-IV: 500 mg PB b.d.; Group-V: 5000 IU vitamin D_3 o.d. Data expressed as Mean ± Standard Deviation. One Way Analysis of Variance (ANOVA) method was used. Analysis of Co-variance was performed when significant difference was found at entry level. *PB*, Phenylbutyrate; *NAL*, Non-adherent lymphocytes; *b.d.*, Twice daily; *o.d.*, Once daily.

Discussion

In this study we demonstrated that oral supplementation of healthy adult volunteers with 500 mg PB b.d. plus 5000 IU vitamin D_3 o.d. (Group-II) consistently induced LL-37 in both macrophages and lymphocytes, and also exhibited increased MDM derived intracellular killing of *M. tuberculosis*.

In an animal model of shigellosis we have previously shown that *Shigella* infection causes downregulation of the rabbit cathelicidin CAP-18 in the epithelia of rectum, lung and trachea [17,20]. Oral feeding of butyrate (0.14 mmol/dose) or PB (0.14 mmol/dose) up-regulates CAP-18 expression in the lung and rectal epithelia of these rabbits and reduces shedding of *Shigella* in stool [20]. We have also demonstrated that PB, induces the *CAMP* gene expression synergistically with 1,25-dihydroxyvitamin D_3 at both protein and mRNA levels in the VA10 lung epithelial cell line [21]. We have now further shown in humans, that

Table 4 Expression of LL-37 peptide in non-adherent lymphocytes in healthy adults before and after supplementation

		LL-37 level in ICF (ng/million cells)		
		Day-0	Day-4	Day-8
Group-I	NAL	0.24 ± 0.07	0.23 ±0.11	0.18 ± 0.12
Group-II	NAL	0.28 ± 0.04	0.49 ± 0.16 [1,2]	0.33 ± 0.11
Group-III	NAL	0.31 ± 0.11	0.25 ± 0.02	0.17 ± 0.06
Group-IV	NAL	0.27 ± 0.14	0.21 ± 0.02	0.68 ± 0.32 [3,4]
Group-V	NAL	0.19 ± 0.08	0.37 ± 0.07	0.27 ± 0.15

Note: Group-I: 250 mg PB b.d. + 5000 IU vitamin D_3 o.d.; Group-II: 500 mg PB b.d. + 5000 IU vitamin D_3 o.d.; Group-III: 1000 mg PB b.d. + 5000 IU vitamin D_3 o.d.; Group-IV: 500 mg PB b.d.; Group-V: 5000 IU vitamin D_3 o.d. Data expressed as Mean ± Standard Deviation. One Way Analysis of Variance (ANOVA) method was used for statistical analysis. Differences are significant, when $p < 0.05$. Difference between, [1]Group-II and -I within day-4 (p = 0.05); [2]Group-II and -IV within day-4 (p = 0.03); [3]Group-IV and -I within day-8 (p = 0.04); [4]Group-IV and-III within day-8 (p = 0.036). *ICF*, Intracellular fluid; *PB*, Phenylbutyrate; *NAL*, Non-adherent lymphocytes; *b.d.*, Twice daily; *o.d.*, Once daily.

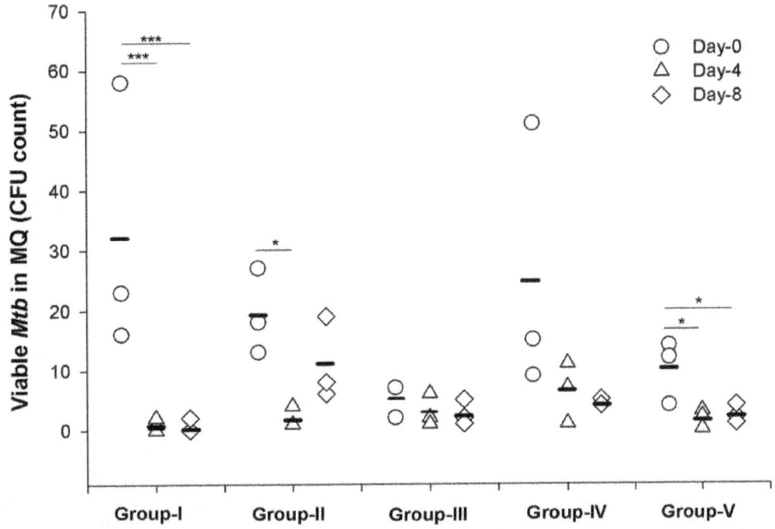

Figure 2 Viable *Mtb* CFU count in Monocyte derived macrophages (MDM). MDM from different group of volunteers were incubated with *Mtb* H37Rv strain for 2 h, after that extracellular bacteria were removed and cultured for 3 days, cells were lysed and plated for variable colony (CFU) count. Group-I: 250 mg PB b.d. + 5000 IU vitamin D_3 o.d.; Group-II: 500 mg PB b.d. + 5000 IU vitamin D_3 o.d.; Group-III: 1000 mg PB b.d. + 5000 IU vitamin D_3 o.d.; Group-IV: 500 mg PB b.d.; Group-V: 5000 IU vitamin D_3 o.d.. PB: Phenylbutyrate. b.d.: twice daily. o.d. : once daily. The straight horizontal line indicates means. Data were analyzed by two-way (treatment and time) repeated measures ANOVA. * $p < 0.05$, and *** $p < 0.001$.

oral intake of PB alone or in combination with vitamin D_3 can also induce LL-37 in immune cells. In this study, three potential doses of PB were selected for healthy adults. Group I (250 mg b.d. with 5000 IU vitamin D_3 o.d.) showed significant increase in LL-37 transcript but not peptide in MDM; no changes in peptide or transcript was noted in NAL. Group-II (500 mg b.d. plus 5000 IU vitamin D_3 o.d.) showed increase in both peptide and transcript in MDM and peptide in NAL. In Group-III with the higher dose of PB (1 g b.d.) along with vitamin D_3 there was no increase in LL-37 transcript or peptide in cells after PB supplementation. Butyrate is known to inhibit RNA and protein synthesis at high concentrations [24-26]. We may speculate that in a similar fashion PB at high doses is inhibitory to the expression of LL-37 both at transcriptional and translational levels. The dose of Group-II appears superior in inducing both peptide and mRNA concentrations in MDM and peptide in lymphocytes.

Various cell types including T lymphocytes are known to express LL-37 [27,28]. However, to our knowledge this is the first study to report enhanced *in vivo* induction of LL-37 in lymphocytes after oral supplementation with PB alone or in combination with vitamin D_3. This finding thus underscores the significance of PB therapy in TB infection since T cells play a major role in the host defense against tuberculosis [29].

The present study showed that oral intake of vitamin D_3 (Group-V) alone or in combination with PB (Group-I and -II) exhibited a marked increase in intracellular killing of *Mtb*. Vitamin D_3-induced LL-37 expression is an important factor in fighting TB [11,12]. Killing of *Mtb* by macrophages is directly correlated with *CAMP* gene expression encoding LL-37 and plasma levels of 25-hydroxyvitamin D_3 [12]. Furthermore, it was shown that activation of Toll-Like Receptor 2/1 in human macrophages up-regulated expression of the genes encoding vitamin D receptor and vitamin D-hydroxylase, leading to induction of LL-37 with subsequent killing of intracellular *Mtb* [11]. Recent studies have shown that human cathelicidin is a key mediator of 1,25-dihydroxyvitamin D_3-induced autophagy and hence provide a mechanistic insight into the role of cathelicidin in combating *Mtb* [30,31]. Interestingly, *in vitro* studies have shown that short chain fatty acids, butyrate and propionate can induce both apoptosis and autophagy [32]. PB is an analogue of butyrate and it is quite likely that PB in combination with Vitamin D_3 may also induce autophagy and LL-37 mediated killing of *Mtb ex vivo*.

The major limitation of this study is the small sample size and the short duration of the PB and vitamin D_3 supplementation. The lack of increase in plasma 25-hydroxyvitamin D_3 level after 4 days supplementation was not unexpected since 1–2 months supplementation is needed to reach steady state vitamin D_3 levels.

Conclusion

In conclusion, oral combination dose of 500 mg PB b.d. with 5000 IU vitamin D_3 o.d. appears to be the optimum dose to induce both LL-37 peptide and transcript expression in functional immune cells as well as enhance intracellular *Mtb* killing in macrophages. The dose of 250 mg PB b.d. with 5000 IU vitamin D_3 o.d. also increased intracellular killing however it enhanced only LL-37 transcript levels (not peptide) in macrophages but not in lymphocytes. This pilot study has generated results for a potential dose in a clinical trial of adults with active pulmonary TB (NCT01580007).

Abbreviations

AMPs: Antimicrobial peptides; b.d.: Twice daily; CFU: Colony forming units; ECF: Extracellular fluid; HDAC: Histone deacetylase; ICF: Intracellular fluid; MDM: Monocyte-derived macrophages; *Mtb*: *Mycobacterium tuberculosis*; o. d.: Once daily; PB: 4-Phenylbutyrate; PBMCs: Peripheral blood mononuclear cells; TB: Tuberculosis.

Competing interests

Birgitta Agerberth, Gudmundur H. Gudmundsson and Rubhana Raqib have a pending patent application for the use of phenylbutyrate to the treatment of infections. There is no financial arrangement between any of the authors.

Authors' contributions

RR, BA contributed to the conception and design of the study; AM, RSR, EA and PS performed laboratory analysis, AM, RSR and RR performed the statistical analysis; AM, RSR and RR prepare the first draft of the manuscript. BA, GHG, ZR, SMMK and PS revised the manuscript. All authors read and approved the final version of the manuscript.

Acknowledgement

The study was supported by icddr,b, 'the Swedish Agency for Research Cooperation with Developing Countries (Sida/SAREC Agreement support; grant 384, SWE-2008-065)'; 'The Swedish Research Council, (grant 58X-11217-14-3)'; 'The Swedish Strategic Foundation (SSF)'; Swedish Cancer Society; 'Karolinska Institutet'; 'The Icelandic Centre for Research (RANNIS)' and 'University of Iceland research fund'. icddr,b acknowledges with gratitude the commitment of all donors' to it's research efforts. GHG is a visiting scientist supported by 'The Wenner-Gren Foundations'. We thank the volunteers for participating in this study.

Author details

[1]International Centre for Diarrheal Disease Research, Bangladesh (icddr,b), Mohakhali, Dhaka 1212, Bangladesh. [2]Department of Medical Biochemistry and Biophysics, Karolinska Institutet, Stockholm 17177, Sweden. [3]National Institute of the Diseases of the Chest and Hospital, Mohakhali, Dhaka 1212, Bangladesh. [4]Institute of Biology, University of Iceland, Reykjavik 101, Iceland.

References

1. Smith PE, Moss AR: **Tuberculosis: pathogenesis, protection, and control, epidemiology of tuberculosis.** *Epidemiol Tuberc* 1994, **1**:47–60.
2. Parsons LM, Driscoll JR, Taber HW, Salfinger M: **Drug resistance in tuberculosis.** *Infect Dis Clin North Am* 1997, **11**(4):905–928.
3. Bradford WZ, Daley CL: **Multiple drug-resistant tuberculosis.** *Infect Dis Clin North Am* 1998, **12**(1):157–172.
4. Gandhi NR, Shah NS, Andrews JR, Vella V, Moll AP, Scott M, Weissman D, Marra C, Lalloo UG, Friedland GH: **HIV coinfection in multidrug- and extensively drug-resistant tuberculosis results in high early mortality.** *Am J Respir Crit Care Med* 2010, **181**(1):80–86.
5. Wejse C, Gomes VF, Rabna P, Gustafson P, Aaby P, Lisse IM, Andersen PL, Glerup H, Sodemann M: **Vitamin D as supplementary treatment for tuberculosis: a double-blind, randomized, placebo-controlled trial.** *Am J Respir Crit Care Med* 2009, **179**(9):843–850.
6. Martins M: **Targeting the human macrophage with combinations of drugs and inhibitors of Ca2+ and K + transport to enhance the killing of intracellular multi-drug resistant Mycobacterium tuberculosis (MDR-TB)–a novel, patentable approach to limit the emergence of XDR-TB.** *Recent Pat Antiinfect Drug Discov* 2011, **6**(2):110–117.
7. Zasloff M: **Antimicrobial peptides of multicellular organisms.** *Nature* 2002, **415**(6870):389–395.
8. Zaiou M, Gallo RL: **Cathelicidins, essential gene-encoded mammalian antibiotics.** *J Mol Med (Berl)* 2002, **80**(9):549–561.
9. Ganz T: **Defensins: antimicrobial peptides of innate immunity.** *Nat Rev Immunol* 2003, **3**(9):710–720.
10. Kai-Larsen Y, Agerberth B: **The role of the multifunctional peptide LL-37 in host defense.** *Front Biosci* 2008, **13**:3760–3767.
11. Liu PT, Stenger S, Li H, Wenzel L, Tan BH, Krutzik SR, Ochoa MT, Schauber J, Wu K, Meinken C, *et al*: **Toll-like receptor triggering of a vitamin D-mediated human antimicrobial response.** *Science* 2006, **311**(5768):1770–1773.
12. Liu PT, Stenger S, Tang DH, Modlin RL: **Cutting edge: vitamin D-mediated human antimicrobial activity against *Mycobacterium tuberculosis* is dependent on the induction of cathelicidin.** *J Immunol* 2007, **179**(4):2060–2063.
13. Salahuddin N, Ali F, Hasan Z, Rao N, Aqeel M, Mahmood F: **Vitamin D accelerates clinical recovery from tuberculosis: results of the SUCCINCT study [supplementary cholecalciferol in recovery from tuberculosis]. A randomized, placebo-controlled, clinical trial of vitamin D supplementation in patients with pulmonary tuberculosis.** *BMC Infect Dis* 2013, **13**:22.
14. Martineau AR, Wilkinson RJ, Wilkinson KA, Newton SM, Kampmann B, Hall BM, Packe GE, Davidson RN, Eldridge SM, Maunsell ZJ, *et al*: **A single dose of vitamin D enhances immunity to *mycobacteria*.** *Am J Respir Crit Care Med* 2007, **176**(2):208–213.
15. Martineau AR, Timms PM, Bothamley GH, Hanifa Y, Islam K, Claxton AP, Packe GE, Moore-Gillon JC, Darmalingam M, Davidson RN, *et al*: **High-dose vitamin D(3) during intensive-phase antimicrobial treatment of pulmonary tuberculosis: a double-blind randomised controlled trial.** *Lancet* 2011, **377**(9761):242–250.
16. Nnoaham KE, Clarke A: **Low serum vitamin D levels and tuberculosis: a systematic review and meta-analysis.** *Int J Epidemiol* 2008, **37**(1):113–119.
17. Raqib R, Sarker P, Bergman P, Ara G, Lindh M, Sack DA, Nasirul Islam KM, Gudmundsson GH, Andersson J, Agerberth B: **Improved outcome in shigellosis associated with butyrate induction of an endogenous peptide antibiotic.** *Proc Natl Acad Sci U S A* 2006, **103**(24):9178–9183.
18. Islam D, Bandholtz L, Nilsson J, Wigzell H, Christensson B, Agerberth B, Gudmundsson G: **Downregulation of bactericidal peptides in enteric infections: a novel immune escape mechanism with bacterial DNA as a potential regulator.** *Nat Med* 2001, **7**(2):180–185.
19. Bergman P, Johansson L, Asp V, Plant L, Gudmundsson GH, Jonsson AB, Agerberth B: ***Neisseria gonorrhoeae* downregulates expression of the human antimicrobial peptide LL-37.** *Cell Microbiol* 2005, **7**(7):1009–1017.
20. Sarker P, Ahmed S, Tiash S, Rekha RS, Stromberg R, Andersson J, Bergman P, Gudmundsson GH, Agerberth B, Raqib R: **Phenylbutyrate counteracts *Shigella* mediated downregulation of cathelicidin in rabbit lung and intestinal epithelia: a potential therapeutic strategy.** *PLoS One* 2011, **6**(6):e20637.
21. Steinmann J, Halldorsson S, Agerberth B, Gudmundsson GH: **Phenylbutyrate induces antimicrobial peptide expression.** *Antimicrob Agents Chemother* 2009, **53**(12):5127–5133.
22. Yoshio H, Tollin M, Gudmundsson GH, Lagercrantz H, Jornvall H, Marchini G, Agerberth B: **Antimicrobial polypeptides of human vernix caseosa and amniotic fluid: implications for newborn innate defense.** *Pediatr Res* 2003, **53**(2):211–216.
23. Edfeldt K, Liu PT, Chun R, Fabri M, Schenk M, Wheelwright M, Keegan C, Krutzik SR, Adams JS, Hewison M, *et al*: **T-cell cytokines differentially control human monocyte antimicrobial responses by regulating vitamin D metabolism.** *Proc Natl Acad Sci U S A* 2010, **107**(52):22593–22598.

24. Soliman MM, Ahmed MM, Salah-Eldin AE, Abdel-Aal AA: **Butyrate regulates leptin expression through different signaling pathways in adipocytes.** *J Vet Sci* 2011, **12**(4):319–323.
25. de Haan JB, Gevers W, Parker MI: **Effects of sodium butyrate on the synthesis and methylation of DNA in normal cells and their transformed counterparts.** *Cancer Res* 1986, **46**(2):713–716.
26. Soliman M, Kimura K, Ahmed M, Yamaji D, Matsushita Y, Okamatsu-Ogura Y, Makondo K, Saito M: **Inverse regulation of leptin mRNA expression by short- and long-chain fatty acids in cultured bovine adipocytes.** *Domest Anim Endocrinol* 2007, **33**(4):400–409.
27. Kin NW, Chen Y, Stefanov EK, Gallo RL, Kearney JF: **Cathelin-related antimicrobial peptide differentially regulates T- and B-cell function.** *Eur J Immunol* 2011, **41**(10):3006–3016.
28. Agerberth B, Charo J, Werr J, Olsson B, Idali F, Lindbom L, Kiessling R, Jornvall H, Wigzell H, Gudmundsson GH: **The human antimicrobial and chemotactic peptides LL-37 and alpha-defensins are expressed by specific lymphocyte and monocyte populations.** *Blood* 2000, **96**(9):3086–3093.
29. Ottenhoff TH, Kaufmann SH: **Vaccines against tuberculosis: where are we and where do we need to go?** *PLoS Pathog* 2012, **8**(5):e1002607.
30. Campbell GR, Spector SA: **Autophagy induction by vitamin D inhibits both *Mycobacterium tuberculosis* and human immunodeficiency virus type 1.** *Autophagy* 2012, **8**(10):1523–1525.
31. Yuk JM, Shin DM, Lee HM, Yang CS, Jin HS, Kim KK, Lee ZW, Lee SH, Kim JM, Jo EK: **Vitamin D3 induces autophagy in human monocytes/ macrophages via cathelicidin.** *Cell Host Microbe* 2009, **6**(3):231–243.
32. Lee JS, Lee GM: **Effect of sodium butyrate on autophagy and apoptosis in Chinese hamster ovary cells.** *Biotechnol Prog* 2012, **28**(2):349–357.

Permissions

All chapters in this book were first published in PM, by BioMed Central; hereby published with permission under the Creative Commons Attribution License or equivalent. Every chapter published in this book has been scrutinized by our experts. Their significance has been extensively debated. The topics covered herein carry significant findings which will fuel the growth of the discipline. They may even be implemented as practical applications or may be referred to as a beginning point for another development.

The contributors of this book come from diverse backgrounds, making this book a truly international effort. This book will bring forth new frontiers with its revolutionizing research information and detailed analysis of the nascent developments around the world.

We would like to thank all the contributing authors for lending their expertise to make the book truly unique. They have played a crucial role in the development of this book. Without their invaluable contributions this book wouldn't have been possible. They have made vital efforts to compile up to date information on the varied aspects of this subject to make this book a valuable addition to the collection of many professionals and students.

This book was conceptualized with the vision of imparting up-to-date information and advanced data in this field. To ensure the same, a matchless editorial board was set up. Every individual on the board went through rigorous rounds of assessment to prove their worth. After which they invested a large part of their time researching and compiling the most relevant data for our readers.

The editorial board has been involved in producing this book since its inception. They have spent rigorous hours researching and exploring the diverse topics which have resulted in the successful publishing of this book. They have passed on their knowledge of decades through this book. To expedite this challenging task, the publisher supported the team at every step. A small team of assistant editors was also appointed to further simplify the editing procedure and attain best results for the readers.

Apart from the editorial board, the designing team has also invested a significant amount of their time in understanding the subject and creating the most relevant covers. They scrutinized every image to scout for the most suitable representation of the subject and create an appropriate cover for the book.

The publishing team has been an ardent support to the editorial, designing and production team. Their endless efforts to recruit the best for this project, has resulted in the accomplishment of this book. They are a veteran in the field of academics and their pool of knowledge is as vast as their experience in printing. Their expertise and guidance has proved useful at every step. Their uncompromising quality standards have made this book an exceptional effort. Their encouragement from time to time has been an inspiration for everyone.

The publisher and the editorial board hope that this book will prove to be a valuable piece of knowledge for researchers, students, practitioners and scholars across the globe.

List of Contributors

Scott K Heysell, Tania A Thomas and Eric R Houpt
Division of Infectious Diseases and International Health, University of Virginia, Charlottesville, VA 29908-1337, USA

Costi D Sifri
Office of Hospital Epidemiology/Infection Prevention and Control, University of Virginia Health System, Charlottesville, USA

Patrice K Rehm
Department of Radiology and Medical Imaging, University of Virginia, Charlottesville, USA

Pierre Le Palud, Romain Magnier, Karine Campbell and Youssef Oulkhouir,
CHU de Caen, Service de Pneumologie et Oncologie thoracique, F-14000 Caen, France

Brigitte Malbruny
CHU de Caen, Service de Microbiologie, F-14000 Caen, France

Vincent Cattoir, Gérard Zalcman and Karine Campbell
Université de Caen-Basse Normandie, F-14000 Caen, France

Emmanuel Bergot
Groupe pour la Recherche et l'Enseignement en Pneumo-Infectiologie (GREPI) de la Société de Pneumologie de Langue Française (SPLF), F-75000 Paris, France

Zhi Chen, Wei Wang, Jianqin Liang, Jinhe Wang, Shisheng Feng and Guangyu Zhang
Department of Tuberculosis, The 309th hospital of PLA, No. 17, Heishanhu Road, Haidian District, Beijing 100091, China

Dewald A. Barnard, Elvis M. Irusen and Coenraad F. N. Koegelenberg
Divisions of Pulmonology, Department of Medicine, Stellenbosch University, 7505 Cape Town, South Africa

Johannes W. Bruwer
Tygerberg Academic Hospital, Cape Town, South Africa

Danté Plekker
Kuils River Hospital, Cape Town, South Africa

Andrew C. Whitelaw
Division of Medical Microbiology and Immunology, Department of Pathology, Stellenbosch University, Cape Town, South Africa
National Health Laboratory Services, Cape Town, South Africa

Jacobus D. Deetlefs
Ampath Laboratories, Cape Town, South Africa

Adrian Chan, Anantham Devanand, Su Ying Low and Mariko Siyue Koh
Department of Respiratory and Critical Care Medicine, Singapore General Hospital, Singapore, Singapore

Anantham Devanand, Su Ying Low and Mariko Siyue Koh
Duke- NUS Graduate Medical School, Singapore, Singapore

S. Maguire, V. Parihar and C. Smyth
Department of Gastroenterology, Connolly Hospital, Blanchardstown, Dublin Dublin 15, Ireland

S. H. Chotirmall
Lee Kong Chian School of Medicine, Nanyang Technological University, Singapore, Singapore

L. Cormican
Department of Respiratory Medicine, Connolly Hospital, Blanchardstown, Dublin Dublin 15, Ireland

C. Ryan and C O'Keane
Department of Histopathology, Mater Misericordiae Hospital, Dublin Dublin 7, Ireland

Tahir Saeed
Gulab Devi Chest Hospital, Lahore, Pakistan

K. Redmond
Department of Cardiothoracic Surgery, Mater Misericordiae Hospital, Dublin Dublin 7, Ireland

Jingtao Gao, Yan Ma, Jian Du, Liang Li and Qi Li
Clinical Center on Tuberculosis, Beijing Chest Hospital, Capital Medical University, Beijing Tuberculosis and Thoracic Tumor Research Institute, Beijing, China

Guofeng Zhu
State Key Laboratory for Molecular Virology and Genetic Engineering, Institute of Pathogen Biology, Chinese Academy of Medical Sciences & Peking Union Medical College, Beijing, China

Shouyong Tan
Department of TB Control, Guangzhou Chest Hospital, Guangzhou, Guangdong, China

Yanyong Fu
Department of TB Control, Tianjin Centers for Disease Control and Prevention, Tianjin, China

Liping Ma
Department of TB Control, Henan Center for Disease Control and Prevention, Zhengzhou, Henan, China

Lianying Zhang
Department of TB Control, Hebei Center for Disease Control and Prevention, Shijiazhuang, Hebei, China

Feiying Liu
Department of TB Control, Guangxi Center for Disease Control and Prevention, Nanning, Guangxi, China

Daiyu Hu
Department of TB Control, Chongqing Anti-tuberculosis Institute, Chongqing, China

Yanling Zhang
Department of TB Control, Yunnan Center for Disease Control and Prevention, Kunming, Yunnan, China

Xiangqun Li
Department of TB Control, Shanghai Municipal Center for Disease Control and Prevention, Shanghai, China

Mohamed Faisal, Tidi M. Hassan and Andrea Y. L. Ban
Department of Medicine, Respiratory Unit, Universiti Kebangsaan Malaysia Medical Centre, Jalan Yaacob Latiff, Bandar Tun Razak, 56000 Cheras, Kuala Lumpur, Malaysia

Hafaruzi Harun and Jamalul Azizi Abdul Rahaman
Respiratory Unit, Serdang Hospital, Jalan Puchong, 43000 Kajang, Selangor Darul Ehsan, Malaysia

Sanjay H. Chotirmall
Lee Kong Chian School of Medicine, Nanyang Technological University, Singapore, Singapore

Mohamed Manji, Grace Shayo and Ferdinand Mugusi
Department of Internal Medicine, Muhimbili University of Health and Allied Sciences (MUHAS), Dar es Salaam, Tanzania

Simon Mamuya
Department of Environmental Occupational Health, Muhimbili University of Health and Allied Sciences (MUHAS), Dar es Salaam, Tanzania

Rose Mpembeni
Department of Epidemiology and Biostatistics, Muhimbili University of Health and Allied Sciences (MUHAS), Dar es Salaam, Tanzania

Ahmed Jusabani
Department of Radiology, The Aga Khan Hospital, Dar es Salaam, Tanzania

Daniel Franzen, Lutz Freitag and Macé M. Schuurmans
Division of Pulmonology, University Hospital Zurich, University of Zurich, Raemistrasse 100, Zurich 8091, Switzerland

Andreas H. Diacon
Department of Internal Medicine, Lung Unit, Tygerberg Academic Hospital, University of Stellenbosch, Cape Town, South Africa

Pawel T. Schubert and Colleen A. Wright
Division of Anatomical Pathology, Tygerberg Academic Hospital, University of Stellenbosch, Cape Town, South Africa
NHLS, Port Elizabeth and Tygerberg Hospital, Cape Town, South Africa

Kashaf Junaid and Abdul Rehman
Department of Microbiology and Molecular Genetics, University of the Punjab, Quaid-e-Azam Campus, Lahore 5400, Pakistan

David A. Jolliffe and Adrian R. Martineau
Centre for Primary Care and Public Health, Barts and The London School of Medicine and Dentistry, Queen Mary University of London, London E1 2AB, UK

Kristie Wood
Genome Centre, Barts and the London School of Medicine and Dentistry, Queen Mary University of London, London EC1M 6BQ, UK

Paul K. Drain
Department of Medicine, University of Washington, Seattle, WA, USA
Department of Surgery, Massachusetts General Hospital, Harvard Medical School, Boston, USA
Department of Epidemiology, University of Washington, Seattle, WA, USA

Elena Losina
Medical Practice Evaluation Center, Harvard Medical School, Boston, USA

Ingrid V. Bassett
Division of Infectious Diseases, Harvard Medical School, Boston, USA
Division of General Internal Medicine, Harvard Medical School, Boston, USA

Jeffrey N. Katz
Department of Orthopedic Surgery, Brigham and Women's Hospital, Harvard Medical School, Boston, USA

Sharon M. Coleman
Boston University School of Public Health, Boston, USA

Janet Giddy
Department of Medicine, McCord Hospital, Durban, South Africa

Douglas Ross
Department of Medicine, St. Mary's Hospital, Durban, South Africa

Andrés Noé and Peter le Souef
School of Paediatrics and Child Health, University of Western Australia, Crawley, Australia

Rafaela M. Ribeiro, Rui Anselmo and Maria Maixenchs
Centro de Investigação em Saúde de Manhiça (CISM), CP 1929 Maputo, Mozambique

Layce Sitole
Maternal and Infant Health Service, Manhiça District, Maputo, Mozambique

Khatia Munguambe
Faculdade de Medicina, Eduardo Mondlane University (UEM), Maputo, Mozambique

Silvia Blanco
ISGlobal, Barcelona Ctr. Int. Health Res. (CRESIB), Hospital Clínic - Universitat de Barcelona, Barcelona, Spain

Alberto L. García-Basteiro
Amsterdam Institute for Global Health and Development (AIGHD), Amsterdam, The Netherlands

Chun-Wei Wu and Jiunn-Yih Wu
Department of Emergency Medicine, Chang Gung Memorial Hospital, Keelung, Taiwan and Chang Gung University College of Medicine, Taoyuan, Taiwan

Meng-Tse Gabriel Lee
Department of Emergency Medicine, National Taiwan University Hospital, Number 7, Chung-Shan South Road, Taipei 100, Taiwan

Chih-Cheng Lai
Department of Intensive Care Medicine, Chi Mei Medical Center, Liouying, Tainan, Taiwan

I-Lin Wu
Department of Emergency Medicine, Taoyuan Armed Forces General Hospital, Taoyuan, Taiwan

Yi-Wen Tsai
Department of Family Medicine, Chang Gung Memorial Hospital, Keelung and Chang Gung University College of Medicine, Taoyuan, Taiwan

Babafemi Taiwo, Robert Leo Murphy and Chad Achenbach
Department of Medicine, Northwestern University, Chicago, IL, USA

Shy-Shin Chang
Department of Family Medicine, Taipei Medical University Hospital and School of Medicine, Taipei Medical University, Taipei 110, Taiwan
Department of Family Medicine, Taipei Medical University Hospital, No.252, Wuxing St, Xinyi District, Taipei, Taiwan

Maxwell Oluwole Akanbi
Institute of Public Health and Medicine, Northwestern University, Chicago, IL, USA

Oche Agbaji, Christiana Ukoli and John Idoko
Department of Medicine, University of Jos, Jos, Nigeria

Agatha Ani
Department of Medical Microbiology, University of Jos, Jos, PL, Nigeria

Yetunde Isa
AIDS Prevention Initiative in Nigeria (APIN) Center, Jos University Teaching Hospital, Jos, PL, Nigeria

Patrick Akande
AIDS Prevention Initiative in Nigeria (APIN), Abuja, Nigeria

Mamoudou Maiga
Department of Biomedical Engineering, Northwestern University, Evanston, IL, USA

Richard Kwizera, Christine Sekaggya-Wiltshire, Joseph Musaazi, Barbara Castelnuovo and Andrew Kambugu
Infectious Diseases Institute, College of Health Sciences, Makerere University, Uganda

Rosalind Parkes-Ratanshi
Cambridge Institute of Public Health, University of Cambridge, Cambridge, UK

David W. Denning and Iain D. Page
The University of Manchester, Manchester, UK
National Aspergillosis Centre, University Hospital of South Manchester, Manchester, UK

Jan Fehr
Infectious Diseases and Hospital Hygiene, University Hospital, Zurich, Switzerland

Ni Zeng, Chun Wan, Jiangyu Qin, Yanqiu Wu, Ting Yang, Yongchun Shen, Fuqiang Wen and Lei Chen
Department of Respiratory and Critical Care Medicine, West China Hospital of Sichuan University and Division of Pulmonary Diseases, State Key Laboratory of Biotherapy of China, Chengdu 610041, China

Fentabil Getnet
Department of Public Health, College of Medicine and Health Sciences, Jigjiga University, Jigjiga, Ethiopia

Meaza Demissie
Addis Continental Institute of Public Health, Addis Ababa, Ethiopia

Nega Assefa and Bizatu Mengistie
School of Public Health, College of Health and Medical Sciences, Haramaya University, Harar, Ethiopia

Alemayehu Worku
School of Public Health, College of Health Sciences, Addis Ababa University, Addis Ababa, Ethiopia

Toyomitsu Sawai, Takumi Nakao, Satoru Koga, Shotaro Ide, Sumako Yoshioka and Nobuko Matsuo
Department of Respiratory Medicine, Nagasaki Harbor Medical Center, 6-39 Shinchi-machi, Nagasaki 850-8555, Japan

Hiroshi Mukae
Second Department of Internal Medicine, Nagasaki University Hospital, 1-7-1 Sakamoto-machi, Nagasaki, Japan

Kelemework Adane
Department of Medical Microbiology and Immunology, College of Health Sciences, Mekelle University, Mekelle, Ethiopia

Geert-Jan Dinant, Mark Spigt and Kelemework Adane
Department of Family Medicine, Maastricht University/CAPHRI School for Public Health and Primary Care, Maastricht, the Netherlands

Mark Spigt
General Practice Research Unit, Department of Community Medicine, UiT the Arctic University of Norway, Tromsø, Norway

S. K. Singh and Gyan Chandra Kashyap
Department of Mathematical Demography & Statistics, International Institute for Population Sciences, Govandi Station Road, Deonar Mumbai 400088, India

Parul Puri
International Institute for Population Sciences, Govandi Station Road, Deonar Mumbai 400088, India

Abyot Asres
Department of Public Health, College of Health Sciences, Mizan Tepi University, Mizan Aman, Ethiopia

Degu Jerene
Management Science for Health, Addis Ababa, Ethiopia

Wakgari Deressa
Department of Preventive Medicine, School of Public Health, College of Health Sciences, Addis Ababa University, Addis Ababa, Ethiopia

Cuthbert Musarurwa, Doreen Zvipo Mhandire, Kudakwashe Mhandire and Witmore Bayayi Mujaji
Department of Chemical Pathology, University of Zimbabwe, College of Health Sciences, Avondale, Harare, Zimbabwe

Lynn Sodai Zijenah and Maria Mary Chipiti
Department of Immunology, University of Zimbabwe, College of Health Sciences, Avondale, Harare, Zimbabwe

Tsitsi Bandason
Biomedical Research and Training Institute, Harare, Zimbabwe

Marshall Wesley Munjoma
Department of Obstetrics and Gynaecology, University of Zimbabwe, College of Health Sciences, Avondale, Harare, Zimbabwe

Shouquan Wu, Yu Wang, Miaomiao Zhang, Minggui Wang and Jian-Qing He
Department of Respiratory and Critical Care Medicine, West China Hospital, Sichuan University, No. 37, Guo Xue Alley, Chengdu 610041, Sichuan, People's Republic of China

Guo Chen
Division of Geriatrics, Sichuan Provincial People's Hospital, Chengdu, Sichuan, China

Carla Loredo, Michelle Cailleaux-Cezar and Fernanda Carvalho Queiroz de Mello
Institute of Thoracic Diseases of Federal University of Rio de Janeiro, Rio de Janeiro, Brazil

Anne Efron
Center for Tuberculosis Research, Johns Hopkins University, Baltimore, Maryland, USA

Marcus Barreto Conde
Hospital Universitário Clementino Fraga Filho, Cidade Universitária, Rua Professor Rodolpho Paulo Rocco n° 255, 6° andar, Rio de Janeiro 21941-913, Brazil

Hiroshi Ohnishi, Shintaro Miyamoto, Shigeo Kawase, Tetsuya Kubota and Akihito Yokoyama
Department of Hematology and Respiratory Medicine, Kochi Medical School, Kochi University, Oko-cho, Kohasu, Nankoku, Kochi 783-8505, Japan

Richard Meldau, Jonny Peter, Grant Theron, Greg Calligaro, Brian Allwood, Greg Symons, Hoosain Khalfey, Gina Ntombenhle, Ureshnie Govender, Anke Binder and Richard van Zyl-Smit
Lung Infection and Immunity Unit, Division of Pulmonology & UCT Lung Institute, Department of Medicine, University of Cape Town, Cape Town, South Africa

Akhirunnesa Mily, Rokeya Sultana Rekha, Evana Akhtar, Protim Sarker, Zeaur Rahim and Rubhana Raqib
International Centre for Diarrheal Disease Research, Bangladesh (icddr,b), Mohakhali, Dhaka 1212, Bangladesh

Keertan Dheda
Institute of Infectious Diseases and Molecular Medicine, University of Cape Town, Cape Town, South Africa

Birgitta Agerberth, Protim Sarker and Rokeya Sultana Rekha
Department of Medical Biochemistry and Biophysics, Karolinska Institutet, Stockholm 17177, Sweden

S M Mostafa Kamal
National Institute of the Diseases of the Chest and Hospital, Mohakhali, Dhaka 1212, Bangladesh

Gudmundur H Gudmundsson
Institute of Biology, University of Iceland, Reykjavik 101, Iceland

Index

www.ingramcontent.com/pod-product-compliance
Lightning Source LLC
LaVergne TN
LVHW080714210926
848485LV00003B/465